Hyperhidrosis

Marcelo de Paula Loureiro
José Ribas M. de Campos
Nelson Wolosker
Paulo Kauffman
Editors

Hyperhidrosis

A Complete Guide to Diagnosis and Management

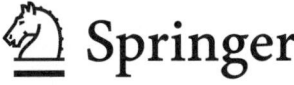

Editors
Marcelo de Paula Loureiro
General Surgery and Biotechnology
Positivo University and INC Hospital
Curitiba, PR
Brazil

Nelson Wolosker
Department of Vascular
and Endovascular Surgery
Hospital Israelita Albert Einstein
São Paulo, SP
Brazil

José Ribas M. de Campos
Thoracic Surgery Division, Heart Institute
Clinics Hospital, University of São Paulo
School of Medicine
São Paulo, SP
Brazil

Paulo Kauffman
Department of Vascular and Endovascular
Surgery
University of São Paulo School of Medicine
São Paulo, SP
Brazil

ISBN 978-3-030-07794-5   ISBN 978-3-319-89527-7   (eBook)
https://doi.org/10.1007/978-3-319-89527-7

© Springer International Publishing AG, part of Springer Nature 2018
Softcover re-print of the Hardcover 1st edition 2018
This work is subject to copyright. All rights are reserved by the Publisher, whether the whole or part of the material is concerned, specifically the rights of translation, reprinting, reuse of illustrations, recitation, broadcasting, reproduction on microfilms or in any other physical way, and transmission or information storage and retrieval, electronic adaptation, computer software, or by similar or dissimilar methodology now known or hereafter developed.
The use of general descriptive names, registered names, trademarks, service marks, etc. in this publication does not imply, even in the absence of a specific statement, that such names are exempt from the relevant protective laws and regulations and therefore free for general use.
The publisher, the authors and the editors are safe to assume that the advice and information in this book are believed to be true and accurate at the date of publication. Neither the publisher nor the authors or the editors give a warranty, express or implied, with respect to the material contained herein or for any errors or omissions that may have been made. The publisher remains neutral with regard to jurisdictional claims in published maps and institutional affiliations.

Printed on acid-free paper

This Springer imprint is published by the registered company Springer International Publishing AG part of Springer Nature
The registered company address is: Gewerbestrasse 11, 6330 Cham, Switzerland

Preface

Hyperhidrosis is a disease that does not kill, but that does disrupt the life of the patient. It not only affects the patient's quality of life but also has a strong influence on the development of their personality. Other aspects of the disease that are rarely thought about, but that can have a great influence on the patient, are the discomfort of the condition and even the impossibility of carrying out some professional activities. It can be dangerous for patients with serious symptoms to carry out certain activities, and in some cases it can even exclude patients from various occupations, such as being electronic technicians or pharmacists, or being members of the military or police forces with jobs that involve a high level of stress.

Hyperhidrosis is not well known generally, although it is present in at least 1% of the global population, and its prevalence could be as high as 3%. Health professionals also don't know a great deal about the condition. In the era of the amazing availability of information—information that can be reliable or false—it is very important to be familiar with the whole picture of this bothersome condition.

To achieve this purpose, "Hyperhidrosis—a Complete Guide to Diagnosis and Management" was conceived as a manual for the thorough understanding of hyperhidrosis. We selected professionals from different fields—psychologists and psychiatrists, dermatologists, endocrinologists, surgeons, and nutritionists—to write the different chapters.

We have paid special attention to the clinical and surgical treatment of the condition. Although surgery is still the most effective treatment for most indications at all sites of hyperhidrosis presentation, as well as for facial blushing, you can find many alternatives in the book. Side effects of treatments like sympathectomy have resulted in the development of other treatments, which are also described here. The purpose of the book is to share as much experience as possible from some of the best specialists worldwide.

We cannot fail to inform about the side effects and complications that can occur not only with clinical treatment, but also with the surgical procedures that are often necessary for the care of these patients. We have chapters devoted to these side effects and chapters devoted to the prevention and treatment of compensatory hyperhidrosis, one of the most frequent problems that can be caused by surgical treatment. This problem is faced with rigor and all the latest information on the subject is included.

In this book we find, for the first time, a desire not only to provide information about hyperhidrosis, but also information on how to select the best indication for treatment and the best treatment; the final results; and the effectiveness of the treatment, whether it is clinical, psychological, or surgical. Several points are considered important in this book, but we highlight the chapters about patient selection, clinical treatment, surgical treatment, compensatory hyperhidrosis, and dietary changes. There is also a chapter written by a patient who underwent surgery on three occasions and a chapter by a physician with legal training, who writes about the medico-legal implications of treatment. Last but not least are two chapters about sympathectomy for plantar hyperidrosis, written by the most experienced surgeons in that field.

To conclude, patients and their relatives, physicians, lawyers, surgeons, or indeed anyone who is eager for knowledge about the subject, will find in this book the most up-to-date and reliable information about hyperhidrosis.

São Paulo, Brazil	José Ribas M. de Campos
Curitiba, Brazil	Marcelo de Paula Loureiro
São Paulo, Brazil	Paulo Kauffman
São Paulo, Brazil	Nelson Wolosker

Contents

Part I The Patient with Hyperhidrosis

1. **Anatomy of the Sudoripar Glands** 3
   Samantha Neves, Dafne Braga Diamante Leiderman,
   and Nelson Wolosker

2. **Secondary Hyperhidrosis: Endocrinopathies and Hyperhidrosis** ... 13
   Marcello D. Bronstein

3. **Hyperhidrosis and Obesity** 19
   Ana Maria Pita Lottenberg and Natália Sanchez Oliveira Jensen

4. **Primary Hyperhidrosis** 27
   Paulo Kauffman

5. **The Prevalence of Hyperhidrosis Worldwide** 33
   Sonia Oliveira Lima and Vanessa Rocha de Santana

6. **Hyperhidrosis in Children** 39
   Samantha Neves, John Robert Pires-Davidson,
   Dafne Braga Diamante Leiderman, and Nelson Wolosker

7. **The Psychological Profile of the Patient
   with Primary Hyperhidrosis** 45
   Ana Rosa Sancovski

8. **Psychiatric Features in Hyperhidrosis** 53
   Marianna Gonzalez de Oliveira Andrade

9. **Anxiety, Depression, and Hyperhidrosis** 57
   Débora Yumi Ferreira Kamikava

10. **Hyperhidrosis and Diet-Induced Thermogenesis** 61
    Najla Elias Farage and Milena Barcza Stockler-Pinto

11. **Constraints Caused by Primary Hyperhidrosis** 65
    Regina Lunkes Diehl

Part II General Treatment of Hyperhidrosis

12 Pharmacological Treatment of Hyperhidrosis 75
Dafne Braga Diamante Leiderman, Samantha Neves,
and Nelson Wolosker

13 Hyperidrosis and Topical Agents 81
Marcia Purcelli

**14 Axillary Hyperhidrosis and Bromhidrosis:
The Dermatologist's Point of View** 89
Roberta Vasconcelos and José Antonio Sanches Jr.

15 Botulinum Toxin for Axillary and Palmar Hyperhidrosis 95
Mônica Aribi, Gabriel Aribi, and Thalita Domingues Mendes

**16 Axillary Hyperhidrosis: Local Surgical
Treatment with Aspiratory Curettage** 107
Ronaldo Golcman, Murillo Francisco Pires Fraga,
and Benjamin Golcman

Part III Sympathectomies for Hyperhidrosis

**17 Anatomy of the Sympathetic Nervous
System in Relation to Surgical Hyperhidrosis Treatment** 117
André Felix Gentil and Arthur W. Poetscher

18 Criteria for Surgical Patient Selection 127
Sérgio Kuzniec and Paulo Kauffman

**19 Surgical Techniques for the Realization
of Thoracic Sympathectomy** 131
Eduardo de Campos Werebe, Carlos Levischi, and Rodrigo Sabbion

20 Bilateral Thoracic Sympathectomy: How I Do It? 147
Davi Wen Wei Kang, Benoit Jacques Bibas, and Mauro Federico
Luis Tamagno

**21 Endoscopic Thoracic Sympathectomy
for Primary Palmar Hyperhidrosis** 155
Alan E. P. Cameron

**22 Evolution of Surgical Methods and Difficulties
Relating to Endoscopic Thoracic Sympathectomy** 163
Paulo Kauffman

**23 Is the Clipping Method for Sympathetic Nerve Surgery
a Reversible Procedure?** 171
Javier Pérez Vélez and Carlos Martinez-Barenys

24	**Surgical Difficulties and Complications of Video-Assisted Thoracoscopic for Thoracic Sympathectomy**.................. Laert de Oliveira Andrade Filho and Fabiano Cataldi Engel	179
25	**Outpatient Clinic Treatment for Patients with Hyperhidrosis**...... Camilo Osorio Barker	189
26	**Management of Compensatory Hyperhidrosis**.................. Dafne Braga Diamante Leiderman, Guilherme Yazbec, and Nelson Wolosker	197
27	**Endoscopic Lumbar Sympathectomy in the Treatment of Hyperhidrosis: Technical Aspects**............ Marcelo de Paula Loureiro, Paulo Kauffman, Rafael Reisfeld, and Roman Rieger	203
28	**Endoscopic Lumbar Sympathectomy in the Treatment of Hyperhidrosis: Results and Complications**................... Marcelo de Paula Loureiro, Rafael Reisfeld, Eraj Basseri, Gregg Kai Nishi, Roman Rieger, and Karina Wurm-Wolfsgruber	215

Part IV Blushing

29	**Facial Blushing: Psychiatric Management**...................... Enrique Jadresic	227
30	**Patient Selection for Endoscopic Thoracic Sympathectomy for Facial Blushing**............................ Claudio Suárez Cruzat and Francisco Suárez Vásquez	235
31	**Endoscopic Thoracic Sympathectomy for Facial Blushing and Craniofacial Hyperhidrosis**............................... Peter B. Licht	243

Part V Final

32	**Quality-of-Life Evaluation During Treatment of Hyperhidrosis**... Hugo Veiga Sampaio da Fonseca and José Ribas M. de Campos	253
33	**Ethical and Legal Aspects of the Management of Hyperhidrosis**.... Irimar de Paula Posso, Daniella Salazar Posso Costa, and Fabiana Salazar Posso	261
34	**Questions and Answers on Hyperhidrosis, Its Treatment and Consequences**.. Miguel L. Tedde, Elias Albino Theophilo, and Flavio Henrique Savazzi	271
Index..		277

Contributors

Laert de Oliveira Andrade Filho Hospital Israelita Albert Einstein, São Paulo, SP, Brazil

Marianna Gonzalez de Oliveira Andrade Hospital Israelita Albert Einstein, São Paulo, SP, Brazil

Gabriel Aribi, MD Department of Dermatology, Ipiranga Hospital, São Paulo, SP, Brazil

Mônica Aribi, MD Department of Dermatology, Ipiranga Hospital, São Paulo, SP, Brazil

Camilo Osorio Barker Universidad Pontificia Bolivariana, Medellín, Antioquia, Colombia

Eraj Basseri, MD The Center for Hyperhidrosis, Beverly Hills, CA, USA

Benoit Jacques Bibas, MD Department of Thoracic Surgery, University of São Paulo, São Paulo, SP, Brazil

Marcello D. Bronstein, MD, PhD Neuroendocrine Unit, Division of Endocrinology and Metabolism, Hospital das Clínicas, University of São Paulo Medical School, São Paulo, SP, Brazil

Alan E. P. Cameron, MCh, FRCS Surgical Department, Ipswich Hospital, Ipswich, UK

José Ribas M. de Campos, MD, PhD Thoracic Surgery, University of São Paulo and Hospital Israelita Albert Einstein, São Paulo, SP, Brazil

Daniella Salazar Posso Costa Posso Costa Associated Lawyers, São Paulo, SP, Brazil

Claudio Suárez Cruzat, MD Thoracic Surgery Department, Clínica Santa María, Santiago, Chile

Thoracic Surgery Program, Universidad de Los Andes, Santiago, Chile

Regina Lunkes Diehl School of Media Communication, Arts and Design - Famecos - Pontifical Catholic University RS, Porto Alegre, Rio Grande do Sul, Brazil

Fabiano Cataldi Engel Hospital Israelita Albert Einstein, São Paulo, SP, Brazil

Najla Elias Farage Nutrition Department, Universidade Veiga Almeida, Rio de Janeiro, RJ, Brazil

Medical Sciences, Universidade Federal Fluminense, Niterói, RJ, Brazil

Hugo Veiga Sampaio da Fonseca, MD Royal Thoracic Surgery Clinic – Royal Portuguese Hospital of Beneficense in Pernambuco, Recife, Brazil

Murillo Francisco Pires Fraga Brazilian Society of Plastic Surgery, São Paulo, SP, Brazil

Faculty of Medical Sciences of Santa Casa of São Paulo, São Paulo, SP, Brazil

André Felix Gentil Neurosurgeon of the Hospital Israelita Albert Einstein in São Paulo, São Paulo, SP, Brazil

School of Medicine, University of São Paulo, São Paulo, SP, Brazil

Benjamin Golcman University of São Paulo, São Paulo, SP, Brazil

Brazilian Society of Plastic Surgery, São Paulo, SP, Brazil

Ronaldo Golcman University of São Paulo, São Paulo, SP, Brazil

Brazilian Society of Plastic Surgery, São Paulo, SP, Brazil

Hospital Israelita Albert Einstein, São Paulo, SP, Brazil

Enrique Jadresic Department of Psychiatry, Faculty of Medicine, University of Chile, Santiago, Chile

Natália Sanchez Oliveira Jensen Collaborator at the Diabetes Control League of the Hospital das Clínicas, University of São Paulo, São Paulo, SP, Brazil

Debora Yumi Ferreira Kamikava Mackenzie Presbyterian University, São Paulo, SP, Brazil

General Hospital, HCFMUSP, São Paulo, SP, Brazil

Psychology Division of Central Institute, HCFMUSP, São Paulo, SP, Brazil

Davi Wen Wei Kang Thoracic Surgeon at Hospital Israelita Albert Einstein, São Paulo, SP, Brazil

Paulo Kauffman Department of Vascular and Endovascular Surgery, University of São Paulo School of Medicine, São Paulo, SP, Brazil

Sérgio Kuzniec Hospital Israelita Albert Einstein, São Paulo, SP, Brazil

Dafne Braga Diamante Leiderman Department of Vascular and Endovascular Surgery, Hospital Israelita Albert Einstein, São Paulo, SP, Brazil

Carlos Levischi Hospital Israelita Albert Einstein, São Paulo, SP, Brazil

Peter B. Licht, MD, PhD Department of Cardiothoracic Surgery, Odense University Hospital, Odense, Denmark

Sonia Oliveira Lima School of Medicine, Tiradentes University, Aracaju, SE, Brazil

University of São Paulo, São Paulo, SP, Brazil

Ana Maria Pita Lottenberg Laboratório de Lípides (LIM-10), Hospital das Clínicas HCFMUSP, Faculdade de Medicina, Universidade de São Paulo, São Paulo, University of São Paulo (HCFMUSP), São Paulo, SP, Brazil

Faculdade Israelita de Ciências da Saúde Albert Einstein, Hospital Israelita Albert Einstein, São Paulo, SP, Brazil

Marcelo de Paula Loureiro General Surgery and Biotechnology, Positivo University and INC Hospital, Curitiba, PR, Brazil

Carlos Martinez-Barenys Thoracic Surgery Department, University Hospital Germans Trias i Pujol, Barcelona, Spain

Thalita Domingues Mendes, MD Department of Dermatology, Ipiranga Hospital, São Paulo, SP, Brazil

Samantha Neves Brazilian Society of Dermatology, São Paulo, SP, Brazil

School of Medicine, ABC, Santo André, SP, Brazil

Gregg Kai Nishi, MD The Center for Hyperhidrosis, Beverly Hills, CA, USA

John Robert Pires-Davidson Hospital Universitário Maria Aparecida Pedrossian–UFMS, Campo Grande, Brazil

Arthur W. Poetscher Neurosurgeon of the Hospital Israelita Albert Einstein, São Paulo, SP, Brazil

School of Medicine, University of São Paulo, São Paulo, SP, Brazil

Albert Einstein Institute for Teaching and Research, São Paulo, SP, Brazil

Fabiana Salazar Posso Clínic Rhinoderma, Santo André, São Paulo, SP, Brazil

Irimar de Paula Posso Hospital Israelita Albert Einstein, São Paulo, SP, Brazil

Study and training center, School of Medicine ABC, Santo André, São Paulo, SP, Brazil

Marcia Purcelli Hospital Israelita Albert Einstein, São Paulo, SP, Brazil

Rafael Reisfeld, MD The Center for Hyperhidrosis, Beverly Hills, CA, USA

Roman Rieger Surgical Department, Salzkammergut-Klinikum Gmunden, Gmunden, Austria

Rodrigo Sabbion Hospital Israelita Albert Einstein, São Paulo, SP, Brazil

José Antonio Sanches Jr., MD, PhD Department of Dermatology, School of Medicine, University of São Paulo, São Paulo, SP, Brazil

Ana Rosa Sancovski PhD in Experimental Physiopathology Sciences from School of Medicine, University of São Paulo, São Paulo, SP, Brazil

Psychosomatic Specialist from Sedes Sapientiae Institute, São Paulo, SP, Brazil

General Medical Clinic, Hospital das Clínicas de São Paulo, São Paulo, SP, Brazil

Hyperhidrosis Outpatient Clinic, Hospital das Clínicas de São Paulo, São Paulo, SP, Brazil

Psychoanalytical Theory, Clinic in Neuropsychology, Neuropsychological Residence of the National Center for Specialization Courses – CENACES, São Paulo, SP, Brazil

Vanessa Rocha de Santana School of Medicine of Bahia, Tiradentes University, Aracaju, SE, Brazil

Flavio Henrique Savazzi Hospital Alemão Oswaldo Cruz, São Paulo, Brazil

Milena Barcza Stockler-Pinto School of Nutrition, Universidade Federal Fluminense, Niterói, RJ, Brazil

Mauro Federico Luis Tamagno, MD Thoracic Surgeon, São Paulo, SP, Brazil

Miguel L. Tedde Department of Thoracic Surgery, Heart Institute (InCor), Hospital das Clínicas, University of São Paulo and Hospital Samaritano, São Paulo, SP, Brazil

Elias Albino Theophilo Hospital Santa Catarina, São Paulo, SP, Brazil

Roberta Vasconcelos, MD, PhD Department of Dermatology, São Paulo Cancer Institute—ICESP, São Paulo, SP, Brazil

Francisco Suárez Vásquez Thoracic Surgery Department, Clínica Santa María, Santiago, Chile

Thoracic Surgery Program, Universidad de Los Andes, Santiago, Chile

Javier Pérez Vélez Thoracic Surgery Department, University Hospital Vall d'Hebron, Barcelona, Spain

Eduardo de Campos Werebe Hospital Israelita Albert Einstein, São Paulo, SP, Brazil

Nelson Wolosker Department of Vascular and Endovascular Surgery, Hospital Israelita Albert Einstein, São Paulo, SP, Brazil

Karina Wurm-Wolfsgruber Surgical Department, Salzkammergut-Klinikum Gmunden, Gmunden, Austria

Guilherme Yazbec Department of Vascular and Endovascular Surgery, A.C. Camargo Cancer Center, Liberdade, São Paulo, SP, Brazil

Part I

The Patient with Hyperidrosis

Anatomy of the Sudoripar Glands

Samantha Neves, Dafne Braga Diamante Leiderman, and Nelson Wolosker

Origin and Location

The sweat glands are formed and located on the skin (Fig. 1.1). The skin, in turn, is the largest organ of the human body, and is formed by three layers:

1. Epidermis
2. Derme
3. Hipoderme

S. Neves (✉)
Brazilian Society of Dermatology, São Paulo, SP, Brazil

School of Medicine, ABC, Santo André, São Paulo, SP, Brazil
e-mail: samantha@samanthaneves.com.br

D. B. D. Leiderman
Department of Vascular and Endovascular Surgery, Hospital Israelita Albert Einstein, São Paulo, SP, Brazil

N. Wolosker
Department of Vascular and Endovascular Surgery, Hospital Israelita Albert Einstein, São Paulo, SP, Brazil

© Springer International Publishing AG, part of Springer Nature 2018
M. P. Loureiro et al. (eds.), *Hyperhidrosis*,
https://doi.org/10.1007/978-3-319-89527-7_1

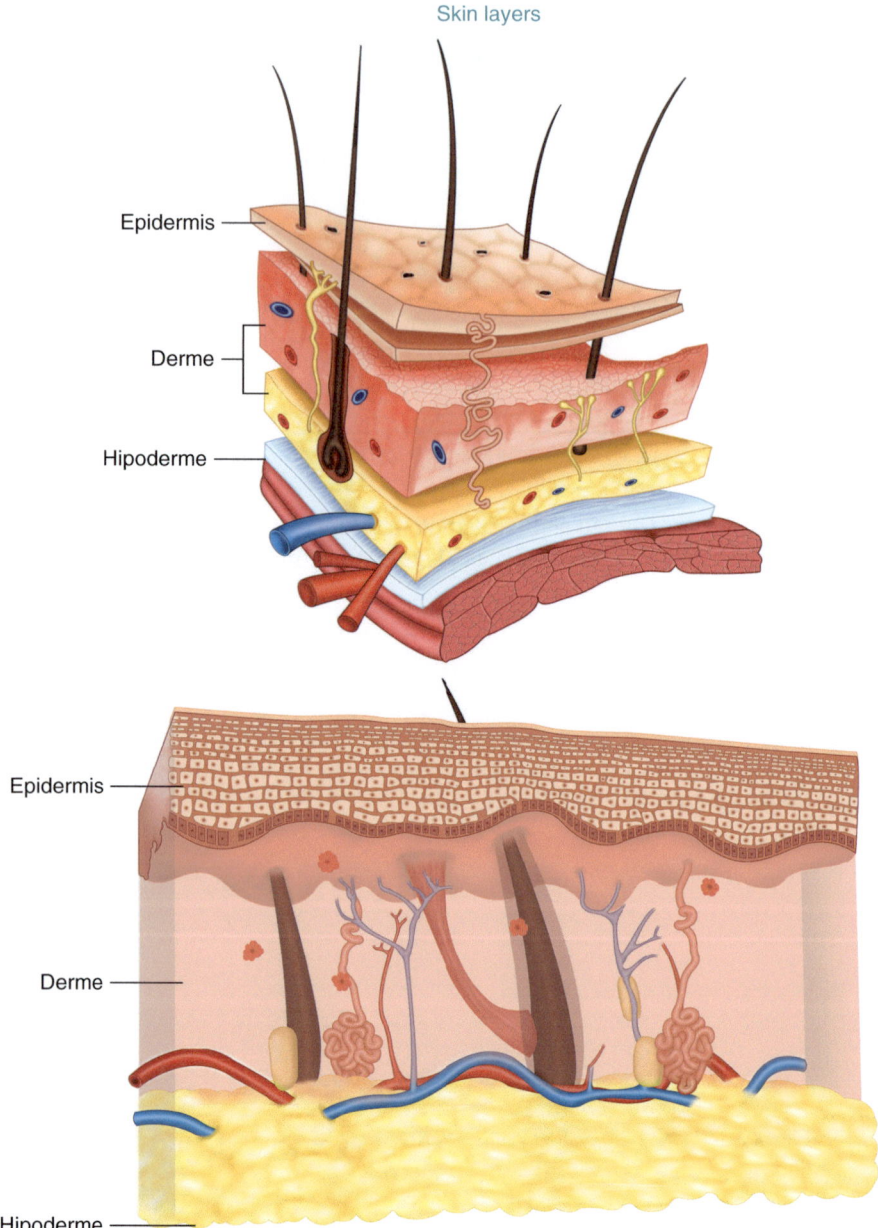

Fig. 1.1 Skin Layers

The first two layers are closely adhered. The epidermis layer, which is in constant regeneration, is the outermost surface of the skin, formed by a stratified and keratinized squamous epithelium. This layer is supported and nourished by a thick layer of richly vascularized fibroelastic connective tissue that has numerous sensory receptors—the dermis [1]. In turn, the dermis is attached to the underlying tissues

1 Anatomy of the Sudoripar Glands

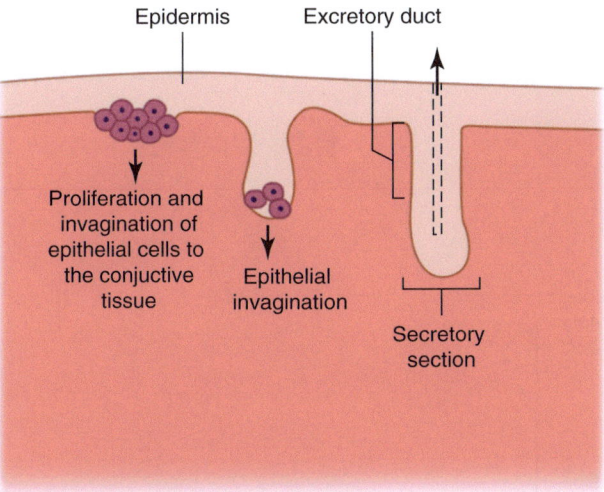

Fig. 1.2 Sweat Gland

by a layer with a variable amount of adipose tissue called the hypodermis, or subcutaneous layer.

The skin has several functions, including protection against chemical, thermal, and mechanical damage [2]. Its surface acts as a barrier to the invasion of microorganisms and, because of its relatively impermeable character, it prevents excessive loss of water. Due to the variety of receptors it possesses, the skin is a sensory organ of paramount importance.

The epidermis, derived from the cutaneous ectoderm, starts from the third week of life of the embryo, and the accumulation of epidermal cells and the increase in underlying mesenchymal cells leads to an invagination and deepening of these structures, thus forming the so-called cords (Fig. 1.2). It is in the protuberances of these strands that the formation of the cutaneous appendages will be formed. These, in turn, are divided into sweat glands, sebaceous glands, and hairs [3]. Thus, hair follicles and sweat and sebaceous glands are epidermal derivatives present at various levels of the dermis.

Types and Functions

The skin glands include:

1. Sebaceous glands
2. Sweat glands (Fig. 1.3)
   (a) Eccrines
   (b) Apocrine
3. Mammary glands.

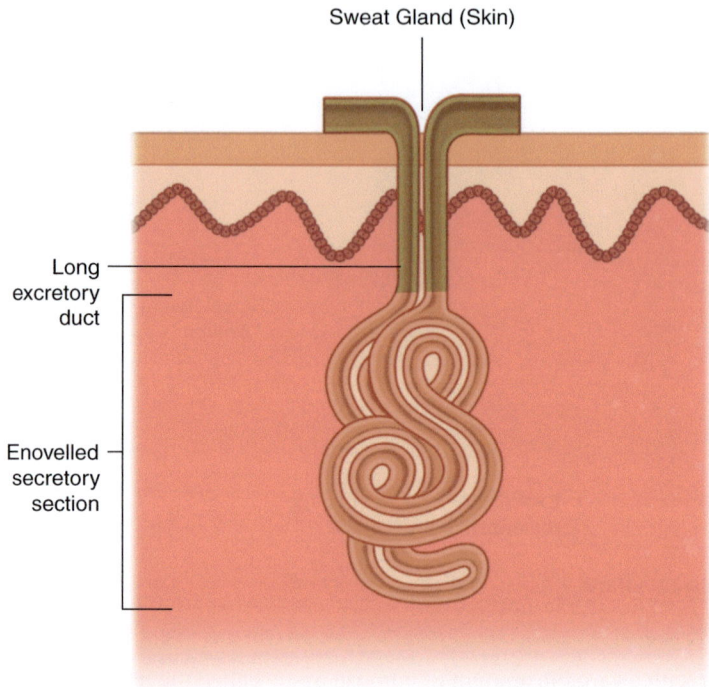

Fig. 1.3 Sweat Gland

(Illustration 3: source: medical literature—copyrighted)

1 Anatomy of the Sudoripar Glands

Eccrine Sweat Glands

Eccrine sweat glands (or meroccrins) are simple enovelous tubular glands (Fig. 1.4).

The main function of these eccrine sweat glands is to exercise body thermoregulation through the formation and excretion of the sweat secretion.

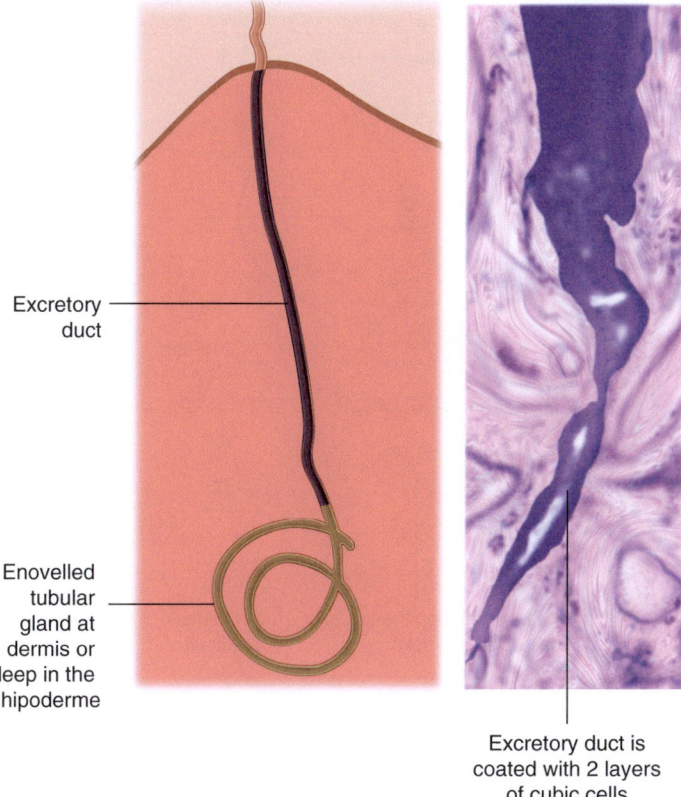

Fig. 1.4 Sweat Gland

The secretory portion is formed by three types of cells (Figs. 1.5 and 1.6):

1. Clear cells
2. Dark cells
3. Myoepithelial cells.

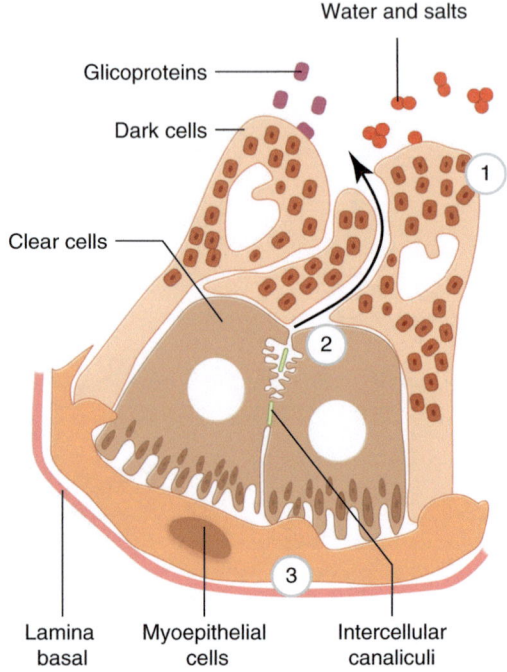

Fig. 1.5 Sweat Gland Secretory Portion

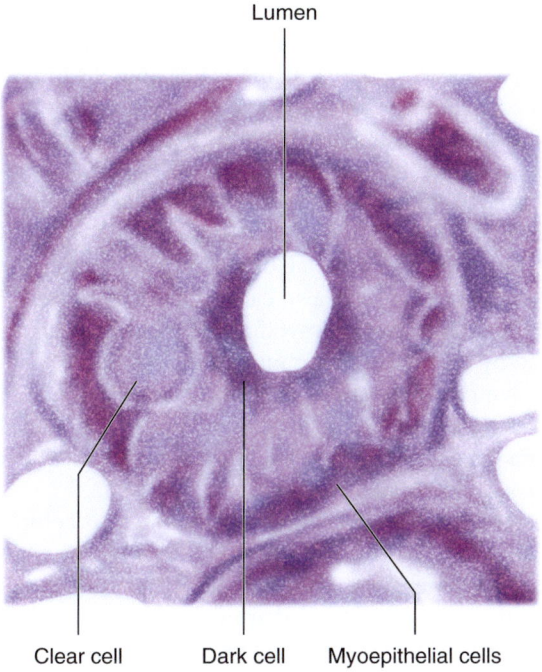
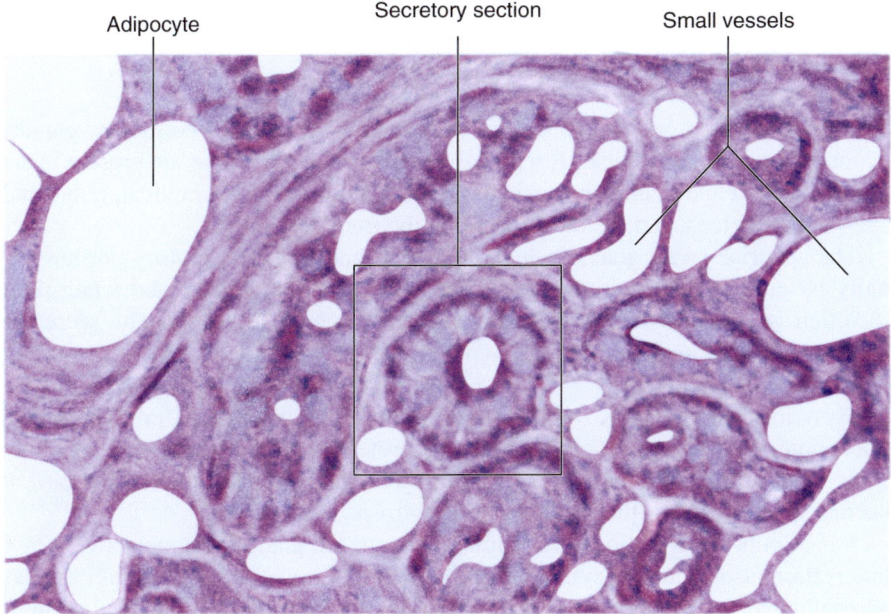

Fig. 1.6 Microscopy of secretory portion of sweat gland (Illustration 6)

The clear cells are separated from each other by intercellular canaliculi, which are present in the basal region of their epithelium invaginations and a large amount of mitochondria. These secrete most of the water and electrolytes (Na^+ and Cl^-) from sweat. Dark cells lean on clear cells and secrete glycoproteins.

Myoepithelial cells are found between the basal lamina and the clear cells responsible for the secretion of sweat.

The intraepidermal excretory portion of the sweat duct is composed of a layer of lining tissue and a layer of epithelial cells, composing the peridural, bilayer sheath of cubic cells that partially reabsorb NaCl and water under the influence of aldosterone. The orifice of the sweat gland, also called the acrosyringeal, is surrounded by keratinocytes [4]. Innervated by non-myelinated postganglionic sympathetic fibers, they are controlled by parasympathetic mediators, but they respond, although to a lesser extent, to sympathomimetic mediators. Therefore, parasympathomimetic drugs, such as acetylcholine, acetyl-β-methylcholine, and pilocarpine, stimulate sweating and parasympatolytic drugs, such as atropine, inhibit it. However, the eccrine glands are also stimulated by adrenaline.

The type of secretion eliminated by the eccrine glands is colorless, odorless, and hypotonic [5].

The eccrine glands are never associated with the hair follicle and are more developed and larger in the palms, plants, and armpits, which justifies the fact that they are present on all body surfaces except the lips, nail bed, small lips, glans, and inner face of the foreskin. These areas are the most affected in cases of localized hyperhidrosis [5].

Apocrine Sudoripar Glands

The apocrine sweat glands, as well as the eccrines, are enveloped tubular glands, which lead to the hair follicles just above the sebaceous duct. They are present in the armpits, areola and mammary papillae, in the pre-sternal, periumbilical, pubic and ano-genital regions, and are rarely found in the trunk and scalp.

The apocrine sweat glands, which are compound in their secretory portion initially by cuboid cells, progressively have their height increases, and when their secretion is promptly eliminated, they become low and flat again. The secretory portion is located in the dermis and hypodermis.

(Illustration 7)

Secretion from apocrine sweat glands has a milky appearance, consisting of a thick liquid, initially odorless, containing proteins, sugars, ammonia, and fatty acids. When this secretion is broken down by microorganisms, such as bacteria, it becomes malodorous—the so-called bromhidrosis.

It is at puberty, with hormonal stimulus, that these glands become active. Their innervation also occurs by sympathetic fibers; therefore, adrenergic stimuli such as adrenaline and noradrenaline produce apocrine secretion. From a practical point of view, this type of sweat gland basically serves as scent glands, and in animals are responsible for the so-called "heat".

References

1. Kierszenbaum AL, Tres LL. Histology and cell biology. 3rd ed. Philadelphia: Elsevier; 2012.
2. Rechardt L, Waris T, Rintala A. Innervation of human axillary sweat glands. Histochemical and electron microscopic study of hyperhidrotic and normal subjects. Scand J Plast Reconstr Surg. 1976;10(2):107–12.
3. Lonsdale-Eccles A, Leonard N, Lawrence C. Axillary hyperhidrosis: eccrine or apocrine? Clin Exp Dermatol. 2003;28(1):2–7.
4. Sato K, Kang WH, Saga K, Sato KT. Biology of sweat glands and their disorders. II. Disorders of sweat gland function. J Am Acad Dermatol. 1989 May;20(5 Pt 1):713–26.
5. Gontijo G.T., Gualberto G.V., Madureira N.A.B. Atualização no tratamento de hiperidrose axilar. Surgical and Cosmetic Dermatology, 2011; 2jun.

Secondary Hyperhidrosis: Endocrinopathies and Hyperhidrosis

Marcello D. Bronstein

Menopause

Menopause has as a landmark the definitive cessation of spontaneous menses. In this way, the onset of menopause can only be considered after 1 year following the last menstrual flow, because in this period, called climacteric, occasional menstruation may still occur. The climacteric represents the passage from the reproductive to the non-reproductive phase, with progressive reduction of the production of estrogens and progesterone.

The age of onset of menopause is variable, usually occurring between 45 and 55 years. If it occurs before the age of 45 years, it is called early menopause and, although it may be physiological, is often linked to pathophysiological processes, such as autoimmune oophoritis, drugs, surgical or radiotherapy iatrogenesis, and pituitary diseases such as hyperprolactinemia/prolactinomas and clinically non-secretory macroadenomas.

The symptomatology includes, in addition to menstrual absence, hot flashes, reduction of libido, vaginal dryness, changes in body composition, insomnia, reduced memory, increased cardiovascular risk, and loss of bone mass.

The hot flashes are present in about 80% of menopausal women, and may already be present during the climacteric period. They are characterized by an intense sudden and transitory sensation of heat, usually beginning in the face and chest, accompanied by the activation of mechanisms of heat loss, which include cutaneous vasodilation and sweating. The duration is minutes, and hyperhidrosis can be associated with palpitations and tremors. Hot flashes can occur several times a day and also at night, leading to sleep disorders. In untreated women, the hot flashes usually last for 5–6 years, with decreasing intensity and frequency, but in some cases they may persist for longer.

M. D. Bronstein
Neuroendocrine Unit, Division of Endocrinology and Metabolism, Hospital das Clínicas, University of São Paulo Medical School, São Paulo, SP, Brazil

It is assumed that the pathophysiology of hot flashes is associated with estrogen-modulated hypothalamic body temperature control dysfunction, which presents a marked decline in menopause. Some studies have shown that hot flashes occur simultaneously with the release of luteinizing hormone (LH), but patients with central cause hypogonadism and those with pituitary tumors also have hot flashes despite low LH levels.

Laboratory diagnosis of menopause is made by the low levels of estrogens and progesterone, accompanied by elevation of gonadotrophins (follicle-stimulating hormone [FSH] and LH). When gonadotrophin levels are normal or low, we should think of hypothalamic–pituitary causes as responsible for amenorrhea.

The treatment of choice is estrogen replacement, since, besides improvement of the hot flashes, the other clinical aspects of the menopause also benefit. For those women with a contraindication to estrogen therapy, due to personal or familial history of gynecological neoplasia or coagulation disorders, other therapies are available. These include use of phytoestrogens such as isoflavones, and medications such as the selective serotonin reuptake inhibitors, clonidine, and gabapentin.

Men who have hypogonadism or undergo anti-androgen therapy for prostate cancer may also present hot flashes, with a high incidence in the latter. Psychotherapy and the use of progestagens, gabapentin, and serotonin reuptake inhibitors are measures that may ease the discomfort of these patients.

Hyperthyroidism

Hyperthyroidism is the most prevalent dysfunction in hyperhidrosis secondary to endocrine causes. It consists of a syndrome that results from excessive exposure to thyroid hormones, with a classic clinical picture, usually accompanying adrenergic manifestations: palpitations, tachycardia, tremors of extremities, and sweating, in addition to heat intolerance and diarrhea. Its most common cause, toxic diffuse goiter (Graves' disease) may or may not be accompanied by ocular manifestations such as exophthalmos (Fig. 2.1).There are, however, other causes of hyperthyroidism, often with less exuberant clinical manifestations. This is the case of toxic

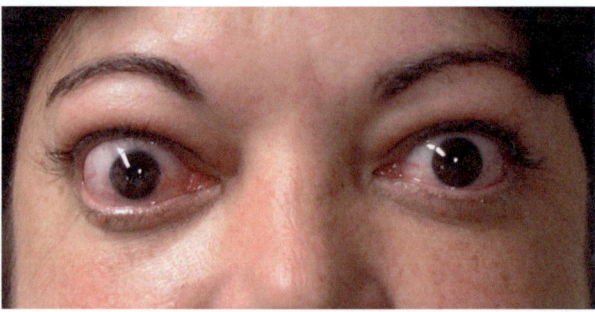

Fig. 2.1 Bilateral proptosis and eyelid retraction in a patient with Graves' orbitopathy

uni- or multinodular goiter, which usually affects older patients. Treatment of hyperthyroidism is performed with thyroid-blocking drugs, radioiodine therapy, or surgery, depending on the case. Blocking drug therapy with thioureas, such as tapazole and propylthiouracil, is used as the initial treatment, especially in more severe cases, such as preparation for surgery or radioiodine therapy. In the case of Graves' disease with small goiter and no ocular signs, there is a good chance of remission of hyperthyroidism without the need for other procedures. The indication of radioiodine therapy or subtotal thyroidectomy will depend on the volume of the goiter and the presence or absence of exophthalmos.

Subacute thyroiditis also leads to thyrotoxicosis by releasing thyroid hormones stored in the glandular colloid. It is usually accompanied by cervical pain and evening fever, but it can be painless (silent thyroiditis) and its diagnosis is often confused with classic hyperthyroidism. The treatment for subacute thyroiditis, usually lasting 2–3 months, is with non-hormonal anti-inflammatories or glucocorticoids and β-blockers. There are extremely rare conditions associated with thyrotoxicosis, such as pituitary tumors producing thyroid-stimulating hormone (TSH), pituitary resistance to thyroid hormone, hydatidiform mole, and struma ovarii. Finally, we must remember factitious thyrotoxicosis, a condition resulting from the ingestion of high doses of thyroid hormone for the general purpose of weight loss. This is a deplorable practice that must be fought.

Pheochromocytoma

Hyperhidrosis is one of the clinical manifestations of pheochromocytomas. These tumors originate from chromaffin cells of the sympathetic nervous system, which release norepinephrine and/or epinephrine and, more rarely, dopamine and other active peptides, and account for about 0.1% of the causes of arterial hypertension. All ages and both sexes are affected, although they are more common in the fourth and fifth decades. Although paroxysmal episodes of hypertension are typical of pheochromocytoma, about half of the cases exhibit maintained hypertension. The triad of headache, diffuse sweating, and pallor in the presence of hypertension is classic and highly suggestive of pheochromocytoma. The location of pheochromocytomas is almost always abdominal (95% of cases) and 85% are in the adrenal glands; 5% are extra-abdominal (e.g., in the mediastinum). Laboratory diagnosis is made by serum or urinary catecholamines or their metabolites, such as metanephrines and vanilmandelic acid. In cases where a laboratory diagnosis is not confirmed, so-called provocative tests, such as the clonidine or glucagon test, are indicated. Diagnosis by magnetic resonance imaging (MRI) is now considered the gold standard: the presence of hyperintense signal in T2 is highly suggestive of pheochromocytoma. Computed tomography is also useful, as is scintigraphy with metaiodobenzylguanidine, which is a more functional assessment because it is based on the uptake of a catecholamine precursor. The treatment of pheochromocytoma is surgical, and requires preparation to avoid serious pressure accidents. This preparation is usually done only with α-adrenergic blockers, in combination with β-adrenergics in cases with tachyarrhythmias. Patients with pheochromocytomas may be carriers of type 2 multiple endocrine neoplasia, in which case these tumors are associated with hyperparathyroidism and with medullary thyroid carcinoma or neurofibromatosis.

Hypoglycemia

Hypoglycemic syndrome has several causes and usually presents the Whipple triad as a clinical feature: (1) adrenergic manifestations, such as tachycardia and generalized hyperhidrosis, and neuroglycopenic symptoms, such as changes in behavior and loss of consciousness; (2) low plasma levels of glucose; and (3) clinical reversibility with glucose administration. The manifestations usually occur with blood glucose lower than 50 mg/dL, but if the fall is rapid they can occur with higher blood glucose levels. Its causes are several, the main ones being (1) tumors of the pancreatic islets, insulinomas, whose most important manifestations usually occur in prolonged fasting—insulinomas may be associated with multiple endocrine neoplasia type 1, which is also characterized by the presence of hyperparathyroidism and pituitary tumors; (2) reactive hypoglycemia, occurring postprandially; (3) iatrogenic hypoglycemia, especially in diabetic patients taking insulin or oral hypoglycemic agents, particularly chlorpropamide; and (4) hypoglycemia linked to specific conditions, such as alcohol abuse, liver failure, or adrenal insufficiency.

Acromegaly

Acromegaly is a rare disease, with an estimated prevalence of 60 cases per million. It is caused in 99% of cases by a growth hormone (GH)-producing pituitary adenoma, leading to the hypersecretion of this hormone, which in turn induces excessive production of insulin-like growth factor-1 (IGF-1), which leads to facial and extremities deformities and visceromegaly. In addition to somatic changes, which generally make the clinical diagnosis quite clear, patients with acromegaly have a high prevalence of co-morbidities such as high blood pressure, heart disease, and diabetes mellitus, which reduce their life expectancy by about 10 years. Acromegalic patients are hypermetabolic, with hyperhidrosis, mainly palmar and plantar, being a common manifestation of this disorder. Clinical diagnosis is confirmed by baseline GH (elevated), glucose tolerance test (non-suppressible), and IGF-1 (elevated). MRI of the sellar region almost invariably shows the presence of a pituitary tumor, usually macroadenoma. The most commonly used initial treatment is pituitary surgery via the transsphenoidal approach. Alternatively, for non-cured cases, those with a low possibility of surgical cure, or with contraindications for general anesthesia, drug treatment with somatostatin analogs, dopaminergic agonists, or GH receptor antagonists plays an important role. Finally, conventional or stereotaxic radiotherapy is indicated for cases of resistance to or impossibility of drug treatment. Hyperhidrosis yields rapidly in efficiently treated cases.

Carcinoid Syndrome

Carcinoid syndrome, a relatively rare condition, is caused by hypersecretion of serotonin, usually by neuroendocrine tumors that may be located in various regions, such as the lung, pancreas, intestine, appendix, and so on. Although it is associated with hyperhidrosis, sweating in patients with carcinoid syndrome is generally relatively modest compared with other symptoms such as flushing, diarrhea, and bronchoconstriction. The main screening test is the determination of 5-hydroxyindolacetic acid. This assay is very affected by food, requiring a fundamental preparatory diet guided by the laboratory. The treatment can be surgical and/or clinical with somatostatin analogs, and should be individualized.

Suggested Reading

Abreu A, Tovar AP, Castellanos R, Valenzuela A, Giraldo CM, Pinedo AC, Guerrero DP, Barrera CA, Franco HI, Ribeiro-Oliveira A Jr, Vilar L, Jallad RS, Duarte FG, Gadelha M, Boguszewski CL, Abucham J, Naves LA, Musolino NR, Rossato d FME, Bronstein MD. Challenges in the diagnosis and management of acromegaly: a focus on comorbidities. Pituitary. 2016;19(4):448–57.

Cryer PE, Axelrod L, Grossman AB, Heller SR, Montori VM, Seaquist ER, Service FJ, Endocrine Society. Evaluation and management of adult hypoglycemic disorders: an Endocrine Society clinical practice guideline. J Clin Endocrinol Metab. 2009;94(3):709–28.

Hamed Ahmadi H, Daneshmand S. Androgen deprivation therapy for prostate cancer: long-term safety and patient outcomes. Patient Relat Outcome Meas. 2014;5:63–70.

Kaunitz AM, Manson JE. Management of menopausal symptoms. Obstet Gynecol. 2015;126(4):859–76.

Maia AL, Scheffel RS, Meyer EL, Mazeto GM, Carvalho GA, Graf H, Vaisman M, Maciel LM, Ramos HE, Tincani AJ, Andrada NC, Ward LS; Brazilian Society of Endocrinology and Metabolism. The Brazilian consensus for the diagnosis and treatment of hyperthyroidism: recommendations by the thyroid department of the Brazilian Society of Endocrinology and Metabolism. Arq Bras Endocrinol Metabol. 2013;57(3):205–32.

Massironi S, Sciola V, Peracchi M, Ciafardini C, Spampatti MP, Conte D. Neuroendocrine tumors of the gastro-entero-pancreatic system. World J Gastroenterol. 2008;14(35):5377–84.

Pacak K, Wimalawansa SJ. Pheochromocytoma and paraganglioma. Endocr Pract. 2015;21(4):406–12.

Hyperhidrosis and Obesity

Ana Maria Pita Lottenberg and
Natália Sanchez Oliveira Jensen

Obesity is a chronic disease characterized by an excessive amount of body fat, which increases the risk of health-related problems [1]. Adults can be considered obese when their body mass index (BMI) is ≥ 30 kg/m^2 [2]. Currently, over 1.9 billion adults are overweight (BMI ≥ 25 kg/m^2) and, of these, more than 600 million are obese [3].

Body fat accumulation in obesity can occur both in the subcutaneous adipose tissue, which is located under the skin, and in the visceral adipose tissue (VAT). VAT, characterized by the accumulation of intra-abdominal fat, has different morphology and characteristics than the subcutaneous adipose tissue: VAT adipocytes are larger, more metabolically active, and more sensitive to lipolysis; also, VAT is associated with a chronic low-grade inflammation due to the release of proinflammatory cytokines (tumor necrosis factor [TNF]-α, interleukin [IL]-1β, IL-6) by the adipocytes and as a consequence of macrophage infiltration and activation [4–6].

Obesity is associated with an increased risk of diseases such as type 2 diabetes mellitus, coronary heart disease, stroke, hypertension, dyslipidemia, sleep apnea, and some types of cancer [6].

In addition, overweight and obesity are also among the main conditions related to hyperhidrosis, probably due to the reduced heat loss caused by the thick subcutaneous adipose tissue layer, which may lead to a compensatory response characterized by the excessive production of sweat [7, 8].

A. M. P. Lottenberg (✉)
Laboratório de Lípides (LIM-10), Hospital das Clínicas HCFMUSP, Faculdade de Medicina, Universidade de São Paulo, University of São Paulo (HCFMUSP), São Paulo, SP, Brazil

Faculdade Israelita de Ciências da Saúde Albert Einstein, Hospital Israelita Albert Einstein, São Paulo, SP, Brazil
e-mail: ana.lottenberg@hc.fm.usp.br

N. S. O. Jensen
Collaborator at the Diabetes Control League of the Hospital das Clínicas, University of São Paulo, São Paulo, SP, Brazil

Obese individuals sweat more profusely in conditions of heat, increasing both the frictional and moisture components [9]. Common locations include the genitocrural, subaxillary, gluteal, and submammary areas and areas between the folds of skin of the abdominal wall [9].

Obesity is associated with changes in skin barrier function, sebaceous glands, sebum production, and sweat glands [10]. Obese individuals present higher transepidermal water loss, due to increased sweat gland activity, than normal-weight individuals [11].

In addition, obesity is associated with physiological changes in response to exercise, such as excessive sweating. One of the reasons for this might be the fact that obese individuals present an increased number of sweat glands and larger body area [12]. A study that assessed the impact of obesity on physiological responses during prolonged exercise showed that obese individuals demonstrated increased sweat and reduced urinary output than overweight and normal-weight subjects [13]. In the overweight BMI range, the amount of sweat produced is already greater than that of normal-weight individuals. The decreased urinary output was associated with higher plasma sodium levels and decreased plasma volume, conditions related to greater water reabsorption by the kidneys mediated by arginine vasopressin secretion [14]. Concurrently, obese individuals also present higher fluid intake associated with greater thirst stimulus, probably because of the increased serum osmolality [13].

Overweight, obesity, and hyperhidrosis are conditions that can affect psychosocial aspects of the patient, exerting a negative impact on quality of life. A study of 559 patients with excess weight [8] reported that the medical treatment of hyperhidrosis was associated with significant improvement in quality of life. Therefore, it is possible that the dietary treatment of obesity, based on lifestyle changes, can contribute to the improvement of hyperhidrosis and to the promotion of patient health and well-being.

Nutrition therapy is a cornerstone of obesity management. The importance of behavioral changes has been increasingly recognized since, being a chronic disease, its treatment needs long-term adherence, overcoming the difficulties faced by the patients in their day-to-day reality for the maintenance of healthy habits. Family, community, and all segments of society, also play an important role in this process [15].

In the following sections we discuss aspects that must be considered in diet planning for overweight and obese individuals.

Macronutrient Composition of the Diet

An energy deficit of 500 kcal/day is recommended for the purpose of weight loss [16]. A study that compared diets of varying macronutrient amounts in a sample of 424 patients aged 30–70 years old found that energy restriction was the main factor responsible for weight loss and body fat reduction, regardless of the amounts of carbohydrates, protein, and fat in relation to total energy [17]. Even though energy restriction can be considered a determinant factor for weight loss, it is acknowledged that the adoption of a healthy diet during the weight-loss period minimizes the chance of weight regain. For years, most international guidelines have been recommending a balanced diet with appropriate macronutrient distribution (55% of total energy intake from carbohydrates, 15% from proteins, and 25–35% from fats). However, recent findings suggest that dietary recommendations should not be based solely on the percentages of energy derived from macronutrients. Important studies have shown that eating patterns (such as the Mediterranean diet pattern) that combine different foods from various food groups are effective for the management of obesity [18, 19]. This model also encompasses diets with controlled amounts of fats, reduced saturated fat intake, the aim of contributing to the normalization of plasma lipids and lipoproteins, as well as those aimed at reducing endotoxemia.

Energy Density and Portion Size

Energy density can be defined as the amount of energy (kcal or kJ) by unit of weight (g). Foods low in energy density usually have high water and fiber content (e.g., fruits, vegetables, whole grains), while foods high in energy density are generally rich in fat and sugar. In a recent meta-analysis with a total of 3628 individuals aged 18–66 years, the intake of foods with low energy density was associated with significant body weight reduction [20].

Further consideration must be given to portion sizes, which have steadily increased over recent decades. A study in a restaurant setting showed that individuals who were served 50% more of a dish ate 43% more than those served a standard portion [21]. In a representative sample of adults in the city of São Paulo, Brazil, researchers have found an association between excess weight and intake of larger portions of pizza, red meat, rice, savory snacks, and soft drinks [22].

A randomized trial of 65 obese patients conducted by Kesman et al. [23] examined the effects of the use of a portion-control plate on weight management. After 3 months, patients in the intervention group had greater weight loss (−2.4% vs. −0.5%) than those who received usual care.

Therefore, strategies encouraging people to eat larger portions of low-energy-dense foods, such as fruits and vegetables, while limiting their intake of high-energy-dense foods might be beneficial for weight management [21].

Extent of Food Processing

The classification of foods according to the extension and purpose of food processing, as defined by Monteiro et al. [24], categorizes all foods and food products into four groups: unprocessed or minimally processed foods; culinary ingredients; processed foods; and ultra-processed food and drink products.

Unprocessed or minimally processed foods include fruits, vegetables, rice and other cereals and grains, beans and other legumes, meat, milk, eggs, mushrooms, and the like. These are foods obtained directly from plants or animals and/or altered by processes such as removal of inedible parts, drying, and freezing [24, 25].

Culinary ingredients include oils, sugar, and salt, which must be used with moderation to make varied and tasteful dishes without compromising nutritional balance. Processed foods, in turn, are unprocessed or minimally processed foods to which processed culinary ingredients were added in order to increase their durability and make them more palatable. Some examples of processed foods are canned or bottled vegetables, fruit in syrup, canned fish, and cheeses [25].

The fourth group is ultra-processed food and drink products. These are industrial formulations typically with refined flour, sugar, fat, and with use of modified ingredients (e.g., modified starch, inverted sugar) and additives such as artificial colors, flavors, food preservatives, bulking agents, acidulants, and flavor enhancers. Examples of ultra-processed foods are diverse cookies and savory snacks, soft drinks, instant soups, noodles and sauces, yoghurts and fruit drinks, sausages, and many ready-to-heat products, including pasta and pizza dishes [25].

Ultra-processed foods have several characteristics that promote excessive eating: they are formulated to be highly palatable due to great amounts of sugar, salt, and flavor enhancers; they are made to be eaten at any place and occasion, even without the need of cutlery, so they can be eaten unmindfully in front of the television, at the work desk, or while walking; also, they are sold in large packages with attractive prices and normally have a high energy density [25].

In Brazil, an analysis of data from the 2008–2009 Household Budget Survey indicated that household availability of ultra-processed foods was positively associated with the prevalence of excess weight and obesity. Individuals in the upper quartile of household consumption of ultra-processed foods were 37% more likely to be obese than those in the lower quartile [26].

Thereby, the control of the production and intake of ultra-processed foods has become one of the main recommendations for the prevention and management of obesity. This recommendation is in agreement with the international guidelines, that recommend healthy eating patterns.

Eating Pattern

Adequate nutrient intake is essential for achieving optimal health. However, the effect of isolated nutrients is insufficient to explain the relationship between food intake and health. This is likely because the health benefits of foods are related to the combination of nutrients and other chemical compounds that are part of the food matrix [25].

The importance of the study of eating patterns has been increasingly recognized. Eating patterns can be defined as combinations of foods or food groups that characterize relationships between dietary intake and health promotion and disease prevention. Eating patterns naturally occurring within populations are based on food availability, culture, and tradition, among other factors [27].

One of the most studied dietary patterns is the Mediterranean diet, which is characterized by high consumption of fruits, vegetables, nuts, legumes, and unprocessed cereals, as well as by low consumption of dairy products (except for some types of cheeses) and by alcohol intake in moderation and generally during meals [19].

Esposito et al. [28] performed a meta-analysis of 16 randomized trials and found a positive effect of the Mediterranean diet on weight loss, especially when associated with energy restriction, increased physical activity, and follow-up longer than 6 months. Other studies have also shown that when the level of adherence to the Mediterranean diet is high, this dietary pattern is associated with the prevention of obesity-related co-morbidities, including type 2 diabetes [29] and cardiovascular diseases [30].

In its current edition, the *2015–2020 Dietary Guidelines for Americans* focus on the encouragement of healthy eating patterns to help individuals to achieve and maintain a healthy body weight and reduce the risk of chronic diseases, embodying the idea that a healthy eating pattern is not a rigid prescription. Instead, it is an adaptable framework in which people can enjoy foods in accordance with their preferences, culture, and tradition. Additionally, the guidelines state that all segments of society have a role to play in supporting healthier food choices [31].

According to the guidelines, a healthy eating pattern includes a variety of colored vegetables, whole grains, low-fat dairy, and various sources of protein, including fish, lean meats and poultry, eggs, legumes, fruits and nuts. On the other hand, a healthy eating pattern limits the amount of saturated fats and trans fats, added sugars, and sodium. If alcohol is consumed, it should be consumed in moderation, that is, up to one drink per day for women and up to two drinks per day for men [31].

Conclusions

Obesity is a chronic disease characterized by the accumulation of body fat, which increases the risk of health-related problems. Increased adiposity is related to factors that cause excessive sweating, with potential impact on patients' quality of life. Therefore, the nutritional management of overweight and obesity could be useful to improve hyperhidrosis-related symptoms. Recent evidence suggests the benefits of dietary treatment based on long-term lifestyle changes, including energy deficit resulting from portion size control, decreased consumption of ultra-processed foods, and the adoption of a healthy eating pattern, with higher consumption of fruits, vegetables, whole grains, low-fat dairy, and lean meats, along with reduced intake of saturated and trans fat, sugars, and sodium.

References

1. World Health Organization. Obesity: preventing and managing the global epidemic. Report of a WHO consultation group on obesity. In: WHO Technical Report Series, vol. 894. Geneva: WHO; 2000.
2. World Health Organization. Diet, nutrition, and the prevention of chronic diseases. In: WHO Technical Report Series, vol. 797. Geneva: WHO; 1990.

3. World Health Organization. Obesity and overweight fact sheet. Updated 2016. http://www.who.int/mediacentre/factsheets/fs311/en/.
4. Castoldi A, de Souza CN, Câmara NOS, Moraes-Vieira PM. The macrophage switch in obesity development. Front Immunol. 2015;6:637.
5. Ibrahim MM. Subcutaneous and visceral adipose tissue: structural and functional differences. Obes Rev. 2010;11(1):11–8.
6. Tchernof A, Després JP. Pathophysiology of human visceral obesity: an update. Physiol Rev. 2013;93(1):359–404.
7. Lecerf JM, Reitz C, de Chasteigner A. Evaluation of discomfort and complications in a population of 18,102 patients overweight or obese patients. Presse Med. 2003;32(15):689–95.
8. Wolosker N, Krutman M, Kauffman P, Paula RP, Campos JR, Puech-Leão P. Effectiveness of oxybutynin for treatment of hyperhidrosis in overweight and obese patients. Rev Assoc Med Bras. 2013;59(2):143–7.
9. Garcia HL. Dermatological complications of obesity. Am J Clin Dermatol. 2002;3(7):497–506.
10. Yosipovitch G, DeVore A, Dawn A. Obesity and the skin: skin physiology and skin manifestations of obesity. J Am Acad Dermatol. 2007;56(6):901–16.
11. Löffler H, Aramaki JU, Effendy I. The influence of body mass index on skin susceptibility to sodium lauryl sulphate. Skin Res Technol. 2002;8(1):19–22.
12. Havenith G, van Middendorp H. The relative influence of physical fitness, acclimatization state, anthropometric measures and gender on individual reactions to heat stress. Eur J Appl Physiol Occup Physiol. 1990;61(5–6):419–27.
13. Eijsvogels TM, Veltmeijer MT, Schreuder TH, Poelkens F, Thijssen DH, Hopman MT. The impact of obesity on physiological responses during prolonged exercise. Int J Obes. 2011;35(11):1404–12.
14. Ball SG. Vasopressin and disorders of water balance: the physiology and pathophysiology of vasopressin. Ann Clin Biochem. 2007;44:417–31.
15. Freedhoff Y, Hall KD. Weight loss diet studies: we need help not hype. Lancet. 2016;388(10047):849–51.
16. Carels RA, Young KM, Coit C, Clayton AM, Spencer A, Hobbs M. Can following the caloric restriction recommendations from the Dietary Guidelines for Americans help individuals lose weight? Eat Behav. 2008;9(3):328–35.
17. de Souza RJ, Bray GA, Carey VJ, Hall KD, LeBoff MS, Loria CM, Laranjo NM, Sacks FM, Smith SR. Effects of 4 weight-loss diets differing in fat, protein, and carbohydrate on fat mass, lean mass, visceral adipose tissue, and hepatic fat: results from the POUNDS LOST trial. Am J Clin Nutr. 2012;95(3):614–25.
18. Garvey WT, Mechanick JI, Brett EM, Garber AJ, Hurley DL, Jastreboff AM, Nadolsky K, Pessah-Pollack R, Plodkowski R, Reviewers of the AACE/ACE Obesity Clinical Practice Guidelines. American Association of Clinical Endocrinologists and American College of Endocrinology comprehensive clinical practice guidelines for medical care of patients with obesity. Endocr Pract. 2016;22(Suppl 3):1–203.
19. Trichopoulou A, Martínez-González MA, Tong TY, Forouhi NG, Khandelwal S, Prabhakaran D, Mozaffarian D, de Lorgeril M. Definitions and potential health benefits of the Mediterranean diet: views from experts around the world. BMC Med. 2014;12:112.
20. Stelmach-Mardas M, Rodacki T, Dobrowolska-Iwanek J, Brzozowska A, Walkowiak J, Wojtanowska-Krosniak A, Zagrodzki P, Bechthold A, Mardas M, Boeing H. Link between food energy density and body weight changes in obese adults. Forum Nutr. 2016;8(4):229.
21. Rolls BJ. What is the role of portion control in weight management? Int J Obes. 2014;38(Suppl 1):S1–8.
22. Pereira JL, Mendes A, Crispim SP, Marchioni DM, Fisberg RM. Association of overweight with food portion size among adults of São Paulo – Brazil. PLoS One. 2016;11(10):e0164127.
23. Kesman RL, Ebbert JO, Harris KI, Schroeder DR. Portion control for the treatment of obesity in the primary care setting. BMC Res Notes. 2011;4:346.
24. Monteiro CA, Cannon G, Levy RB, et al. NOVA. The star shines bright. World Nutrition. 2016;7:28–38.

25. Brasil. Ministério da Saúde. Secretaria de Atenção à Saúde. Departamento de Atenção Básica. Guia alimentar para a população brasileira. 2 edn. Brasília: Ministério da Saúde; 2014.
26. Canella DS, Levy RB, Martins AP, Claro RM, Moubarac JC, Baraldi LG, Cannon G, Monteiro CA. Ultra-processed food products and obesity in Brazilian households (2008-2009). PLoS One. 2014;9(3):e92752.
27. Evert AB, Boucher JL, Cypress M, Dunbar SA, Franz MJ, Mayer-Davis EJ, Neumiller JJ, Nwankwo R, Verdi CL, Urbanski P, Yancy WS Jr. Nutrition therapy recommendations for the management of adults with diabetes. Diabetes Care. 2014;37(Suppl 1):S120–43.
28. Esposito K, Kastorini CM, Panagiotakos DB, Giugliano D. Mediterranean diet and weight loss: meta-analysis of randomized controlled trials. Metab Syndr Relat Disord. 2011;9(1):1–12.
29. Koloverou E, Esposito K, Giugliano D, Panagiotakos D. The effect of Mediterranean diet on the development of type 2 diabetes mellitus: a meta-analysis of 10 prospective studies and 136,846 participants. Metabolism. 2014;63(7):903–11.
30. Tektonidis TG, Åkesson A, Gigante B, Wolk A, Larsson SC. A Mediterranean diet and risk of myocardial infarction, heart failure and stroke: a population-based cohort study. Atherosclerosis. 2015;243(1):93–8.
31. U.S. Department of Health and Human Services and U.S. Department of Agriculture. 2015–2020 dietary guidelines for Americans. 8th ed; December 2015. http://health.gov/dietaryguidelines/2015/guidelines/

Primary Hyperhidrosis

Paulo Kauffman

Introduction

Physiologically, sweat production by the sweat glands, which is highly developed in humans, is an important survival factor for organisms in high-temperature environments, allowing heat loss by evaporation through the skin. Hyper-function of these glands also occurs physiologically in menopause, when we are under the effect of intense emotions, and when we perform physical exercises, conditions under which there is greater production of heat in the body.

The relationship between body and spirit has been studied since the time of Hippocrates. More recently, study of the psychosomatic illnesses, which addresses this relationship in a deeper way, has gained increasing importance. The hustle and bustle of modern life, which accompanies the social revolution of modern times, raises emotional conflicts that cause somatic disorders when reaching certain thresholds, affecting, in particular and with greater intensity and ease, those individuals with the so-called "hyper-emotive" constitution.

These disorders often manifest themselves in the glandular sphere, especially in the sweat glands, without any underlying disease responsible for them, resulting in excessive sweat production that has no relation to the thermoregulation needs of the organism, featuring primary or essential hyperhidrosis, also called "emotional" by some authors.

Pathogenesis

There is no satisfactory explanation for hyperhidrosis; it is assumed that there is, in certain individuals, stimulation of the sympathetic nervous system, possibly at the central level, causing excessive sweating in the extremities, beyond that required for

P. Kauffman
Department of Vascular and Endovascular Surgery, University of São Paulo School of Medicine, São Paulo, SP, Brazil

thermoregulatory requirements. There would then be an increase in the nerve impulses that originate in the central nervous system, releasing excessive amounts of acetylcholine and increased sudoral response; while sleeping, there is cessation or significant decrease of emotional sweating, supporting this theory. It is also possible that normal-intensity stimuli produce an increased nervous tone of the sympathetic fibers that innervate the sweating glands.

However, it should be emphasized that, although the emotional stimulus is necessary to trigger the hyperhidrosis, we cannot characterize it as a purely psychosomatic disease, as it is considered by some authors to be a physiological disorder. These patients present with a hypothalamic center sweat controller more sensitive to emotional stimuli from the cortical areas of the brain than the general population. The greatest evidence of this fact is the occurrence of hyperhidrosis in the neonatal period. Some babies have excessive sweating in the hands and feet at an age at which emotional factors are not significant. This would, therefore, characterize a genetic disorder with greater sensitivity of the controlling centers or greater frequency of the cerebral impulses.

Epidemiology

Hyperhidrosis has a reported incidence of about 1–4.5% in studied populations, being more common in adolescents and young adults; that is, it is a feature of the early years of life. It is also important to mention that hyperhidrosis has family characteristic, which is described in the literature as being 57% and in Brazil has been shown to be around 46%.

Recently, a representative sample of the US population was studied via a questionnaire, which aimed to establish public perception in relation to the amount of sweat that they presented. The authors found that the prevalence of hyperhidrosis was 2.8%, or an estimated 7,800,000 Americans considered their amount of perspiration abnormal. Approximately 38% of these patients had already discussed this problem with a health professional.

Hyperhidrosis affects male and female patients equally. Women, due to their temperament, seem to accept this condition less, seeking treatment more often than men do, hence the apparent prevalence of the disease in women.

Clinical Aspects

Hyperhidrosis occurs predominantly in the palmar, plantar, and axilla regions where it has a symmetric character. It may also occur in the craniofacial segment. It can appear in childhood, but manifests itself with greater intensity in adolescence, a stage of life in which there is great instability because the patient, in this transitional period, presents hormonal and sexual maturation; no longer considered a child but not considered an adult, their aspirations and desires often outweigh their emotional reality. Thus, conflicts occur that trigger or aggravate conditions under which there is a significant psychosomatic component, such as hyperhidrosis, which may persist

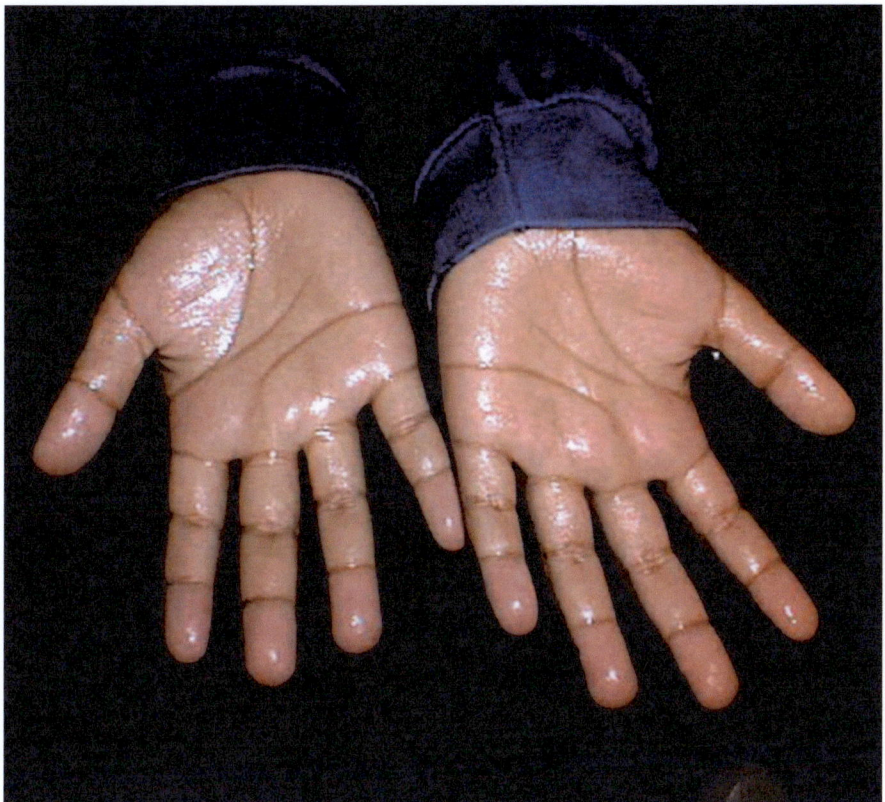

Fig. 4.1 Appearance of the hands in patient with palmar hyperhidrosis

into adulthood. However, in some patients, it improves during this period, especially after marriage.

Palmar hyperhidrosis (Fig. 4.1), in the vast majority of cases, is of greater clinical importance than the plantar or axillary forms, creating problems in the educational, social, affective, and professional spheres, and worsening existing personality changes in these patients. Thus, these individuals moisten all structures that they touch, making writing, reading, and school activities in general more difficult. Parents and even teachers ignorant about the real health conditions of the patient can punish the child or student by thinking they are wetting their notebooks and books on purpose, as we have had the opportunity to observe. From a social and affective point of view, these patients retreat, avoiding handshakes and social situations such as parties, dancing, and dating; they often use, almost permanently, scarves on their hands in order to dry them. Professionally, palmar hyperhidrosis can make patients incapable of carrying out work in various fields of human activity; for example, industrial workers with this disorder who handle metals have been labeled "rust makers" because of the corrosive action of their sweat. Other activities can become dangerous under these circumstances, such as for workers who deal with electrical and electronic equipment.

Fig. 4.2 Appearance of the foot with hyperhidrosis

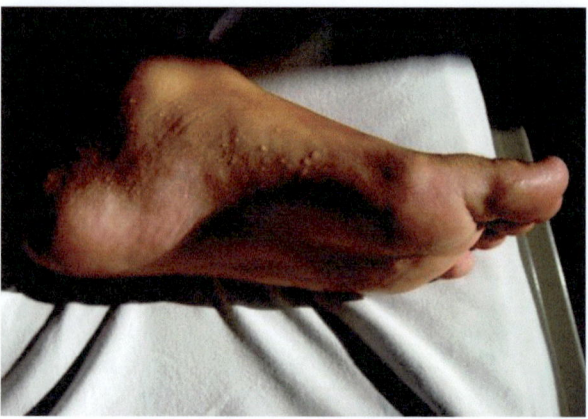

Fig. 4.3 Axillary hyperhidrosis in patient with colorful clothing

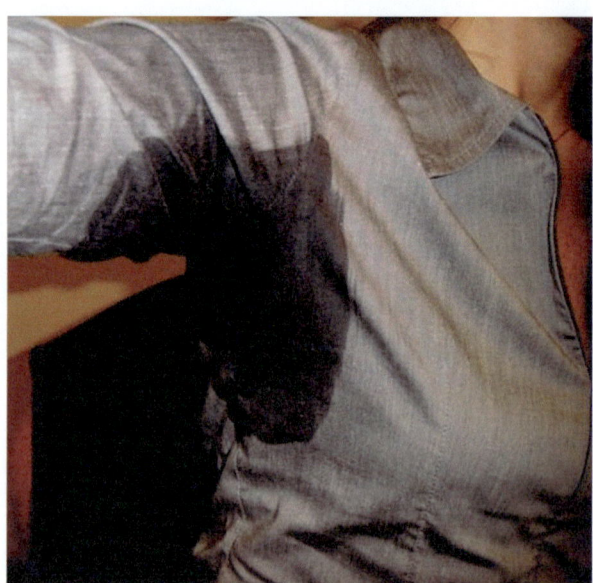

Plantar hyperhidrosis (Fig. 4.2), often associated with the palmar form, is exacerbated by the use of closed shoes as these hinder evaporation and aid the maceration of the skin. The constant humidity promotes the appearance of fungal or bacterial infections, causing an unpleasant odor not only in the feet but also in socks and shoes.

Axillary hyperhidrosis (Fig. 4.3) usually manifests itself at puberty, with increased production of sex hormones; it also causes social embarrassment as sweat pours down the body, wetting and damaging clothes. Patients often avoid wearing colorful clothes, preferring to always wear white and/or black and, sometimes, use tricks such as rolls of paper or even sanitary napkins in the armpits.

Similarly, craniofacial hyperhidrosis (Fig. 4.4) can become an embarrassing problem for the patient, as much socially as professionally, because it gives

Fig. 4.4 Craniofacial hyperhidrosis in a male patient

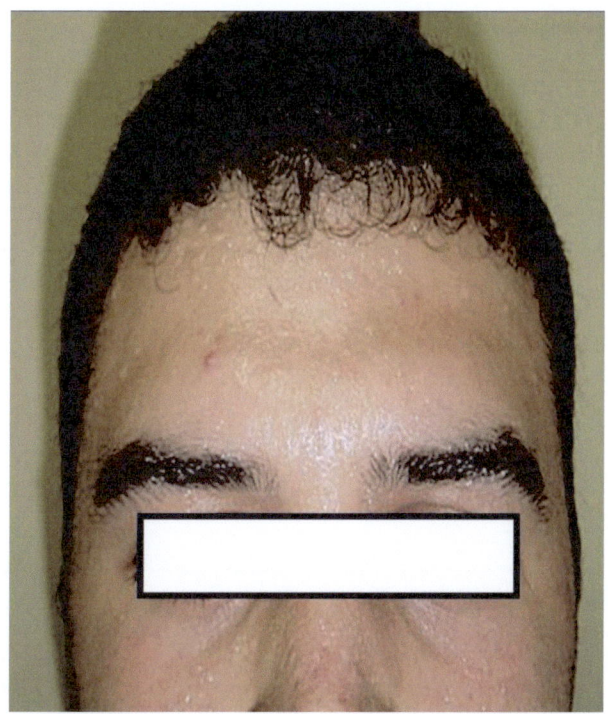

Fig. 4.5 Patient with facial flushing

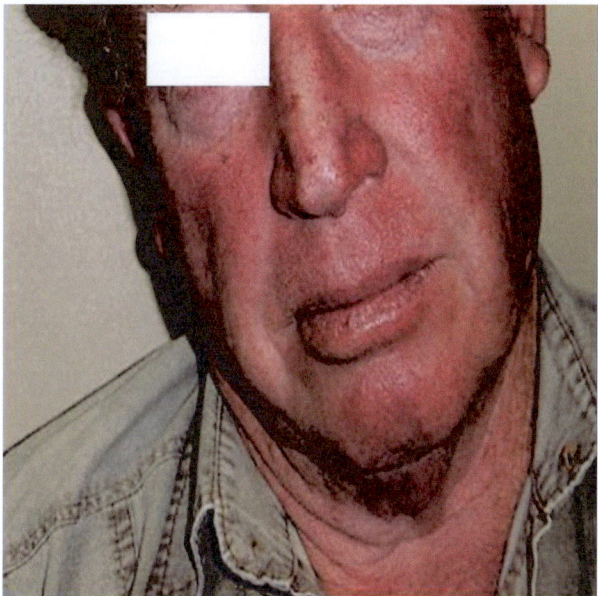

the impression of insecurity to the patient's interlocutor. Patients with facial flushing (Fig. 4.5)—which is usually related to social phobia—in isolation or in association with craniofacial hyperhidrosis, can also benefit from thoracic sympathectomy.

Diagnosis

The diagnosis of hyperhidrosis is highly clinical, being carried out by anamnesis and physical examination. Patients with palmar hyperhidrosis usually present with cold and clammy hands, with coloration that can vary from pale to redness.

The following criteria identify and facilitate correct diagnosis of hyperhidrosis:

- Visible sweat, which is exaggerated and localized, with a duration of at least 6 months, without apparent cause and with at least two of the following features:
  - Bilateral and symmetrical sweat.
  - Frequency: at least one episode per week.
  - Impairment of daily activities.
  - Age of onset <25 years.
  - Family history.
  - Absence of sweat during sleep.

Suggested Reading

Drott C, Claes G, Olsson-Rex L, Dalman P, Fahlén T, Göthberg G. Succesful treatment of facial blushing by endoscopic transthoracic sympathectomy. Br J Dermatol. 1998;138:639–43.

Haider A, Solish N. Focal hyperhidrosis: diagnosis and management. CMAJ. 2005;172:69–75.

Hurley HJ. Diseases of the eccrine sweat glands. In: Moschella SL, Hurley HJ, editors. Dermatology. 3rd ed. Philadelphia: WB Saunders; 1992. p. 1514–37.

Kauffman P, de Campos JRM, Wolosker N, Kuzniec S, Jatene FB, Puech-Leão P. Thoracoscopic cervicothoracic sympathectomy: an eight-year experience. Braz Vasc Surg. 2003;2:22–8.

Wolosker N, Kauffman P. Upper extremity sympathectomy. In: Cronenwett & Johnston, editor. Rutherford's vascular surgery. 8th ed. USA: Saunders; 2014. p. 1923–33.

The Prevalence of Hyperhidrosis Worldwide

Sonia Oliveira Lima and Vanessa Rocha de Santana

Introduction

Primary hyperhidrosis (PH) is a chronic disease that negatively affects the daily activities of the carrier. The presence of excessive sweating causes the individual to realize there is something wrong and embarrassing; however, they do not always recognize this as a symptom of a curable disease. When the patient discovers PH, he does not know which medical specialist to consult or even whether the disease is treatable. Some patients suffer without seeking help, refusing to consult a doctor in search of treatment, and avoiding revealing their discomfort, even in their immediate surroundings, like they are carriers of a shameful disease.

PH can cause biopsychosocial problems, by causing discomfort and disability, resulting in anxiety and depression with high rates of isolation among those affected. Although the diagnosis of hyperhidrosis is highly clinical, little is known and valued by health professionals, as it is not seen as a disease itself, but rather as a patient's emotional response. Even physicians and teachers have scarce access to information, as it is not being sufficiently debated in academia, although it is classified in the *International Classification of Diseases* (ICD–R61.0).

S. O. Lima (✉)
School of Medicine, Tiradentes University, Aracaju, SE, Brazil

University of São Paulo, São Paulo, SP, Brazil

V. R. de Santana
School of Medicine of Bahia, Tiradentes University, Aracaju, SE, Brazil

Prevalence of Hyperhidrosis

An article published in the International Society of Paraplegia's journal in 1922 is a historic landmark in PH research [1]. In this article, the presence of irritating hyperhidrosis in patients with spinal cord injury was investigated by means of a questionnaire given to 192 patients, of whom 154 participated in an interview. Forty-one reported unbearable sudoresis, of whom 13 showed an underlying somatic cause. Twenty-eight patients mentioned having hyperhidrosis at that time (and described it as annoying), without a contributing somatic cause, i.e., PH.

Studies on PH are mostly directed at diagnosis, treatment, and quality of life. In our review of the literature, covering the period from 1997 to 2017, we found only ten articles whose objective was to evaluate the prevalence of PH, and this prevalence varied from 0.6% to 16.7% (Table 5.1).

A pilot study, carried out in 1997, in a young population from Israel, estimated a prevalence of 0.6–1.0% of PH in all body sites and levels of severity. Of these, 53% presented axillary PH and 19% in its severe form. All of the interviewed patients were submitted for a surgical procedure.

In 2004, research was conducted in the USA by Strutton and colleagues, with a sample of 150,000 families. These families were questioned about unusual or excessive sweating through a validated questionnaire that was mailed to them. It verified the prevalence of PH of 2.9%; 50.8% of carriers reported axillary hyperhidrosis symptoms and 35.7% of the symptomatic patients reported it as interfering in their daily activities. In this study, only 38% of patients with hyperhidrosis had reported their problems to a health professional.

In Fuzhou, in the People's Republic of China, in 2007, research was conducted in two stages involving 13,000 high school and university students aged 15–22 years. A questionnaire was applied by professionals, with later individual medical assessment for likely cases of palmar PH. It was found that the rate of palmar hyperhidrosis prevalence was 4.59% and that it affected the sexes in a similar manner. The onset of symptoms occurred between 4 and 22 years and peaked between 6 and 16 years of age. Of those patients, 6.12% were classified as severe cases and 15.3% presented a positive family history.

Table 5.1 World prevalence of primary hyperhidrosis from 1977 to 2017

Country	Study	Year of publication	Prevalence of PH (%)
Israel	Adar et al.	1997	0.6–1.0
USA	Strutton et al.	2004	2.9
China	Yuan-Rong et al.	2007	4.59
Brazil	Fenili et al.	2009	9.0
Brazil	Westphal et al.	2011	5.5%
Poland	Stefanieak et al.	2013	16.7
Germany	Augustin et al.	2013	16.6
Japan	Fujimoto et al.	2013	12.76
Brazil	Lima et al.	2015	14.76
Brazil	Santana	2017	15.9

In Poland in 2013, the prevalence of PH was evaluated in medicine and dentistry students though a questionnaire that used the visual analog scale (VAS). PH was subsequently confirmed in 16.7% of the students by medical professionals during a consultation using gravimetry. In Germany in the same year, 14,336 employees from 51 firms were examined by dermatologists and interviewed with regards to PH. Amongst the workers, 16.6% had PH and 6.1% referred to it as serious. Only 27% of those with PH had consulted a doctor, but 28% had used some type of medication, prescribed or not.

In Japan in 2013, specific questionnaires on PH were sent to schools and commercial firms in various locations from Hokkaido to Okinawa. In total, 5807 individuals between 5 and 64 years of age were evaluated, obtaining a PH prevalence of 12.76%. Of those with PH, 15.3% reported having a family history, 5.33% reported palmar hyperhidrosis, 2.79% plantar, 5.75% axillary, and 4.7% craniofacial, with negative effects on quality of life. Only 6.2% of the patients with hyperhidrosis had consulted with health professionals and some reported the treatment as inappropriate, even after visiting a medical institution.

In Brazil in 2009, the prevalence of hyperhidrosis in the southern region of Blumenau-SC was found to be 9.0%. For convenience, the research was conducted by interview with 500 individuals in urban transportation terminals. Of those interviewed who mentioned having PH, 60% reported compromised daily activities. In this research, the authors did not assess the severity of PH or report the percentage of confirmed diagnoses by qualified professionals.

In the northern region of Brazil, in Manaus-AM, a study was conducted in 2011 of a population of 293 medical students at the Federal University of Amazonas (UFAM) were interviewed. A standard questionnaire from the Hyperhidrosis International Society was used, and 5.5% of these students were observed to be excessive sweating carriers, 31.3% of whom reported negative effects on their daily activities. A family history was present in half of the hyperhidrosis carriers and no one reported known causes of the disease.

In Sergipe, Brazil, in 2015, a study was conducted, through individual interviews, by researchers previously trained in the use of a validated questionnaire specific for PH diagnosis. The study evaluated 760 medicine students from two universities who were chosen randomly by lottery. A PH prevalence of 14.76% was found, with positive family history in 45%. The onset of symptoms occurred between 15 and 20 years of age and the body sites most commonly affected were the palms, soles, and armpit, with academic, social, and occupational activities compromised. The diagnosis of PH was given by a doctor in only 22.72% of respondents, although in this study the carriers were medical students involved in health practice.

In an additional study in 2017, which involved 300 medical students from a private university in Sergipe, it was found that 54 (18%) students fulfilled the diagnostic criteria for PH. They were classified as grade 1 (3.7%), 2 (12%), 3 (2%), and 4 (0.3%). According to the scale of severity of hyperhidrosis, grade 1 is considered imperceptible sweat which does not impede daily activities; grade 2 is tolerable sweat which sometimes impedes daily activities; grade 3 is almost unbearable sweat which frequently impedes daily activities; and grade 4 is intolerable sweat which always impedes daily activities. Grades 3 and 4 may be associated with considerable morbidity, including skin lesions and secondary skin infections, and it may be edematous, macerated, or even cracked. In this study, therefore, there was a predominance of moderate PH (grades 2 and 3; 14%). With respect to self-assessment of quality of life, six (11.1%) classified it as excellent, 13 (24%) as very good, 20 (37%) as good, and 15 (27.8%) as bad. Of the medical student carriers of PH, 43 (79.6%) reported that they consider excessive sweating to be a disease and, of these, six (11.1%) had already had surgical treatment and five (9.2%) clinical treatment. This indicates the importance of the classification of the severity of PH, its effect on quality of life, and, in future, the treatment rationale.

In further research conducted in the state of Sergipe in Brazil and presented as a doctoral thesis in 2017, 1330 volunteers were chosen at random from five districts of the city of Aracaju. Interviews were conducted individually at home, with the help of a public community health agent. A valid questionnaire was used, and medical students were the interviewers, trained by professional doctors on the specific content of every question. The prevalence of PH was 15.9%, with a sex prevalence of 17% among males and 14.9% among females. The onset of PH symptoms occurred during childhood and adolescence in 82.5%, and family history was reported in 38% of carriers.

These studies did not report the severity of the PH uniformly: some considered the PH in degrees according to the Hyperhidrosis Disease Severity Scale (HDSS) classification and others classified severe PH cases in relation to reports regarding negative effects on daily activities and the quality of life of the patient. Table 5.2 presents the percentage of severe cases among those reported as having PH, family history, and those with PH who sought medical attention.

Table 5.2 Prevalence of severe cases of primary hyperhidrosis between 1977 and 2017

Country	Year	Severe cases (grades 3 and 4)	Family history	Patients who sought medical attention
Israel	1997	19%	53%	All were interviewed at the surgery
USA	2004	35.7%	Not mentioned	38%
China	2007	6.12%	15.3%	Not mentioned
Brazil	2009	60%	Not mentioned	Not mentioned
Brazil	2011	31.3%	50%	Not mentioned
Poland	2013	Not mentioned	Not mentioned	16.7%
Germany	2013	6.1%	Not mentioned	27%
Japan	2013	Not mentioned	15.3%	6.2%
Brazil	2017	2.3%	45%	22.72%
Brazil	2017	Not mentioned	38%	Not mentioned

Conclusion

Between 1977 and 2017, scientific research conducted around the world on the epidemiological prevalence of PH shows high variation, with values ranging from 0.6% to 16.7%. The occurrence of PH cannot be determined in some studies, since they are based exclusively on data collected using questionnaires, which may lead to false results. The majority of people know at least someone who presents excessive sweating, which leads us to believe that the prevalence of PH may have been underestimated by previous studies. The Variation of Prevalence may also depend on the population group analyzed. It is important for the development of actual knowledge on the prevalence of PH to use validated instruments, with individual interviews, in addition to clinical recognition of the disease being made by prepared professionals.

Onset of PH symptoms occurs in childhood and adolescence, the transitional phase characterized by mental changes, an additional aggravating factor in this condition. Although some studies indicate a higher prevalence of the disease between the ages of 25 and 64 years old, it is possible that these data have the bias of most patients seeking medical attention when they are adults. It is of great importance that PH be recognized as a curable disease and that it is understood that treatment in childhood avoids difficulties that individuals may encounter during their life.

The age of onset of PH symptoms is probably influenced by the affected region of the body, with palmar and plantar PH arising predominantly during childhood, axillar during adolescence, and craniofacial in adult ages. PH affects patients of both sexes similarly, and melanodermic individuals are less affected. A family history is frequently described in PH carriers, which points to autosomal dominant inheritance.

The low incidence of diagnosis by physicians reported in the studies reaffirms the importance of early diagnosis and treatment, to minimize and/or avoid damage to the patients' quality of life. By increasing publicity on PH, it allows patients and doctors to accept this disorder as a valid and curable condition.

The wider the awareness of this disorder, the better the improvement in the quality of life of many people will be who feel excluded from society because of PH, as well as aiding in the assessment of the actual prevalence of the disease.

Reference

1. Andersen LS, Biering-Sørensen F, Müller PG, Jensen IL, Aggerbeck B. The prevalence of hyperhidrosis in patients with spinal cord injuries and an evaluation of the effect of dextropropoxyphene hydrochloride in therapy. Paraplegia. 1992;30(3):184–91.

Suggested Reading

Lima SO, Aragão JFB, Neto JM, Almeida KBS, Menezes LMS, Santana VR. Research of primary hyperhidrosis in students of medicine of the state of Sergipe, Brazil. An Bras Dermatol. 2015;90(5):661–5.

Stefaniak T, Tomaszewski KA, Proczkomarkuszewska M, Idestal A, Royton A, Abi-Khalil C. Is subjective hyperhidrosis assessment sufficient enough? Prevalence of hyperhidrosis among young polish adults. J Dermatol. 2013;40:819–23.

Yuan-Rong T, Xu L, Min L, Fan-Cai L, Yue-Ping L, Jian-Feng C, Jian-Gang Y. Epidemiological survey of primary palmar hyperhidrosis in adolescente in Fuzhou of People's Republic of China. Eur J Cardiothorac Surg. 2007;31:737–9.

Hyperhidrosis in Children

Samantha Neves, John Robert Pires-Davidson,
Dafne Braga Diamante Leiderman, and Nelson Wolosker

Introduction

Hyperhidrosis in children, as well as in adults, is characterized by excessive sweating. However, diagnosis before the age of 18 years is more delicate. Nevertheless, in addition to meeting criteria such as being localized, visible, and excessive, with a minimum duration of 6 months and no apparent cause, it must be accompanied by at least two other criteria, such as bilateral and symmetrical distribution, impairment of daily activities, at least one weekly episode, family history, or focal sweating that ceases during sleep. The major problems that this disease can cause are the implications and emotional repercussions of social rejection. Over the years these problems can be aggravated and the child can become an adult with behavioral, self-esteem, and relationship problems. The treatment of hyperhidrosis may involve multiple approaches that are isolated, combined, or even superimposed in cases of non-adherence, intolerance, or failure. The main ones are topical antiperspirant

S. Neves (✉)
Brazilian Society of Dermatology, São Paulo, SP, Brazil

School of Medicine, ABC, Santo André, SP, Brazil
e-mail: samantha@samanthaneves.com.br

J. R. Pires-Davidson
Hospital Universitário Maria Aparecida Pedrossian–UFMS, Campo Grande, Brazil

D. B. D. Leiderman
Department of Vascular and Endovascular Surgery, Hospital Israelita Albert Einstein, São Paulo, SP, Brazil

N. Wolosker
Department of Vascular and Endovascular Surgery, Hospital Israelita Albert Einstein, São Paulo, SP, Brazil

treatment, iontophoresis, botulinum toxin, laser, microwave, surgical treatment, and systemic treatment with oxybutynin.

Definition and Diagnosis

Primary focal hyperhidrosis (PFH) in children and adolescents is probably underdiagnosed. Approximately 1.6% of adolescents are affected as well as 0.6% of prepubescent children.

PFH in children and adolescents, as well as in adults, usually affects the armpits, palms of the hands, soles of the feet, and craniofacial region. In some cases, more than one area can be affected. It is observed in practice that palmar–plantar involvement is generally significantly earlier than the axillary, although little has been published regarding this fact, just as the craniofacial involvement seems to be the latest to occur. In addition, patients in whom the complaint began in pre-puberty most commonly have a diagnosis of isolated palmoplantar hyperhidrosis.

The presence of generalized sweating suggests some alteration other than PHF. Excessive heat is one of the most common causes of sweating. Other causes include systemic diseases and medications, in which case it often continues during sleep. Differential diagnoses of secondary sweating and their causes are as follows:

- *Generalized hyperhidrosis*: medications, illicit drugs, cardiovascular alterations, respiratory failure, infections, malignant tumors, endocrine–metabolic changes (thyrotoxicosis, hypoglycemia, pheochromocytoma, acromegaly, carcinoid tumor), neurological changes (Parkinson disease).
- *Regional*: cerebrovascular accident, peripheral nerve injury, central or peripheral nervous system injury causing anhydrosis can cause compensatory hyperhidrosis in other areas (stroke, spinal cord injury, neuropathy, Ross syndrome).
- *Focal*: Frey's syndrome, gustatory sweating, eccrine nevus, anxiety disorders, unilateral focal hyperhidrosis.

The diagnosis of PFH is clinical. Tests used to quantify the production of sweat are not needed in clinical practice and are particularly useless and difficult when it comes to the child's daily routine. It is fundamental to understand how much the quality of life (QoL) of the patient is affected, as well as how their emotional health is affected in this condition, especially when dealing with children and adolescents. Although we observe in daily practice how deeply the child's life is affected due to hyperhidrosis, literature is scarce in establishing the negative psychosocial impact of the child's QoL.

In addition, although there is little reported in the literature, there is also a relationship with increased cutaneous infections in patients with PFH. Fungal infections are common in the areas of hyperhidrosis, particularly dermatophytes (tinea pedis, tinea corporis, tinea cruris). Likewise, the risk of bacterial infections also increases, particularly grooved plantar keratolysis. Finally, the risk of viral skin infections, especially plantar and verruca vulgaris, also increases.

Individuals under the age of 18 years are never alone during medical appointments. It is important to try to separate the anxiety of the parents (or companions) and the history of the child (or adolescent). Frequent complaints are wetting clothes and having to change them, wetting the paper while writing, being ashamed to hold hands with people, or slipping when walking barefoot. Trying to use the same language as the child is fundamental and, depending on the intensity of the response, it is possible to quantify and make the evaluation of sweating a bit more objective. Children under 6 years of age should be approached in a subtle manner: observation of the simple fact of supporting the hand while writing (palmar hyperhidrosis) and walking and leaving footprints (plantar hyperhidrosis) often confirms diagnoses that are impossible to elucidate through laboratory tests or mathematical quantifications.

Children and adolescents with PFH often have a type of phobia regarding sweat and, not infrequently, this "panic" affects their relatives. Therefore, the greater expectation revolves around wanting to "sweat absolutely nothing".

The differential diagnosis that differentiates between excessive non-pathological sweating and hyperhidrosis is due to the psychological, emotional, social, school, and sports impact. The biggest problems with PFH are the emotional—implications of the social rejection that it can cause due to the withdrawal/denials from friends and even from more intimate relationships. This worsens over the years and the child can become an adult with behavioral disorders, low self-esteem, and a difficulty in interpersonal relationships.

Treatment

Local Treatment

Topical options for hyperhidrosis are limited in children and adolescents. Topical aluminum chloride is usually used as the first choice of treatment. However, other therapies deserve mention here, especially for use in adolescents, whose skin is already more resistant and presents a lower risk of sensitization.

Iontophoresis

Iontophoresis is an alternative for palmoplantar hyperhidrosis. Dogruk Kacar et al. published an article in which 21 patients younger than 18 years were treated with iontophoresis for palmoplantar hyperhidrosis, the youngest patient in this study being 7 years old. Iontophoresis of "tap water" was given at regular intervals, starting with five times a week and decreasing to once a week in the fifth week. Maintenance with weekly sessions for 6 weeks was recommended. Nineteen patients completed the 21 sessions. Side effects were well-tolerated. Only seven patients were free of excessive sweating in the third month after treatment. In a ranking from 0 (persistence of excessive sweating) to 10 (absence of excessive sweating), the mean was almost 6 at the end of the fifteenth session and almost 6.4 at the end of treatment. The average satisfaction was approximately 5.

Iontophoresis with tap water is an effective primary treatment method for primary palmoplantar and axillary hyperhidrosis in pediatric patients. But unanswered questions remain about the mechanisms of action, ideal ranges between sessions, and protocols for maximum effectiveness. Nevertheless, there are a very limited number of studies in the literature investigating the effectiveness of this treatment in children and adolescents.

The German Dermatology Society guideline, published in 2010, recommended that children who received iontophoresis with tap water should be at least 5 years old to ensure that they can understand the instructions.

Botulinum Toxin

To date, botulinum toxin use has restricted US Food and Drug Administration (FDA) and ANVISA (the Brazilian Health Surveillance Agency) approval only for the treatment of axillary PFH and in adults (over 18 years of age); however, there are several publications regarding its use for PFH in pediatric patients.

The first use of botulinum toxin for palmar hyperhidrosis in a pediatric patient was published in 2002, in a 13-year-old child. In 2005, the first use of botulinum toxin was reported in a patient under 18 years of age for the treatment of axillary hyperhidrosis.

Dos Santos et al. published a study in pediatric patients with palmar hyperhidrosis treated with botulinum toxin A (BTX-A) in 2009, showing an improvement in PFH with an average duration of 7 months. BTX-A injections are less invasive than surgical procedures, since they are done on an outpatient basis under topical or local anesthesia; however, the patient's acceptance of this procedure, especially in pediatric patients, is very variable.

Systemic Treatment

The use of anticholinergics for childhood hyperhidrosis, although documented in the medical literature, is still off-label. Therefore, both glycopyrrolate and oxybutynin hydrochloride are not approved by ANVISA or the FDA for treatment of hyperhidrosis, but several publications are based on its safety in children and adolescents with PFH.

Paller et al., in 2012, observed that of 90 children with hyperhidrosis intolerant or resistant to aluminum salts, a group of 31 children with an average age of 14 years showed improvement with glycopyrrolate use.

Oxybutynin is the drug of choice for the treatment of hyperhidrosis, as well as for patients under 18 years of age. Early reports on safety and adverse effects of oxybutynin in children were based on its use for the treatment of nocturnal enuresis.

The proposed protocol for oxybutynin, for children weighing more than 40 kg, is 2.5 mg once daily at night for 7 days, then twice daily for 7–21 days, followed by 5 mg twice daily, as in adults. Patients weighing less than 40 kg receive the same treatment for the first 3 weeks, but the dose is not increased after the twenty-first day.

Wolosker et al., in 2014, evaluated 45 children aged 7–14 years with palmar hyperhidrosis 6 weeks after protocol treatment (as proposed above) with oxybutynin. QoL was assessed before and after treatment using a validated questionnaire. More than 85% of children with palmar hyperhidrosis treated with oxybutynin experienced moderate or intense improvement in the level of sweating and 80% experienced improvement in QoL.

Children who initially had a very poor QoL benefited most from oxybutynin treatment. Adverse effects occurred in 25 children (55.5%) and were mostly dry mouth (considered mild in 13, moderate in seven, and severe in four patients). This effect was manifested in patients receiving doses >0.125 mg/kg and the only neurological effect occurred in one patient receiving 0.2 mg/kg. The authors concluded that oxybutynin is an effective treatment for children with palmar hyperhidrosis because it improves clinical symptoms and QoL.

In a more recent study (2015), the same authors observed 97 patients, an average of 19.6 months, with particular attention being given to 59 children aged 4–14 years with palmoplantar hyperhidrosis who were treated for more than 6 months. More than 91% presented moderate or high improvement in self-perception of sweating, and 94.9% experienced improvement in QoL. More than 90% of the children reported improvement in hyperhidrosis at other sites.

It is worth mentioning that anticholinergic adverse effects are more frequent in children under 5 years of age receiving doses higher than 10 mg/day. All children (in the study) were 5 years or older. It is mentioning that chilren in general under 5 years of age present more adverse effects when the dose exceeds 10mg/day. This may explain the adverse effect rate of the 2014 study (55.5%), which was lower than in previous studies.

Oxybutynin is contraindicated in children with glaucoma.

Surgical Treatment

Videothoracoscopic sympathectomy is the therapy of choice for hyperhidrosis after failure of other treatments, especially after treatment with oxybutynin in children. In particular, it is an option for palmar and/or axillar hyperhidrosis and is widely described in the literature for both adults and children. The most common adverse effect of this surgery is compensatory hyperhidrosis, and other less frequent complications include Horner's syndrome, neuralgia, or pneumothorax.

In 2012, Neves et al. published results of the follow-up of 45 children younger than 14 years, comparing 30 who underwent sympathectomy for hyperhidrosis with 15 who had not received treatment after 4 years. Children undergoing surgical treatment had a greater improvement in QoL, and the authors concluded that this treatment is the most appropriate in children with hyperhidrosis.

Conclusion

Hyperhidrosis in children is a well-established disease in the medical literature and various treatments are available. Recognition by family members, appropriate and accurate diagnosis by professionals dealing with children under 18 years of age, and referral to qualified professionals for evaluation and establish the best therapy are essential to initiate treatment as early as possible, so that social harm is minimized.

Systemic treatment with anticholinergics has a sound scientific basis and should be considered the treatment of choice for children with PFH. Today, PFH in children and adolescents no longer has to shape their personality.

Suggested Reading

Bakheit AM, Severa S, Cosgrove A, et al. Safety profile and efficacy of botulinum toxin A (Dysport) in children with muscle spasticity. Dev Med Child Neurol. 2001;43(4):234–8.

Bellet JS. Diagnosis and treatment of primary focal hyperhidrosis in children and adolescents. Semin Cutan Med Surg. 2010;29(2):121–6.

Buraschi J. Videothoracoscopic sympathicolysis procedure for primary palmar hyperhidrosis in children and adolescents. Arch Argent Pediatr. 2008;106(1):32–5.

Coutinho dos Santos LH, Gomes AM, Giraldi S, et al. Palmar hyperhidrosis: long-term follow-up of nine children and adolescents treated with botulinum toxin type A. Pediatr Dermatol. 2009;26(4):439–44.

Dogruk Kacar S, Ozuguz P, Eroglu S, et al. Treatment of primary hyperhidrosis with tap water iontophoresis in paediatric patients: a retrospective analysis. Cutan Ocul Toxicol. 2014;33(4):313–6.

Neves S, Uchoa PC, Wolosker N, et al. Long-term comparison of video-assisted thoracic sympathectomy and clinical observation for the treatment of palmar hyperhidrosis in children younger than 14. Pediatr Dermatol. 2012;29(5):575–9.

Paller AS, Shah PR, Silverio AM, et al. Oral glycopyrrolate as second-line treatment for primary pediatric hyperhidrosis. J Am Acad Dermatol. 2012;67(5):918–23.

Steiner Z, Cohen Z, Kleiner O, et al. Do children tolerate thoracoscopic sympathectomy better than adults? Pediatr Surg Int. 2008;24(3):343–7.

Wolosker N, Schvartsman C, Krutman M, et al. Efficacy and quality of life outcomes of oxybutynin for treating palmar hyperhidrosis in children younger than 14 years old. Pediatr Dermatol. 2014;31(1):48–53.

Wolosker N, Teivelis MP, Krutman M, et al. Long-term efficacy of oxybutynin for palmar and plantar hyperhidrosis in children younger than 14 years. Pediatr Dermatol. 2014;32(5):663–7.

The Psychological Profile of the Patient with Primary Hyperhidrosis

Ana Rosa Sancovski

According to the Hippocratic Doctrine, medicine has as its object the sick man in his totality, including understanding his illness, temperament, and life history. Disease is conceived as a global reaction of the subject that involves both his body and spirit, and the therapeutic intervention must seek to re-establish the lost harmony of man with his environment and with himself. However, what characterizes the body with which science confronts us is the exclusion of desire as the cause of its functioning and as a causal explanation of its destiny and its death. We have to take into account the subjective representation of this body that has a singular discourse, and that its successive psychic representations will accompany the evolution of somatic life, and that this body will function, increasingly, under the aegis of its unconscious motivations that decide the causalities attributed to the striking events of its existence.

The mind–body dichotomy proposed by Descartes in the seventeenth century gave way to a rationalist, mechanistic, and reductionist conception in which the human body came to be thought of as a machine. Descartes argued that clear and distinct ideas should not be mixed with the senses emanating from the body.

Although positivist science has achieved so many advances and modern therapies that it has often helped human beings to suffer less, the Cartesian way of thinking still affects current medical therapy, which leads many physicians to undertake a partial treatment, disregarding the presence and strength of the unconscious. Many scientists still think of man as they have for some centuries, disregarding the fact that the head and

---

A. R. Sancovski
PhD in Experimental Physiopathology Sciences from School of Medicine of USP, São Paulo, SP, Brasil

Psychosomatic Especialist from Sedes Sapientiae Institute, Boonton, NJ, USA

General Medical Clinic, Hospital das Clínicas de São Paulo, São Paulo, SP, Brasil

Hyperhidrosis Outpatient Clinic, Hospital das Clínicas de São Paulo, São Paulo, SP, Brasil

Psychoanalytical Theory, Clinic in Neuropsychology, Neuropsychological Residence of the National Center for Specialization Courses – CENACES, São Paulo, SP, Brasil

© Springer International Publishing AG, part of Springer Nature 2018
M. P. Loureiro et al. (eds.), *Hyperhidrosis*,
https://doi.org/10.1007/978-3-319-89527-7_7

body are not separated and that what occurs in one sector has a significant impact on the other. If not, how do you explain the changes that occur in our body when it is subjected to a strong emotional experience? One can even think of the physiological trajectory of the emotions to explain and rationalize what causes the manifestation of a symptom.

Mello Filho points out that in every emotion there is an "integrated configuration of emotional expression, properly speaking, hormonal and physiological responses and consequent motor actions; however, all this integrated standard is put into operation in function of the evaluation that the subject makes of the lived situation in correlation with the pulsional possibilities of answer". But one cannot fail to consider that these reactions will come later in the interpretation of what has occurred—whether they have been felt and understood as positive or negative—thus giving the tonality and direction of the responses in physiological, motor, or emotional responses. Therefore, it is very important to emphasize and consider that the reaction and the physical symptom are subsequent to the subjective experience of a given situation, based on the pre-existing emotional and psychic repertoire of that moment. Thus, there is a trauma, characterized as an excess, which triggers the disease as a phenomenon, an explosion in the body, with a discharge function as a wordless response to a primitive, non-verbal conflict, provoking a "short circuit" in the person's psychic workings, where part of the body is called to express what is prevented from being said; that is, the subject has an ego, an area that functions as a mediator of the pulsional areas and the environment, which does not support this excess. Freud defines this as a fact that causes too much excitement. He pointed to the psychic apparatus as a protective structure against the excesses of excitement coming from outside and from within the body.

In this way, the representations and symbols of the ego are constituted from:

- Earliest childhood
- Physical and psychic characteristics
- The parents' speech about them
- Family and domestic environment
- The respect and care received
- The family support received during their identity construction
- The healthy organization of sexuality
- The love
- The limits
- The values
- The role models
- The coherence of the parents' commands and attitudes
- The traumas and losses of early childhood
- The affective experiences in the psychological repertoire
- Parental illness
- Parental attitudes (aggressive, cold, unruly, excessively affective and invasive)
- Country or city changes (restrictions of full verbal expression, such as language barriers and cultural differences) and countless other such factors

These will be the catalysts of pulsional excitations circulating in the organism. Thus, considering the mentioned factors, one should not seek the causes of illness just in the organ, or in the symptom by severing sympathetic nerves that would apparently alleviate the patient's suffering, disregarding that the symptom may be an explicit, unintelligible effect of pains, difficulties, and soul sufferings.

According to Zimerman (1992), the onset of organic disease is compounded by deep psychic symbolic meanings that are invested in the formation of body image and, in addition to physical suffering, this may cause the patient to be invaded by feelings of helplessness, fear, confusion, anxiety, guilt, shame, and even humiliation for having "failed" or "weakened" by having fallen ill or for the original human pain of having to acknowledge that he is a mortal like any other. On the other hand, it is common for psychosomatic diseases to be triggered by the loss of beloved people, objects of love, affections, or values to which the individual reacts with the feeling of abandonment and hopelessness.

The human being is marked by the parents' words like invisible tattoos. What parents say influences their impressions about themselves. If the parents said good words, they will trust and internalize themselves, but if they said bad words, the same process will occur. The body and the psyche are a single, indissoluble whole. For Capisano, "the human being is essentially psychosomatic". According to psychoanalyst Joyce McDougall, body and mind "are born from the same somatopsychic matrix", which slowly differentiates into distinct but always interconnected fields, one possibility being psychosomatic sickness. This same author points out that somatic disease always represents an inability of the mind to process psychic conflicts, producing a regression in which the individual falls into the somatopsychic indifferentiation of the baby (the subject regresses and part of his personality begins to function as if he were a baby). She emphasizes that the passage of the body to the psyche is the result of the baby's initial attempts to overcome physical pain, empty experiences, frustrations, and fears, and that psychosomatic patients require too much of the physical body or even ignore the signs of the helpless body, as if the body could not be represented as a psychic object. On the other hand, Piera Aulagnier (1985) emphasized that the raw material of the psychic representations is found in the corporal functions. Other authors consider that body and mind or psyche are like two dialects—two languages—that express, at the same time, the same vital phenomenon, which is untranslatable. It is known that in psychosomatic disease there is a failure in the channel of psychic expression, but messages continue to flow in an abrupt, primitive, disorganized, or organized way according to unknown rules, and the only possible expression is the body. The psychosomatic symptom can be represented as a part of the subject's history that cannot be written psychically and ends up presenting itself as a hieroglyph that is inscribed in the body. Considering this, decoding needs to be done and voice and expression to verbal language needs to be given, with the possibility of symbolization and psychic representation; that is, to have an imaginative life of fantasies, dreams, and daydreams so these patients do not have to present failures in the process of emotional development.

Protocol for the Psychological Evaluation of Patients

In view of these findings, a protocol was developed for the psychological evaluation of patients who came to the Hyperhidrosis Outpatient Clinic of the Hospital das Clínicas of the Medical School of the University of São Paulo (USP) for surgery and to treat compensatory hyperhidrosis resulting from this surgical procedure.

After medical screening, the sample included 376 subjects aged between 7 and 50 years with no previous psychiatric illnesses who had primary hyperhidrosis and who were considered, according to the French school of psychosomatics, as being poorly mentalized (symbolic poverty) or with uncertain mentation (excessive repression and affective repression) leading to a fragile psychic structure that resulted in difficulties in the affective, social, and professional areas. In addition, more than 80% of the sample had an urgent desire to solve the problem as quickly as possible, almost magically, through sympathectomy to try and reduce their suffering. However, following the psychological evaluations performed, these patients were found to be in crisis; they were distressed and depressed, with difficulties in the personal and social spheres, and sought out the Hyperhidrosis Outpatient Clinic to request help, and not necessarily surgery, given that they were unaware of compensatory hyperhidrosis or, even in those who knew about it, lacked clarity or deep understanding of the surgery results, effectivness.

The general objectives were as follows:

1. Evaluate the quality of life and influence of the psychic dynamics in action on hyperhidrosis.
2. Evaluate the psychic effects the surgery has on patients' lives.

The specific objective was as follows:

1. Communicate to the patient and the team the results of the evaluations, the main difficulties raised, and whether the requirement was surgical or psychological.

The sample consisted of 51% female patients, 72% were single, 35% had axillary hyperhidrosis, 15% had palmar, 10% had palmar and axillary, 35% had palmar, axillary and plantar, and 5% had diffuse sweating.

Psychological Assessments

The following psychological assessments were carried out:

1. *Semi-directed psychological interview.* This is a fundamental instrument of the clinical method, being a technique of scientific investigation in psychology, involving the patient's life history, psychosexual development, family relationships, social, affective, and professional factors, and the environment in which they developed. Through listening to the patient, we can evaluate their ability to associate ideas and symbols and to express affections without "verbiage".
2. *World Health Organization Quality of Life–BREF (WHOQOL–BREF).* This quality-of-life questionnaire has 26 questions that assess the physical,

psychological, social, and environmental fields. The concept of life that each person possesses is what will influence the evaluation that she makes of her quality of life. Life belongs to her exclusively and can make her what she pleases. For Szalai, quality of life is an indivisible concept, and it is necessary to attribute to it clear and specific content, through greater investigation and reflection. This instrument for assessing overall quality of life was chosen as the quality-of-life questionnaire used in medical screening and was very directive and specific for patients with hyperhidrosis, almost inducing and expecting positive responses from them to the truisms provided.

3. *Murray's (Projective) Thematic Apperception Test (TAT) [partial, with the use of four boards]*.[1] Proponents of the technique assert that the subject's responses, in the narratives they make up about ambiguous pictures of people, reveal their underlying motives, concerns, and the way they see the social world.
4. *Pigid Desiderative Questionnaire*. A clinical instrument used to understand the psychic phenomena, allowing the development of intervention measures, which is often indispensable, soon after its application (therapeutic consultations). It consists of proposing to the subject that he first make three positive choices and then three negative choices: "If you could not be a person, what would you most like to be? Why?" (Expecting responses from the animal, plant, and inanimate world, regardless of the order presented.)
5. *Patient psychological feedback about the evaluation results*. This refers to explaining to the patient, in a delicate and amicable way, the results of the tests. The report should begin by emphasizing the positive aspects of his personality, what was found and verified in his answers to the applied tests, integrating these answers to his life history, and helping him to make a link (link-points) to what was lived, but not integrated, felt, and understood within that context. It is as if his inner world has a series of loose facts and affections, which the patient does not know and cannot fit to form a symbol in order to give meaning to what has occurred in his life, and which has overwhelmed his capacity to elaborate, causing psychic excitement and arousing much anxiety and triggering archaic depressive nuclei, which probably led to the presentation of hyperhidrosis, as a form of expression of something that was not inscribed in the subjective field of his being, represented, felt, thought, or said. The results found in the psychological assessment show that affective–emotional aspects, evidently altered by current and past life situations, preponderated over surgical demand.

The most prevalent psychic characteristics found in the 376 patients tested were ego fragility, low abstraction capacity, concreteness, childishness, immaturity, low articulation of ideas, stereotyped psychodynamics, low capacity for symbolization

---

[1] The TAT clinical instrument was partially used, because they were patients with psychosomatic disorder, in crisis, whose initial demand was not psychological evaluation; in addition, they would not have continuity of psychological treatment, although four other services were offered, after evaluation and devolution.

and continence, psychic rigidity, anxious fantasies, high impulsiveness and destructiveness, repressed aggression, obsessive defenses, isolation, repression, and repression. Self-rejection and social phobia, attribution of all life difficulties to hyperhidrosis, idealizations regarding the solving of all problems after surgery, affective–emotional immaturity, low self-esteem, compromised self-image, social stereotypy, reactive depressions, and major depression were found. In addition, 85% of the sample reported accentuation of hyperhidrosis on hot days and during stress or competitions.

All patients evaluated presented some type of crisis, with diffuse anguish, for which they are unable to detect the cause, depressive symptoms, and difficulty and lack of psychic resources to face and try to solve their conflicts and personal problems. These factors exacerbated their symptoms of hyperhidrosis, prompting them to attend the outpatient clinic for help, but not necessarily for surgery. Therefore, if the request is met without psychological evaluation, the team has to be attentive to the demand that is implicit between the lines of the surgical request; sympathectomy solves hyperhidrosis at the complaint site but may also divert it to other areas, and it also increases the risk of new somatic disorganizations, since the patient's request may not be what has been explained and the sympathetic innervation may have improper surgical intervention because the causes of hyperhidrosis are psychological. Moreover, without evaluation and psychological treatment, it must be understood that the patient may not himself know what he wants because he is repressed, fragmented, or disconnected in his unconscious.

Case Report

Rodrigo, a 20-year-old male patient who presented to the Hyperhidrosis Outpatient Clinic with suicidal ideation and a desire to be reoperated on immediately, hoping to revert the hyperhidrosis surgery he had undergone, was referred to the psychological service. He had been operated on 6 months earlier at another public service and had symptoms worse than his initial hyperhidrosis.

In presenting his life story, the young man reported being an only child who did not remember his father as his parents separated when he was only 2 years old. He said that his mother was affectionate, but because she was very young, she traveled a lot, had several boyfriends, and he was taken care of sometimes by an aunt, sometimes by a neighbor, and sometimes by a more distant relative. He said that because he was very poor, he had to share his school backpack with his mother. When she traveled at weekends, she would take the backpack and put her belongings in it. On Mondays, he would find his backpack and put his school notebooks and books in it, with lessons done. He reported at this very emotional moment that once when he was 8 years old, shortly after a break during school, a student complained to the teacher that he had left his walkman in his backpack and when he returned he could not find it anymore. The teacher then locked the door to the classroom and said that all backpacks would be searched until the walkman was found. This was done; however, when Rodrigo's backpack was emptied, two pairs of women's panties and four intimate absorbents were removed from one of the pockets, causing the entire class to sneer and question his masculinity. Rodrigo reported that since that time he has had intense palmar, axillary, and facial flushing hyperhidrosis when he presents in public, and has a great deal of difficulty in performing professional functions (he has tried to work as a receptionist, salesman, and exhibitor) and the symptoms described have caused him profound malaise. Thus, he underwent surgery at another hyperhidrosis service. He said the following to me: "Doctor, I'm sitting here and wearing an absorbent; because my compensatory hyperhidrosis in the groin area is so intense that wherever I sit, I leave a 'stamp' of perspiration arousing repulsion in people. Besides, I no longer have a social life because every time I feed myself, by chewing, I feel a strong itch in the head and I look like a monkey who scratches his head without stopping". This led him to a social phobia, due to embarrassment, and consequent intense weight loss, leading him to conclude that it was no longer worth living if this surgery were not reversed. Unfortunately, we know this to be impossible.

Would you have operated on this patient if you knew his history?

Conclusions

In this sample, 72% of the patients in the environmental domain, which includes financial aspects, reporting altered and unsatisfactory quality of life, as did 76% with respect to psychological aspects. In the physical domain, surprisingly, 83% of the sample said that their quality of life was very good. Regarding medical explanations provided regarding compensatory hyperhidrosis, 46.7% of the sample did not assimilate them, leading to idealizations and expectations of all life problems being solved following surgery. Regarding the psychological problems found, 92% of the sample has a need for psychotherapy.

Pre-surgical psychological evaluation is indispensable to avoid high levels of frustration, accompanied by depression, decreased quality of life, and complaints of dissatisfaction following surgery.

It is important to investigate the relationship between the onset of the disease and some facts of life, in order to rule out losses, acquisitions, and traumas, current or past, which may have temporarily caused hyperhidrosis as a form of expression of difficulties of adaptation.

When asked about the desire to undergo psychotherapy, 83.2% of the sample admitted needing it and agreed to seek treatment, regardless of the surgery.

The risk of not providing psychotherapy is this: to operate without psychological evaluation may lead to deepened psychic symptoms, new physical illnesses, and aggravation of the psychosomatic balance of the patient.

Suggested Reading

Aulagnier P. Cuerpo, história y Interpretación. Buenos Aires: Paidos; 1985.
Dejours C. O corpo entre a biologia e a psicanálise. Artes Médicas: Porto Alegre; 1988.
Dejours C. Repressão e subversão em psicossomática. Rio de Janeiro: Jorge Zahar; 1991.

Dolto F. A imagem inconsciente do corpo. Perspectiva: São Paulo; 2001.
Ferraz F. Psicossoma – psicossomática psicanalítica. Casa do Psicólogo: São Paulo; 1997.
Freud A. El ego y los mecanismos de defensa. Paidós: Buenos Aires; 1949.
Groddeck G. O livro d 'isso. Perspectiva: São Paulo; 1988.
Kellner R. Psychosomatic syndromes, somatization and somatoform disorders. Psychoter Psychosom. 1994;61:4–24.
Lipowski ZJ. Somatization: the experience and communication of psychological distress as somatic symptoms. Psychoter Psychosom. 1987;47:160–7.
Marty P. Mentalização e psicossomática. Casa do Psicólogo: São Paulo; 1998.
McDougall J. Teatros do corpo. Martins Fontes: São Paulo; 1991.
Sancovski AR. Sentimentos na relação médico-paciente? Rev Bras Clín Terapeut. 2000;26(6): 226–8.
Zimerman DE. "A Formaçao Psicológica do Médico"_ Psicossomática Hoje. Porto Alegre: Artes Médicas; 1992. p. 64–9.

Psychiatric Features in Hyperhidrosis

Marianna Gonzalez de Oliveira Andrade

The relationship between the integumentary system and the nervous system begins in the comum embryonic origin. During the third week of embryonic development the formation of the three primary germinative cell layers occur: ectoderm, mesoderm, and endoderm. The ectoderm then splits into the neuroectoderm (which gives origin to the nervous system) and superficial ectoderm (which originates the epidermis, sweat and sebaceous glands, hair, nails, etc.). In clinical practice we can observe that the interaction between skin and psyche runs both ways: neuropsychiatric pathologies can manifest with dermatologic signs and symptoms (dermatitis, hyperhidrosis, pruritus, alopecia, etc.) and in the opposite direction, primary dermatologic conditions often interfere in self-esteem causing anxiety, mood and behavior disturbances. Afflictions such as vitiligo, acne, primary hyperhidrosis, psoriasis, and alopecia can begin or be aggravated in the context of significant psychological stress.

Considering that skin is the main human interface with the environment, it is understandable that conditions that compromise ones self-image and self-esteem can also compromise individual interactions with the external world.

Primary hyperhidrosis and anxiety have a complex relationship mediated by the dysregulation of the sympathetic nervous system, however the true etiology remains unknown. The autonomous nervous system is an important mediator between the mind and the rest of the body, regulating the release, conservation and loss of energy. When we consciously or unconsciously feel a need to defend ourselves from something that is perceived as dangerous, our sympathetic nervous system makes energy available for defense responses. The homeostatic responses mediated by the autonomic nervous system are reached by a balance between the actions of the sympathetic, parasympathetic, and endocrine systems.

Primary hyperhidrosis is considered to be a form of intermittent dysautonomia characterized by temporary dysregulation of the autonomic function exceeding that

M. G. de Oliveira Andrade
Hospital Israelita Albert Einstein, São Paulo, SP, Brazil

required for thermoregulatory homeostasis. The psychological symptoms experienced in hyperhidrosis are mostly not related to trauma or neurosis but rather by the hypervigilance and anxious apprehension of profuse sweating events generated by the autonomic deregulation. The perception of the profuse sweating aggravates anxiety, which in return pertetuates sweating by promoting a positive feedback.

Excessive sweating in primary hyperhidrosis is often spontaneous (in the absence of thermogenic or psychologic triggers), although it may be exacerbated by anxiety. Excessive sweating leads to significant impairment in basic daily social interactions such as meeting people, shaking hands, and developing intimate personal relationships. Hyperhidrosis patients are constantly and highly concerned on how they present themselves and whether the excessive sweating might be noticed by others, causing embarrassment and negative self-evaluation, and fear of the social stigma of inappropriate sweating. Studies examining the temperament and characteristics of patients with hyperhidrosis indicate that these patients might express greater fatigability and asthenia, having a tendency towards tiredness and to recover slowly from psychological and physical stressors and illness.

Onset of primary hyperhidrosis is typically by late childhood to the mid-teens and has a chronic presentation. Frequently, this early onset negatively influences social skills development, interpersonal interactions and school performance. Beyond social consequences, it can also precipitate chronic psychological or psychiatric disorders. Primary hyperhidrosis patients present higher rates of general anxiety and social anxiety in addition to deficits in emotional processing (characterized by the inability to identify and describe emotions), all leading to a sense of decreased quality of life. They also present somatic hypervigilance regarding thermoregulatory symptoms (sweating, hot flashes and heat perception), likely representing both a vulnerability factor and a maintenance factor for cognitive–affective symptoms. Hyperhidrosis patients are more concerned with how they present themselves, most likely due to the social stigma of inappropriately or profusely sweating. These differential psychopathological findings and consequent emotional disabilities highlight the social burden caused by hyperhidrosis.

Several studies have assessed anxiety features in patients with hyperhidrosis. However, most of them occurred in small samples of patients and lacked multivariable analysis, therefore reporting mixed findings. These studies have in common the agreement that successful treatment of hyperhidrosis improves anxiety, quality of life and social functioning.

Mild and moderate anxiety have a higher prevalence rate in primary hyperhidrosis patients (49.2%). However, depression in this population has a similar prevalence as in general population and is often associated with anxiety symptoms. Studies conducted with dermatological outpatients (with and without hyperhidrosis) examined the correlation between hyperhidrosis, anxiety, and depression. The prevalence of anxiety in patients with primary hyperhidrosis (23%) is significantly higher than in patients with other dermatological diseases (7.5%). The incidence of social anxiety disorder in patients with hyperhidrosis varies between 23% and 47%. Rates of social anxiety disorder in control groups of other dermatological patients without hyperhidrosis (7–13.8%) are similar to the general population. There is a positive correlation between the severity of hyperhidrosis and an increase in the prevalence of anxiety.

The higher prevalence of anxiety in these patients is found to be independent of other variables such as age, gender, age of onset, body mass index, co-morbidity with other dermatologic diagnoses, ethnicity, and body area affected by hyperhidrosis (palmar, axillary, plantar, head, and trunk).

Therapeutic possibilities for psychological symptoms and quality of life include cognitive–behavioral therapy focusing on somatic symptoms in addition to the prescription of serotonin reuptake inhibitor medication (such as sertraline).

On the other hand, secondary hyperhidrosis of clinical severity is present in many anxiety disorders, such as generalized anxiety disorder, panic disorder, post-traumatic stress disorder, and especially social anxiety disorder. An autonomic dysfunction by hyperactivity of the sympathetic nervous system is considered to be the cause of induction of somatic symptoms in anxiety, such as sweating, tachycardia, and tremor. Anxious patients have increased sympathetic tonus, slower adaptation to repeated stimuli, and excessive response to mild or moderate stimuli. Considering all anxious disorders, these findings are more prominent in patients who present social anxiety disorder (also known as social phobia), which presents a life time prevalence of 5–12%. The clinical features are composed of disproportionate fear and marked anxiety triggered by social situations which the patient strongly feels that he can be observed and evaluated by other people. The patient shows excessive concern about being judged negatively, accompanied by somatic signs of autonomic hyperexcitation. This presentation causes significant psychological suffering and loss of social functioning. Patients with social anxiety disorder commonly present excessive fear that others will notice symptoms of autonomic arousal when they are in social or performance exposure situations. The best established treatments for social anxiety disorder are cognitive–behavioral therapy and selective serotonin reuptake inhibitor antidepressants.

Investigation of the presence of hyperhidrosis is quite neglected in the psychiatric care of patients with social anxiety disorder, despite being a prominent feature. Moderate or severe sweating associated with social situations is reported in 25–32% of patients diagnosed with social anxiety disorder. The presence of hyperhidrosis features is associated with higher levels of disability, fear and avoidance of social triggers. This may also indicate that primary hyperhidrosis can result in significant social anxiety and should be ruled out before a diagnosis of primary social anxiety is made. While treating patients with social anxiety, clinicians should always investigate the presence of hyperhidrosis, and vice versa. The distinction between primary hyperhidrosis with secondary social anxiety and primary social anxiety disorder with secondary hyperhidrosis might not be clear in clinical practice. These conditions have early onsets, making it necessary to rely on the patient's retrospective judgment, which might be insufficient to determine this distinction.

For anxiety patients whose social anxiety is triggered predominantly by excessive sweating, treatment targeting primary hyperhidrosis should be considered. Therefore, psychiatrists should be aware of treatment options for hyperhidrosis. Many patients whose anxiety features are benefited by psychopharmacologic treatments for social anxiety disorder are left with residual sweating at the end of the treatment. In these cases, other treatment approaches deserve to be explored (oxybutynin, topical antiperspirants, botulinum toxin A injection, endoscopic thoracic sympathectomy).

Conclusions

Primary hyperhidrosis and anxiety features might share the same pathogenic autonomic dysfunction pathway. Clinical findings in patients with hyperhidrosis go beyond a decrease in quality of life, also pointing to high prevalence rates of anxiety, especially social anxiety disorder.

Patients suffering from this co-morbidity present both discomfort from sweating itself and disproportionate fear of being observed and negatively judged by other people. The development of anxiety features in this context may produce great suffering, leading to the adoption of avoidance behavior even in situations of minimal social contact. In severe cases, patients may seek social isolation, becoming incapable of attending school, work, and other activities that presuppose minimal social contact.

During the follow-up of hyperhidrosis patients, psychiatric evaluation may be important to rule out co-morbid anxiety. Psychotherapeutic (cognitive–behavioral therapy) and psychopharmacological (selective serotonin reuptake inhibitors antidepressants) interventions can increase the chance of the success of dermatological and surgical treatments in improving overall quality of life.

Suggested Reading

Ak M, Dincer D, Haciomeroglu B, Akarsu S, Cinar A, Lapsekili N. Temperament and character properties of primary focal hyperhidrosis patients. Health Qual Life Outcomes. 2013;11(1):5.

Bahar R, Zhou P, Liu Y, Huang Y, Phillips A, Lee T, et al. The prevalence of anxiety and depression in patients with or without hyperhidrosis (HH). J Am Acad Dermatol. 2016;75(6):1126–33.

Bracha H, Lenze S, Chung M. A surgical treatment for anxiety-triggered palmar hyperhidrosis is not unlike treating tearfulness in major depression by severing the nerves to the lacrimal glands. Br J Dermatol. 2006;155(6):1299–300.

Bragança G, Lima S, Pinto Neto A, Marques L, Melo E, Reis F. Evaluation of anxiety and depression prevalence in patients with primary severe hyperhidrosis. An Bras Dermatol. 2014;89(2):230–5.

Davidson J, Foa E, Connor K, Churchill L. Hyperhidrosis in social anxiety disorder. Prog Neuro-Psychopharmacol Biol Psychiatry. 2002;26(7–8):1327–31.

Lessa L, Luz F, de Rezende R, Durães S, Harrison B, de Menezes G, et al. The psychiatric facet of hyperhidrosis. J Psychiatr Pract. 2014;20(4):316–23.

Owens A, Low D, Iodice V, Critchley H, Mathias C. The genesis and presentation of anxiety in disorders of autonomic overexcitation. Auton Neurosci. 2017;203:81–7.

Pohjavaara P, Telaranta T, Väisänen E. The role of the sympathetic nervous system in anxiety: is it possible to relieve anxiety with endoscopic sympathetic block? Nord J Psychiatry. 2003;57(1):55–60.

Schneier F, Heimberg R, Liebowitz M, Blanco C, Gorenstein L. Social anxiety and functional impairment in patients seeking surgical evaluation for hyperhidrosis. Compr Psychiatry. 2012;53(8):1181–6.

Anxiety, Depression, and Hyperhidrosis

9

Débora Yumi Ferreira Kamikava

The association between anxiety, depressive symptomatology, and chronic diseases is not uncommon. The prevalence of anxiety or depression in people with changes in physical health is broad, about 18–35% and 15–61%, respectively. In addition, there is evidence that these emotional repercussions are associated with a decrease in quality of life, generating a significant impact in patients with hyperhidrosis (HH).

It is known that, although it isn't considered a serious disease, the quality of life of patients with HH is considerably affected. The symptoms are manifested through the skin, the body's means of communication with the external world, and it is through it that the individual has his emotions exposed to others, often transforming a common social situation into an embarrassment, generating greater vigilance of the individual in relation to the body itself and their contact with people.

Recent studies indicate that most HH patients classify their quality of life as poor or very poor, and that following treatment they perceive significant benefits, including improvement in quality of life related to physical and mental health. In general, the impact on the patients' quality of life depends not only on the sweat intensity, but also how well patients adapt to this situation, their psychic resources to deal with adverse situations, and the psychosocial context in which they are inserted.

Currently there are specific questionnaires to evaluate quality of life in HH, and although there is still no consensus on the best way to assess the quality of life of these patients, studies show the importance of using these instruments to indicate the most appropriate treatment, whether clinical or surgical, and to verify the efficacy of the treatment performed.

D. Y. F. Kamikava
Mackenzie Presbyterian University, São Paulo, SP, Brazil

General Hospital, HCFMUSP, São Paulo, SP, Brazil

Psychology Division of Central Institute, HCFMUSP, São Paulo, SP, Brazil
e-mail: debora.yumi@hc.fm.usp.br

© Springer International Publishing AG, part of Springer Nature 2018
M. P. Loureiro et al. (eds.), *Hyperhidrosis*,
https://doi.org/10.1007/978-3-319-89527-7_9

Difficulties in adapting to the adverse situations imposed by the clinical manifestations of HH can be reflected in several areas, causing impairment in social life, academic and professional performance, and self-image, in addition to a greater tendency of these patients to develop mood changes associated with anxiety and depression. When exposed to chronic sources of stress, that damage becomes more frequent and requires continuous adaptation, causing subjective suffering to the patient.

Anxiety and stress are conditions commonly triggered by the appearance and development of a disease, and are considered aggravating factors for the degree of sweating.

Although there is little research to prove the cause and effect relationship of co-morbidities and psychological aggravating factors in patients with HH, some authors point out a higher prevalence of anxiety in those patients than in the general population and patients with other chronic diseases. Depressive symptoms are usually less prevalent and, when present, are associated with anxiety. Corroborating this idea, studies show a correlation among the indexes of anxiety, depression, and dermatological diseases, without necessarily establishing a cause and effect relationship.

Since this topic doesn't yet have a large literature, a study is being carried out in the Hyperhidrosis Outpatient Clinic of the Thoracic Surgery Service of Hospital das Clínicas da Faculdade de Medicina da Universidade de São Paulo (HCFMUSP). This research aims to evaluate the presence of anxiety and depression symptoms in patients with HH and its association with the perception of patients related to the degree of sweating, as well as the effect of clinical treatment on HH symptoms and its association with anxious and depressive symptomatology.

Because HH predominantly arises in childhood and adolescence, age groups considered important in the emotional development of the individual, and in which there is a certain predisposition to the development of some types of psychopathologies, it can become responsible for greater damage to the mental health of those younger people and negatively influence the evolution of the disease. However, it is important to note that the emotional repercussions, which may or may not affect HH patients, don't necessarily indicate the presence of a psychiatric disorder.

Due to the fact that, on some occasions, HH is triggered by stress or emotions, patients are often characterized as anxious, timid, and unsafe individuals, eventually leading to diagnostic errors and stereotypes in this regard. However, HH is not only caused by emotional stimulation, so a misunderstanding of this relationship can generate a significant loss of confidence and reduce the capacity of the individual to discriminate between what is physiological and what is emotional, negatively influencing their coping with the condition and treatment of the disease, since many individuals live years believing that excessive sweating is due to anxiety, not the opposite, and because of this, they delay the search for a solution to the HH.

Thus, it is important that differential diagnoses be correctly defined and the indicate treatment is relevant to the needs and demands of the subject, so that the person can have a better quality of life and is better adapted to the social and environmental demands in their life. In addition, early treatment of HH can be considered preventive in order to avoid or aggravate psychic and social disorders, since HH is a risk factor for the development of these conditions, which are often reactive or overlap the process of the disease and are not the primary cause of this condition.

What commonly occurs in the clinic when assessing HH patients who manifest some associated emotional symptom is the diagnosis of adjustment disorders described in the ICD-10 (*International Statistical Classification of Diseases and Related Health Problems, 10th edition*) and DSM (*Diagnostic and Statistical Manual of Mental Disorders*) diagnostic manuals. Adjustment disorders are characterized by the presence of emotional and behavioral symptoms in response to an identifiable stressor. Such a disorder may present as depressed mood; anxiety; anxiety and depression; behavioral disturbance; or even mixed disturbance of emotions and conduct, characterized as a state of subjective suffering and emotional disturbance, which can lead to impairments in the social and professional performance of the individual. According to the DSM-5, symptomatic responses to an identifiable stressor should occur within 3 months of the onset of the stressor event, and do not last more than 6 months after the stressor and its consequences cease.

In cases in which the stressor is persistent, adjustment disorders can progress to the chronic form, causing significant suffering and impairment in the patients' quality of life, and eventually to their family members and people living with them. It is understood that when emotional symptoms fall within the diagnostic criteria of adjustment disorders, patients tend to exhibit emotional and behavioral symptoms in response to the stress of having a medical condition that causes harm in different spheres of the subject's life until the symptoms of HH are treated.

Preliminary data from the study being conducted in our unit has been relevant in supporting this idea, pointing out that 5 weeks after the beginning of clinical treatment for symptoms of HH it is already possible to measure and compare levels of intensity of anxiety and depressive symptomatology before and after treatment, indicating a decrease in the anxious and depressive symptoms, concomitant with the improvement of the clinical symptoms of HH in a significant number of the patients. Based on these data, Table 9.1 shows the main anxious and depressive symptoms reported by patients with HH symptoms.

Currently, there are several instruments available to evaluate emotional symptoms that help professionals to perform better screening and diagnosis processes, which favor the planning of more effective interventions, and with significantly more favorable results to solve the psychic problem presented concomitant with clinical manifestations of HH. For proper choice of the evaluation instrument it is important that the professional considers the characteristics and symptoms presented by the patient and also knows the characteristics of application and correction of the instruments.

Table 9.1 Main anxious and depressive symptoms reported by patients with hyperhidrosis symptoms

Anxiety		Depression
Difficulty in relaxing		Social isolation
Face flushed		Insecurity
Nervousness	Hyperhidrosis	Low self-esteem
Irritability		Sadness
Heat sensation		Pessimism

In addition to the use of instruments, clinical interviews of the patient are also necessary, considering the areas of life that are negatively affected by HH, the individual's understanding of the disease, treatment expectations, and whether the emotional and social damage, eventually presented by the patient, are only reactive to the presence of HH, if the disease is an aggravating factor of the pre-existing emotional symptoms, or if it has triggered more severe emotional losses.

The possibility that emotional symptoms are a transient condition, as in the case of adjustment disorders, doesn't mean that they don't need to be treated. Because these symptoms cause high suffering and loss in the patient's relational life, with his environment and with himself, psychotherapy is an important form of treatment and follow-up of these patients, since it provides host, strengthening, and helps the development of skills for facing the situations experienced by HH patients.

By favoring the emergence of psychic coping resources, the psychologist assists in the development of resilient behaviors, aiming at overcoming crises and adversities to which these individuals are exposed, strengthening individual attributes and environmental resources in a process that results in overcoming and managing these situations. Thus, the relationship between resilience and the disease situation is contextualized as the individual's ability to deal with his diagnosis and its implications, adapting and evolving positively and creatively.

Suggested Reading

Andrade Filho LO, Campos JRM, Jatene FB, Kauffman P, Kusniek S, Werebe EC, Wolosker N. Quality of life, before and after thoracic sympathectomy: report on 378 operated patients. Ann Thorac Surg. 2003;76:886–91.

Campbell TPDA, Campos JRM, Kauffman P, Krutman M, Puech-Leão P, Schvartsman C, Wolosker N. Efficacy and quality of life outcomes of oxybutynin for treating palmar hyperhidrosis in children younger than 14 years old. Pediatr Dermatol. 2014;31:48–53.

Dias LIN, Miranda ECM, Mussi RK, Toro IFC, Mussi RK. Relation between anxiety, depression and quality of life with the intensity of reflex sweating after thoracic sympathectomy by videosurgery for the treatment of primary hyperhidrosis. Rev Col Bras Cir. 2016;43:354–9.

Hyperhidrosis and Diet-Induced Thermogenesis

10

Najla Elias Farage and Milena Barcza Stockler-Pinto

Introduction

Hyperhidrosis is a condition that causes the subject to experience excessive sweating, even when the ambient temperature is low or the body is at rest. It may be of primary origin, affecting about 1% of the population, or secondary, which originates from other causes, such as anxiety, cancer, presence of diabetes, heart disease, hyperthyroidism, and spinal cord injury, among others.

Nutrition does not seem to play a dominant role in increased sweating, but studies that refer to diet-induced thermogenesis (DIT) reveal that there are symptoms that may be alleviated by some nutritional behaviors. DIT is the energy required for digestion, absorption, utilization, and storage of nutrients after ingestion of food.

Some studies have shown that consumption of some foods causes prolonged thermogenesis. Because it is an energetic component, DIT plays an important role in regulating the energy balance, and among the factors that modulate the energy content and composition of the diet. In addition to diet, sensory factors also contribute to increased DIT, such as appearance, aroma, and texture.

Another important fact that also contributes to thermogenesis is the sympathetic nervous system (SNS); stimulation of this system promotes in the body the action of the catabolic systems of energy balance, mobilization of fat stores, weight loss, increase of lipolysis, and consequently thermogenesis. The central nervous system (CNS), particularly the hypothalamus, controls the temperature of the human body and regulates the thirst and hunger processes. It also monitors the

N. E. Farage (✉)
Nutrition Department, Universidade Veiga Almeida, Rio de Janeiro, RJ, Brazil

Medical Sciences, Universidade Federal Fluminense, Niterói, RJ, Brazil

M. B. Stockler-Pinto
School of Nutrition, Universidade Federal Fluminense, Niterói, RJ, Brazil

© Springer International Publishing AG, part of Springer Nature 2018
M. P. Loureiro et al. (eds.), *Hyperhidrosis*,
https://doi.org/10.1007/978-3-319-89527-7_10

amount of calories ingested, and when it is higher than necessary it sends a command for this energy to be burned, thus generating heat. Through this pathway the heat generated is proportional to the rate of body metabolism, which is around 40–60% of the energy coming from the hydrolysis of adenosine triphosphate (ATP) and is lost as heat.

In addition to the thermogenesis from the SNS, there is also cephalic thermogenesis, which is optional, and gastrointestinal thermogenesis, which is mandatory. The cephalic phase is exerted by sensorial stimuli, so it is related to the taste buds, which will stimulate the SNS, mobilizing brown adipose tissue and generating more ATP, and consequently will produce more heat.

Mechanisms that Influence Diet-Induced Thermogenesis

Brown adipose tissue is made up of different types of cells and connective tissue. It is composed mostly of adipocytes, which are cells that store energy, and their excess is stored in form of triglycerides, which constitute fat. Lipids, while providing more energy when oxidized, release less heat than carbohydrates. Brown adipose tissue is composed of brown adipocyte cells; these brown adipocyte cells have a large number of mitochondria, which use ATP to generate heat and maintain thermogenesis. This function is related to uncoupling protein 1 (UCP-1), which increases thermogenesis due to increased oxidative phosphorylation. UCP-1 also allows the oxidation of fatty acids in the form of heat production. This occurs through norepinephrine, one of the catecholamines that is signaled by the SNS when there is a need for heat production, thus performing lipolysis. Therefore, when the release of fatty acids from triglycerides occurs, they enter the mitochondria to undergo oxidation, interact with the UCP-1, and degrade their energy for heat generation.

There are some factors that modulate DIT, such as the macronutrient composition of the diet and total energy content. In a mixed diet composed of carbohydrates, proteins, and fats, DIT can represent an energy expenditure of 10–15% of the total amount of energy consumed; for proteins, carbohydrates, and lipids separately, DIT corresponds to 20%, 30%, and 5% respectively.

Higher DIT was observed after eating a high-carbohydrate diet than after eating a high-fat diet, raising the hypothesis that carbohydrates are capable of activating the SNS by the postprandial insulin response. On the other hand, some studies showed that the intake of diets rich in carbohydrates and lipids did not present a significant change in the DIT. Thus, not only the amount of carbohydrates and lipids offered is important in the thermal effect of the diet, but also its quality, which can be manipulated to obtain a higher postprandial energy expenditure.

Protein-rich diets show higher DIT than diets with higher carbohydrate and lipid content, and this effect seems to be a result of the metabolic cost of binder peptide synthesis, gluconeogenesis, and ureogenesis. Regarding carbohydrates and lipids, there are differences in the results, but it seems that the DIT is higher in carbohydrates when it is related to the size of the glucose load and the reading time of the metabolic response.

Diet Composition and Palatability

The composition of the diet can stimulate or inhibit caloric intake, according to the palatability of the foods and the degree of their satiety. The magnitude of DIT is also influenced by palatability, for example in preparations that include spices such as pepper, garlic, and a higher concentration of sucrose, due to the higher insulin response in this case.

Some review studies also address the influence of meals on DIT. Some studies have shown that the DIT increases significantly when the energy content increases, even in a discrete magnitude. The models showed that for each 24-calorie increase in food intake, it would increase by 0.26 DIT energy. Other studies also evaluated the macronutrient composition of the diet and found that diets rich in carbohydrates, compared with lipid-rich diets, have a significantly higher thermal effect. There is also evidence that even in isocaloric diets with higher protein content, DIT was significantly higher than with carbohydrates and lipids.

In a study of 12-h fasting women, higher DIT was observed in diets with a higher sucrose concentration than in basal diets and with a higher lipid concentration. In relation to fats, medium-chain triglycerides (MCTs), such as coconut oil and palm oil, have a higher DIT than long-chain triglycerides from fish, molluscs, and vegetables. On the other hand, polyunsaturated fatty acids (present in corn oil, soybean, fish, and seaweed) and monounsaturated fatty acids (present in oilseeds) have a higher DIT than saturated fatty acids (present in butter and animal fat). Whole foods also have higher DIT than processed foods. In addition, the volume of meals also appears to influence DIT, and some studies have shown a significant increase in DIT when meals were larger and less frequent when compared with less bulky and more frequent meals.

A meta-analysis has been carried out to evaluate the effect of energy intake on the DIT, the results of which clearly support that the energy content of the meals consumed has a rapid influence on the DIT, even adjusting for age, gender, body mass index, and duration of DIT. Some food components also appear to influence DIT, such as luteolin, a flavonoid from some vegetables and spices such as sweet peppers, celery, spearmint, rosemary, and chamomile. Luteolin increased the thermogenic potential of brown adipose tissue in rats fed with diets supplemented with this flavonoid.

In summary, DIT appears to be strongly influenced by its composition of macronutrients, drawing attention to diets rich in protein and simple carbohydrates. Therefore, to minimize the intensity of hyperhidrosis, it is advisable to consume an appropriate amount of protein and carbohydrates in the diet to generate lower DIT.

Currently, the increase in the demand for physical activity practice leads individuals to consume a higher protein and carbohydrate quota in order to fulfill training programs, which often leads to increased hyperhidrosis, as well as to the higher consumption of thermogenics that promise an energetic expense and weight loss. It is up to professionals to better guide and evaluate the still modest research in this field.

The following is a summary regarding foods that can relieve the intensity of hyperhidrosis:

- Foods that should be avoided in large quantities and eaten less frequently: pork, red meat, viscera (liver, kidney), sausage, cola-based soft drinks, energy drinks, coffee and high-caffeine drinks, chocolates, high-sugar food, guarana powder, ginger, shoyo, black tea, and ketchup.
- Foods that must be included frequently in the diet: fruits, natural juices, mint, white meat, fresh vegetables in the form of salads, cold preparations, or at room temperature, without being too hot, and meals in smaller volume and more frequently.

Suggested reading

Farshchi HR, Taylor MA, Macdonald IA. Beneficial metabolic effects of regular meal frequency on dietary thermogenesis, insulin sensitivity, and fasting lipid profiles in healthy obese women. AJCN. 2005;81(1):16–24.

Hermsdorff HH, Miranda MS. Effect of high-sucrose and high lipid on the energy metabolism in normal weight and overweight women: Universidade Federal de Viçosa; fevereiro 2005.

Constraints Caused by Primary Hyperhidrosis

Regina Lunkes Diehl

Today, it is well-known that the anguish patients with hyperhidrosis is part of a vicious cycle of sweat–suffering–more sweat–more suffering, only capable of ending at the hands of specialists in the correction of hyperhidrosis. The procedure is called bilateral cervicothoracic sympathectomy, and the specialists that are dedicated to understanding this issue and operating safely are thoracic and vascular surgeons. It was because I underwent sympathectomy with the correct professionals—a thoracic surgeon, Dr. José Ribas Milanez de Campos, and a vascular surgeon, Dr. Paulo Kauffman, both living and working in São Paulo—that I can live happily and without the permanent anguish that previously accompanied me. The following collection of testimonials was obtained from the hyperhidrosis communication project known as "Suando em Bicas", which is composed of a book and a website published in 2002 (www.suandoembicas.com.br). Receipt of the testimonials was centralized via the website and reports of patients who had or had not already submitted to surgical treatment or other palliative forms of cure were displayed. I find it impossible not to be moved by the intimate confessions that I still receive to this day, in 2017, via emails from the most diverse places in Brazil and abroad.

Excessive sweating leaves anyone affected by it with a terrible sense of impotence. Imagine with me: when you feel very hot, on those very stifling days, whether you sweat or not, the first ideas that come to your mind range from taking a shower to finding an air-conditioned spot, refreshing yourself with an ice cream, or sitting up in a fresh environment. They all seem simple. If this works for you, good news: consider yourself a non-hyperhidrosis sufferer. For those suffering from this

---

Regina Lunkes Diehl is a journalist and author of the book *Suando em Bicas*, published by Editora Nobel in 2004.

R. L. Diehl
School of Media Communication, Arts and Design - Famecos - Pontifical Catholic University
RS, Porto Alegre, Rio Grande do Sul, Brazil
e-mail: regina@suandoembicas.com.br

© Springer International Publishing AG, part of Springer Nature 2018
M. P. Loureiro et al. (eds.), *Hyperhidrosis*,
https://doi.org/10.1007/978-3-319-89527-7_11

disease—excessive sweating on certain parts of the body, especially at the extremities such as the hands, feet, armpits, and head—these outlets do not solve the problem.

Most sufferers of this disease are astonished when it begins. Primary hyperhidrosis usually manifests itself more strongly from adolescence, to the point of causing people to develop a kind of aversion to living with others ("social phobia"). It is estimated that 1% of the world population suffers from this disorder, for many years considered, erroneous and simply, a reflection of poorly resolved emotions. Until the end of the 1990s, excessive sweating was understood as an anomaly of the involuntary nervous system, the only possibility of permanent cure for which is the surgery that this book deals with.

In this chapter, I use the condition of "ex-suadinha" (ex-sweater) to share the anguish of those who, from birth, sweat in an incredible fashion from their hands and feet, wetting the sheets of the crib. I dreamed—or rather "pined"—for upper and lower extremities of the body (hands and feet) for nearly 30 long and wet years, during which I was diagnosed by doctors as a "nervous", "very dynamic" person. Their recommendation: to be calmer than goes by. The specialists used to be very foccused in their issues, and the different areas of Medicine didn't communicate to each other. So, as an example, the Dermathologists didn't know that a toracic surgeon was becoming able to correct hyperidrosis by an specific treatment called sympatectomy. I consulted dermatologists, gynecologists, endocrinologists, neurologists, and a whole host of other "ists", but none helped, leaving me unhappy, which is why I lived in a state of distress.

There was, however, a trigger for the process of sweating too much for me. Incredibly, it has absolutely nothing to do with an emotional state, but rather with climatic conditions, such as high air humidity, and/or heat above 28 °C. Just as the summer begins to show its face in my hometown, Porto Alegre,[1] I once again experienced hyperhidrosis, mainly on the feet and hands. This also happened in the cold and humid days of the heavy winters that occur in the southern region of Brazil, where even house walls pour water. It was in environments with high relative humidity of the air that I sweated even more, freezing my feet and hands in such a way that I could barely walk or write.

The so-called "emotional factor", diagnosed as the cause of the medical disorder, became dominant only from the moment the hyperhidrosis appeared, but it was definitely not the source of the problem. That was, for me, a certainty, but no one believed me.

The fact is that no specialist had detected, at least until the year 2001 in Brazil, that what I had was a lack of control of the sympathetic nervous system chain. Because of the incredible sweating, soaking my hands and feet, I could not wear sandals or flip-flops (the famous Brazilian rubber shoes), besides being deprived of things as simple as playing games with friends in high school, playing the piano, knitting, and writing.

Before sympathectomy became known, as it is today, the medical recommendations for hyperhidrosis were psychological treatment, coupled with the purchase of some manipulated or soothing creams, which had no positive impact on the cause

---

[1] Porto Alegre is in the south of Brazil, and is the capital of the State of Rio Grande do Sul.

of the disease, and other aberrations such as the use of electric current appliances that were promised to "numb" the problem. This lack of knowledge on the part of the professionals has led thousands of "sweaters" to uselessly expose their ills, spending money and losing hope with specialists who, if on the one hand helped them to solve fundamental questions related to their psyche, on the other hand did not lead them to correct ways to cure the disease. Many professionals from the most varied branches of medicine simply did not know that there was already a specific surgery to correct this malady. The result of this "mismatch" between what was available and what was being recommended in all fields of medicine generated countless exhausted and frustrated patients, and also sucked away their hopes of living in peace.

The excessive sweating that we are discussing here is known as primary hyperhidrosis, which is caused by something that is not yet well-known, but which, because of a "birth defect", causes some people to have a hyperactive sympathetic system. For those who do not know much about the subject, there is an important clarification: sweating too much because of menopause, diabetes, or extra caloric intake during a dinner has nothing to do with the hyperhidrosis we are talking about.

Interviews

"I have been suffering from palmar and plantar sweat since I was a child. Whenever I went to the doctors, they told me this was psychological. I have taken many remedies, but never got results". (B.J., 22 years)

Ø "My name is Caio, I'm from Petrópolis/RJ and I discovered that I have hyperhidrosis. I cannot live this way anymore, I have suffered from this evil since I've known people. I'm 19 years old today. I need help urgently, because I cannot be among friends anymore, for always being the subject of jokes. I'm already saturated with all this. I need to know how and where to treat myself. And also if there is another definitive exit without […] thoracic surgery, since I have undergone another surgery in my life and I was traumatized". (C.)

"Only those who suffer from the problem of hyperhidrosis know what it is. Imagine how I suffer, living in a city where it is horrible heat where, in the winter, I also sweat exaggerated even in an air conditioned environment! I am 24 years old and since adolescence my hands and feet are a river of sweat [laughs]".(C.)

Ø "The city where I lived—Tapiraí—is very cold, and here where I am living—Sorocaba—is very hot, so I transpire even more. My hands and feet are filled with bubbles that burst and peel. This is horrible. Where I study, everyone asks what I have. I only wear closed shoes in this heat. I lost a job because I went to the interview wearing sandals—worse bullshit I could have done! It was a job in my area—Administration—and my salary was better than I was getting. As I sat down, it seemed to form a river around my feet resting on the ground. My foot was dripping, my hands were slipping, I was nervous because I saw that everyone was watching, which made me even more nervous. The manager said he called me—but he did not, of course! It was God who made me watch you giving that program interview! I'm sorry for sending you emails, but as long as you do not heal me you're going to have to put up with me [laughs]". (C.)

Ø "I sweat a lot in my armpits, sometimes it drips. Most of the time I'm not nervous, not exercising or it's not a very hot day. I simply begin to perspire without making the slightest effort. It seems that on cold days it is worse. I'm really upset about this because in my school shirt is a 'pizza slice' [laughs]. I'm ashamed to raise my arm to do anything, even to touch my hair. Clinging, colored and baby-look blouses I love, but I do not use it because it soaks everything under my arm. I feel very distressed and ashamed, thinking that someone can see and find it disgusting. I take two to three baths a day, but it seems that I never feel 100% clean because, I barely got out of the bath and I'm already perspiring (ahh ... for me this is death!). It does not smell very strong, but just being perspiring bothers me too much. I wanted to know which doctor I could go to and what is the best treatment for this excessive sweating? I was very happy and relieved when I saw that I'm not the only one having this problem". (G.P.C., 17 years).

Ø I have suffered from hyperhidrosis since my adolescence, and today I am 23 years old. Only I did not know it was a disease! I always thought the cause was nervous and emotional—in fact, that's what everyone told me. I have sweat on my hands, feet and armpits. I have been a religious for two years and I have to live with this suffering, under a habit that stretches down to my feet. After looking for a doctor and getting to know his history, I would like to know how his recovery was, especially with regard to the feet that, as I understand it, do not stop sweating with the surgery. I am very hopeful to be free of all this". (A nun from Divinópolis/MG)

Ø "Since I live in a very hot place, it's terrible because I barely finish brushing my hair and I'm all wet, like I just got out of the shower". (C., from Cuiabá/MT)

Ø "Whenever someone greets me, comes that remark: 'you seem to be dead with these icy hands' or even those looks as if they were all disgusted with me". (K.M., 15 years)

Ø "I discovered your book when I worked in a bookstore, and a client bought a copy to send it to Japan. It was a find for me. Reading the testimonials I felt like a new person. I was never ashamed to say that my hands were sweating, until the funniest ones began to mock: 'Looks like you spit in the hand ... hahahahah!' They laughed at me, unaware of how annoyed I was. This mainly upsets my affective life, because I do not know how to get close, to caress someone with those wet, icy hands, looking like the hands of a corpse! And I also suffer from facial flushing—I do not need to feel such embarrassment for my face to become a pepper'. Pure social phobia. It is simply dreadful to have to present expository works. Nobody deserves! I'm finishing [studying] history, and I decided to consult after I read your entire book. I'm crazy to use Havaianas [laughs], go hand in hand (ah, what a dream!), drive a car ... I even have habilitation, but I do not drive. Here at home, they think it's incompetence, but it's because people do not understand the drama of driving with the wet steering wheel! If I marry one day, I wonder: I hope the groom does not have to dry my hands with a hair dryer when it's time to put the wedding ring on". (L.M.P., São José do Rio Preto)

Ø "I found your email looking for a solution to my problem and I saw that you had the same thing as me. Today, after the cure, you are another woman, a happier woman. I would love to heal myself. I'm sweating more every day—my problem is in my hands and feet. I'm about to lose my boyfriend because he complains that it's not safe in his hands". (R.S.S., Bahia)

Ø "My name is also Regina, I'm 23 years old, married and currently a housewife who lives in constant depression. I've been suffering a lot for a year now, always canceling myself out of shame for perspiring so much. I quit practically everything. I always wear black blouses to hide my sweating, but most of the time I just quit, especially when it's hot. I feel the greatest shame when I see my back all wet and my face sweating on spouts. I only have my husband as a friend and confidant, and I do not even have the courage to tell my family about my trauma". (R.A.B., Paraná)

Ø "I'm 19 years old and I've always been sweaty. To prove this story, I still keep with me sheets of drawings, which I did in college, completely wrinkled. I've tried all kinds of treatment, but none […] successfully. Today, I see that surgery is the only solution. My mother does not support me to do the surgery, thinking that all this is 'freshness'. Today, I found your site, www.suandoembicas.com.br, and I decided to write. I found the initiative very important. When I read the content, I was more confident of persisting…". (B.P.A. Amazonia)

Ø "I am a doctor specialized in dermatology and medicine and cosmetic surgery. Right now, I'm on my third postoperative day of axillary hyperhidrosis—an evil, an embarrassment, a burden that accompanied me right up to the age of thirty-one, just like your case, as you put it in your book, 'Suando em Bicas'. Exactly at 7:30 AM on August 27, 2007, I was in the operating room, anesthetized and intubated—it was time for my surgery and everything was within the plan, and by that time I was no longer awake or knowing what was going on. It was all ready for me to experience, after the surgery, what it would be like to live and feel free of hyperhidrosis, without further embarrassment. I could finally open my arms and not feel ashamed of myself for being sweaty, and would no longer have to wear coats or use other subterfuges to hide an evil that bothered me greatly. Here I am, telling my story to you, about how I got where I am, and to say that your book was a very important help for me to resolve to be cured of hyperhidrosis. I thank you for this wonderful job and you can be sure that it is already and will continue to help more and more people like you and me to have a better and better quality of life. You were a fighter, did not give up an ideal that was to be cured and this is a great step to seek more and more happiness and the quality of life that we want and deserve. Today, at this very moment when I write to you, I can tell you one thing: I made the right decision in my life. I'm very happy, I feel some pain still, of course, but this is normal. I am recovering very well, already doing some activities that require little of me, and wanting, more than anything, to return to 'work out'. But for that, I will still have to wait a little longer. I'm very happy with the result and, of course, I already bought colored shirts that I could not wear before and I think I even looked prettier [laughs]. I wanted to share with you, who did the same harm I did, my story summarized above, but with a great end in common that is success". (R.L.R.)

Ø "It's been about three years since I saw you on her show at Cultura Network and today I've had surgery for 18 days. I am very happy, Regina, because I have completely dried up! I perspired both in my feet and hands, back, legs and even belly—literally, I also lived 'sweating on spouts.' But, finally, I did: I did the surgery for the medical insurance that I own (and that I did not want to authorize, but I went after my rights…). I'm very happy, and thanks to that show I was watching. I always watched all programs directed to hyperhidrosis, but this one touched me a lot, especially because I saw that I was not alone. I had gone through several professionals and they had me look for psychologists or even psychiatrists, while others said I was 'weak'. Thank you so much for your words, it was they who encouraged me. Today I can say, too, that I was reborn 18 days ago". (M., 37 years old, two children, Franca/SP)

Ø "I did the surgery a year ago, the problem was solved, but I suffered for several months with the effects of compensatory sweating (I began to sweat in the feet, groin and back) that still persist, but reduced. Another very boring thing that happened is that my hands were completely dry and I had no perspiration problem on my hands. And now I depend on moisturizers to keep the hands minimally wet. With that, things get very easy out of my hands and I cannot open grocery bags, turning pages of books and magazines, for example, needing to moisten my fingers with water or saliva. This all bothers me a lot". (C., Santos/SP)

Ø "Two years ago, I underwent hyperhidrosis surgery because I was sweating a lot on my face. Today, I face a much bigger problem—I sweat exaggeratedly on the back and belly, compensating, I think … the part of the face today is totally dry, but I pour water from the breast down". (D.C.S.)

Ø "I need your help in resolving this drama that I am experiencing with compensatory hyperhidrosis. I did the surgery in 2003 and today I am desperate and I see no way out. When I operated I complained that the problem was palmar. In this region, I have no more embarrassment. But today I sweat heavily on the back and belly, wetting all my clothes, which makes me very frustrated and unhappy". (C.L.)

Ø "I live in Brasília, I'm 21 years old. For some time I have suffered from sweating under the armpits and hands. I did the bilateral thoracic sympathectomy surgery in March 2007; I read the testimonials published in his book, but what happened to me was the following:

Perspiration improved only on the right side. My hand and armpit on this side are really frosty, just the way I always wanted it. But the left side continues to present sweating, as before. The doctor said that maybe there was a very small nerve that he did not see at the time and scheduled a new surgery to correct that side. I am willing to do, therefore, despite what has happened, I still trust the doctor. I do not know whether by the desperation to improve the situation or by trusting him, in fact. But anyway. I am willing to be cured and he said that solves the problem with a new surgery. Have you seen something like that? What guidance do you give me, based on all your knowledge of the subject?"

Regina replies: I also have very uncomfortable compensatory sweating, especially since I returned to live in Porto Alegre, where summers are so hot and humid. I take a medicine based on oxybutynin hydrochloride (a recommendation from my surgeon, which greatly improves the picture). I also recommend physical exercise. I think I'm a lot better than if my hands were still dripping, something so restrictive for performing so many activities.

In addition to these statements that I selected with the intention of portraying the pre- and post-surgical life of some patients, I report here the recent experience of a friend from Porto Alegre. Surprisingly, for me, this hyperhidrosis patient had two surgeries performed on different occasions—one that corrected sweat in her hands (2005) and another in her feet (2010). Both were carried out with the authorization of her health plan, without any impediment, which is so different from my situation, in 2001, when everything was paid by me. In addition, she no longer has any symptoms, despite commenting that sometimes she still perspires a little on her legs, in the region below the knees, on really hot days. She considers the results a true success, having completely changed her life. Before the surgery, she lived with wet hands, in summer or winter, and faced dramas in her daily life such as typing on a computer keyboard, driving, and even in getting along with people because of the anguish and embarrassment brought about by sweating. Sheets of paper always got wet. Inside the house she was always in socks, just as she was in the street, in midsummer. The soaked feet in her closed shoes produced a characteristic noise that made her embarrassed, but at least she could walk more comfortably and safely. Just like me.

Seeking the Right Answer: The Importance of Correct Diagnosis

To help patients with hyperhidrosis quickly and surely rid themselves of the agony of constant sweating, there are now more than 500 doctors in Brazil—thoracic and vascular surgeons—who make use of the technique known worldwide: cervicothoracic bilateral sympathectomy for the correction of excessive hyperhidrosis of the feet, hands, armpits, and/or head. Through it, defective nerve endings are resected which, for unknown reasons, send excess stimuli to the sweat glands, producing an unbelievable downpour to the extremities that exceeds the capacity of gloves and shoes in more serious cases of the disease. It is the only definitive way to fix this disease that affects between 1% and 2.4% of the world's population.

Surgery is very effective for hand sweating, and it also helps reduce foot symptoms by up to 70%. Specific foot surgery has been studied in more depth in recent years, as it is known that it can increase compensatory sweating in patients with this predisposition.

Worldwide, the technique correcting primary hyperhidrosis is most frequently performed in China, Israel, England, Spain, and France, as well as Brazil, which is among the most advanced in this area. In Italy and Germany there are a few centers dedicated to the subject.

Over the years, for the sake of those suffering from hyperhidrosis and with the growing interest of the media and patients seeking information about surgery, more professionals have specialized in the technique. The number of specialists in Brazil jumped from three or four pioneers in the 1990s to more than 500 today (2017). Nowadays, there is a great chance that a patient can be treated in his own city, or a nearby center, which is always recommended. After all, in larger centers, there is usually a waiting list in public hospitals. In one of the largest reference centers for surgery in Latin America—Hospital das Clínicas, in São Paulo—the number of patients awaiting this procedure increased by 200% in the first years of surgery, generating an agonizing waiting time of up to 3 years, a situation that has now normalized, with the time between the consultation, preoperative examinations, and surgery taking no more than 2 months. Health plans also now authorize the procedure without major problems.

To facilitate access to information, it should be noted that the complete list of Brazilian specialists in sympathectomy is on the website of the Brazilian Society of Thoracic Surgery (www.sbct.org.br) and the Brazilian Society of Angiology and Vascular Surgery (www.sbacv-nac.org.br). It is fundamental to seek the assistance of one of these two professionals so that the surgery takes place as successfully as possible, since these are the specialists in the diagnosis and surgical recommendations for the correction of hyperhidrosis.

Part II

General Treatment of Hyperhidrosis

Pharmacological Treatment of Hyperhidrosis

12

Dafne Braga Diamante Leiderman, Samantha Neves, and Nelson Wolosker

Introduction

In the last decade, many papers addressing safe and effective hyperhidrosis treatment techniques have been published. Treatments have long been known, from the soaking of hands in tea so that the astringent tannin present in the infusion would decrease sweating for palmar hyperhidrosis to burying the hands or feet in sand to dry them or using atropine-based elixirs, in which the use of anticholinesterases has already shown action.

The non-surgical arsenal used in the treatment of hyperhidrosis currently includes topical drugs, oral medications, iontophoresis, and botulinum toxin.

Topical Use Drugs

Topical agents such as aluminum chloride salts or aluminum hydroxide chloride have been used in the treatment of hyperhidrosis due to their effectiveness, safety, low price, and easy application. Concentrations range from 15% to 35%.

D. B. D. Leiderman
Department of Vascular and Endovascular Surgery, Hospital Israelita Albert Einstein, São Paulo, SP, Brazil

S. Neves (✉)
Brazilian Society of Dermatology, São Paulo, SP, Brazil

School of Medicine, ABC, Santo Andre, São Paulo, SP, Brazil
e-mail: samantha@samanthaneves.com.br

N. Wolosker
Department of Vascular and Endovascular Surgery, Hospital Israelita Albert Einstein, São Paulo, SP, Brazil

Several vehicles are used in an attempt to minimize adverse effects, such as skin irritation and aluminum toxicity, especially in formulations of high concentrations, when systemic absorption occurs. The action of aluminum salts is due to the reaction with mucopolysaccharides and precipitation in the glandular ducts, blocking them and promoting atrophy and glandular vacuolization.

Other drugs can be used in the topical treatment of hyperhidrosis, but with little effectiveness or many adverse effects. Topical anticholinergic agents such as scopolamine, propantheline, defemanyl, methasulfite, atropine sulfate, and glycopyrrolate have been used, and theoretically would be less toxic than the same drugs used orally due to the lower risk of systemic intoxication. What happens, however, is that, as a rule, they do not reach the concentration necessary for local action. Aldehydes of topical use, such as formaldehyde and glutaraldehyde, have limited therapeutic application as they can cause sensitization and localized skin irritation.

Drugs for Oral and Systemic Use

Oral Anticholinergics

As with topical use, many systemic use medications have limited utility, either because of inadequate efficacy or the systemic toxicity it triggers. Anticholinergics are widely used and allow treatment of generalized forms. The most commonly used anticholinergics are glycopyrrolate, oxybutynin, and propantheline. Their therapeutic effect is due to the competitive blockade of the muscarinic receptors in the neuroglandular junction, thus blocking sweat production.

Oxybutynin

The specific use of oxybutynin for the treatment of hyperhidrosis was first performed at Hospital das Clinicas—School of Medicine—University of São Paulo in 2009, and since then several articles have been published in this regard. It has been observed in daily practice that treatment with lower doses of oxybutynin (<10 mg daily) has fewer adverse effects, and is effective in the treatment of hyperhidrosis in its different presentation sites.

Treatment is initiated with low doses of oxybutynin (2.5 mg/day) and progressively increased up to 10 mg daily. This protocol is used because patients with urinary disorders initiate their treatment with doses of 5 mg every 12 h and have a high incidence of dry mouth and headache at the beginning of medication use. This discomfort may lead some patients to abandon treatment. The use of low doses and their progressive increase decreases the occurrence of symptoms.

Oxybutynin has proved to be effective and safe in the treatment of patients with hyperhidrosis, regardless of sex, age, patient weight, and symptom localization.

The use of oxybutynin in the treatment of hyperhidrosis has revolutionized the treatment of the disease. With the "first pharmacological" treatment protocol instituted for patients with hyperhidrosis, some improvement in symptoms was reported in more than 98% of patients after 6 weeks of treatment, and the improvement was moderate or significant in palmar hyperhidrosis in 90.2% of patients on regular medication for at least 6 months. Patients with a body mass index <25 tend to have better treatment outcomes. Similar results were observed for moderate to significant improvement of axillary (82.9%), plantar (84.7%), and facial (94%) hyperhidrosis. Studies have also shown improvement in 89–94% of hyperhidrosis in other associated sites, where the complaint of excessive sweating was secondary.

The most common adverse effects are dry mouth (more than 80% complain of at least mild dry mouth), headache, and drowsiness. Other less frequent effects are blurred vision, hyperthermia, orthostatic hypotension, urinary retention, constipation, tachycardia, and palpitations. Only about 2% of patients undergoing long-term treatment for hyperhidrosis developed such serious adverse effects that oxybutynin treatment was discontinued, but no major adverse effects, such as constipation or bowel obstruction, were reported.

Absolute contraindications to oxybutynin treatment include myasthenia gravis, paralytic ileus, and pylorus stenosis. Relative contraindications are angle-closure glaucoma, urinary obstruction, gastro-esophageal reflux, and heart failure.

Glycopyrrolate

Glycopyrrolate is an approved medication for reduction of gastric secretion, used in preoperative of gastric surgeries, treatment of peptic ulcer, and decrease of excessive oral secretion. The use of this drug to treat hyperhidrosis started in 2007 and it is most commonly used in Europe and Asia, with studies reporting significant improvement in 75–79% of patients with a dose of 2–8 mg/day, with adverse effects in 36–42%, dry mouth being the main one, but without the need to discontinue the use of the medication because of these effects. There are also studies with use in children aged 9–18 years, with satisfactory response in 90% of the cases, and in cases of compensatory sweating.

Glycopyrrolate is contraindicated in cases of myasthenia gravis, pyloric stenosis, and paralytic ileus.

Other Drugs

Other classes of drugs also appear to be used in the treatment of hyperhidrosis, such as benzodiazepines, amitriptyline, gabapentin, paroxetine, clonidine, indomethacin, calcium channel blockers, and β-blockers. Benzodiazepines treat hyperhidrosis triggered by emotional causes. Paroxetine acts by an intrinsic cholinergic action or by an anxiolytic effect through central mechanisms. Clonidine is indicated in the craniofacial and generalized forms. Indomethacin acts in a generalized way by inhibiting the formation of prostaglandin E2 that has been shown to reduce hyperhidrosis in in vitro studies. Calcium channel blockers act on the primary form through the inhibition of calcium-mediated acetylcholine secretion.

Iontophoresis

Introduced for the treatment of hyperhidrosis in 1952, iontophoresis is now regarded as the first-line treatment by the US Food and Drug Administration (FDA) due to the efficacy and safety it presents. Its action derives from the passage of an electric current in water through intact skin, and is especially indicated in the focal forms in areas that can be submerged in the containers containing the liquid; thus, the axillary form is difficult to treat using this method. The mechanism is uncertain, but it seems that the electrical current prevents the action of the sweat gland, perhaps by inducing hyperkeratosis of the pores of these glands and acting as horny buffers in the eccrine sweat glands, interrupting the ionic channels in the secretory glomerulus and obstructing them. It is assumed that there is a possible derangement of the glandular electrochemical gradient. The therapeutic success of iontophoresis depends on the current intensity applied. Sessions of 20–30 min, three to four times a week, with currents of 15–20 mA are considered effective. With the improvement of sweating, treatment is performed once a week and then once every 2 weeks, and maintenance treatment is performed at intervals of 1–4 weeks. Anhydrosis is usually achieved after 6–15 sessions. Currents of 20–25 mA or 0.2 mA/cm^2 are well-tolerated by intact skin. Initially, distilled water is used, but dilutions containing anticholinergics may also be used as an alternative. Children need a lower maximum dose to achieve the therapeutic effect.

Adverse effects are usually mild and include skin irritation, dry and scaly extremities, vesicles at the treated site, erythema and burning, signs and symptoms that add up or decrease with cessation of treatment, use of emollients, or administration of topical corticosteroids. Iontophoresis is contraindicated in pregnant women, patients with pacemakers or metallic implants (metallic orthopedic prostheses and intrauterine devices), heart patients, and epileptics. If combination therapy of iontophoresis with baths containing anticholinergic agents such as glycopyrrolate is being used in order to increase therapeutic efficacy, contraindications to these drugs should also be remembered.

Botulinum Toxin

Taken as an intermediate therapy between conservative measures and surgery, the use of botulinum toxin was approved by the FDA in 2004. Originally produced by *Clostridium botulinum*, it has seven forms, serotypes A–F. Serotype A is more widely used in the treatment of hyperhidrosis. The therapeutic effect is temporary and treatment should be repeated at regular intervals.

As in hyperhidrosis there seems to be hyperstimulation of the eccrine sweat glands, some authors suggest that blocking neurotransmission would be the ideal way to treat the disease. The effect of botulinum toxin A therapy on the treatment of hyperhidrosis lasts on average from 8 to 9 months.

The maximum recommended dose of botulinum toxin A at each administration is 300–400 U and no more than 400 U should be administered every 4 months. In axillary hyperhidrosis, the dose of botulinum toxin A is 1 U/cm^2, in a total of 50–100 U per axilla. In palmar hyperhidrosis, the dose is 1.5–2 U/cm^2, with a total maximum dose of 100–150 U. In the treatment of plantar hyperhidrosis the suggested doses are 2–3 U every 2 cm, with a maximum dose of 250 U per foot. In facial hyperhidrosis the recommended dose is 1 U/cm^2, with a maximum dose of 100 U. As a rule, the higher the dose used, the more pronounced the therapeutic effect is. Clinical response is expected 2–4 days after initiation of treatment and should be complete after 2 weeks.

Adverse effects are rare, but are reported to be transient muscle weakness, pain, local burning, headache, dry mouth, and impaired visual accommodation. In addition to these, loss of effect may occur due to the formation of new synapses, requiring applications at smaller intervals and with a greater quantity of product. There are reports of compensatory hyperhidrosis post-application of botulinum toxin, but its incidence has not been quantified.

Contraindications range from vehicle allergy (albumin), neuromuscular diseases such as myasthenia gravis, pregnancy, lactation, organic causes of hyperhidrosis, infection at the site of application, and use of medications that interfere with neuromuscular transmission such as aminoglycosides, penicillin, quinine, and calcium channel blockers.

Conclusion

Clinical treatment with topical agents, botulinum toxin, and iontophoresis has demonstrated limited efficacy. Surgical treatment, once considered the gold standard for the treatment of hyperhidrosis, despite a low risk and high success rate, has as a drawback in the occurrence of compensatory hyperhidrosis, which is frequently of variable intensity and not predicted in the preoperative period. The use of oxybutynin has revolutionized the treatment and quality of life of these patients, and is a solution for many patients with compensatory hyperhidrosis.

Suggested Reading

Campanati A, Penna L, Guzzo T, et al. Quality-of-life assessment in patients with hyperhidrosis before and after treatment with botulinum toxin: results of an open-label study. Clin Ther. 2003;25(1):298–308.

Eisenach JH, Atkinson JLD, Fealey RD. Hyperhidrosis: evolving therapies for a well-established phenomenon. Mayo Clin Proc. 2005;80(5):657–66.

Ram R, Lowe NJ, Yamauchi PS. Current and emerging therapeutic modalities for hyperhidrosis, part 1: conservative and noninvasive treatments. Cutis. 2007;79(3):211–7.

Reisfeld R, Berliner KI. Evidence-based review of the nonsurgical management of hyperhidrosis. Thorac Surg Clin. 2008;18(2):157–66.

Solish N, Bertucci V, Dansereau A, et al. Comprehensive approach to the recognition, diagnosis, and severity-based treatment of focal hyperhidrosis: recommendations of the Canadian Hyperhidrosis Advisory Committee. Dermatol Surg. 2007;33(8):908–23.

Wolosker N, de Campos JRM, Kauffman P, Puech-Leão P. A randomized placebo-controlled trial of oxybutynin for the initial treatment of palmar and axillary hyperhidrosis. J Vasc Surg. 2012;55(6):1696–700.

Wolosker N, Teivelis MP, Krutman M, et al. Long-term results of oxybutynin treatment for palmar hyperhidrosis. Clin Auton Res. *2014*;24(6):297–303.

Wolosker N, Teivelis MP, Krutman M, de Paula RP, Kauffman P, de Campos JRM, et al. Long-term results of the use of oxybutynin for the treatment of axillary hyperhidrosis. Ann Vasc Surg. 2014;28(5):1106–12.

Wolosker N, Teivelis MP, Krutman M, et al. Long-term results of oxybutynin use in treating facial hyperhidrosis. An Bras Dermatol. 2014;89(6):912–6.

Wolosker N, Teivelis MP, Krutman M, et al. Long-term results of the use of oxybutynin for the treatment of plantar hyperhidrosis. Int J Dermatol. 2015;54(5):605–11.

Hyperidrosis and Topical Agents

Marcia Purcelli

Introduction

Several dermatological diseases are perceived by those who have them as disgusting, even when they are not contagious. Like the obese, the patient with excessive sweating or hyperhidrosis is perceived by those around him as being guilty of causing their condition:

- "He is very nervous and so does not stop sweating."
- "She does not care, she's fat, so she sweats too much."
- "He is smelly, he does not take a shower."
- "She is rude because she does not perform proper foot hygiene."

Hyperhidrosis sufferers, in turn, feel this constant judgment and their self-esteem is seriously affected. It is common to find patients with hyperhidrosis who have drastically changed their lives because of this condition. This critical situation is easier to understand when we know some phrases of hyperhidrosis obtained in surveys undertaken by consumer services departments of the manufacturers of antiperspirants:

"I just have a dream. Only one. One day I could wear a silk sweater."

"I did not invite anyone to my wedding, I did not get married in the church and there was no party."

"I did not want to be seen on the altar sweating without stopping."

"My dream was to be a dentist like my father. I cannot be a dentist and have palmar hyperhidrosis."

"My boyfriend told me, you stink."

"My boss said, you have to stay hidden from customers. You cannot greet anyone shaking hands."

M. Purcelli
Hospital Israelita Albert Einstein, São Paulo, SP, Brazil

Hyperhidrosis

Hyperhidrosis is a hidrosis, that is a disease of, the eccrine or apocrine sweat glands.
General aspects of the sweat glands.

Eccrine Glands

The eccrine glands and the eccrine bud of the epidermis are found all over the skin, except in the labial mucosa, nail bed, small vulval lips, in the glans, and inner face of the foreskin. They are found in greater numbers and are more developed in the palmar, plantar, and axillary regions (Fig. 13.1).

Eccrine glands are tubular glands, which have a secretory folded part and a duct that, coming out of the dermis, crosses the epidermis (acrosiringium) and opens directly on the surface of the skin. This hole is invisible except on the palms and soles of the feet where they can be recognized with a magnifying glass. The eccrine glands are innervated by cholinergic sympathetic fibers and secrete a variable amount of sweat after exogenous stimuli, such as the heat of the environment, or endogenously by metabolic changes.

The secretions of the eccrine glands are also affected by emotional factors or neurological injuries. Depending on the intensity of the stimuli, the secretion can be localized only in the palmoplantar and/or axillary or generalized regions. In the secretory phase, the glandular cells do not alter their shape and size, the secretion is almost immediate after the stimulus, and takes between 10 and 30 s from the secretory part to the sweat pore. If there is stimulation, it can have several hours of continuous activity. A high-intensity heat stimulus, such as exercise, can produce up to 3 L of sweat per hour.

Sweat

Sweat is a clear, odorless liquid that is 99.5% water. The main components are sodium, potassium, calcium, magnesium, chloride, urea, and lactate. Traces of amino acids, immunoglobulins, prostaglandins, vitamins, and systemically administered drugs can be found.

Secretory Function

The secretory function of the eccrine glands does not replace renal function, even partially. The primordial function of the eccrine glands is thermoregulation, that is, to maintain, through sweating, the temperature of the body.

13 Hyperidrosis and Topical Agents

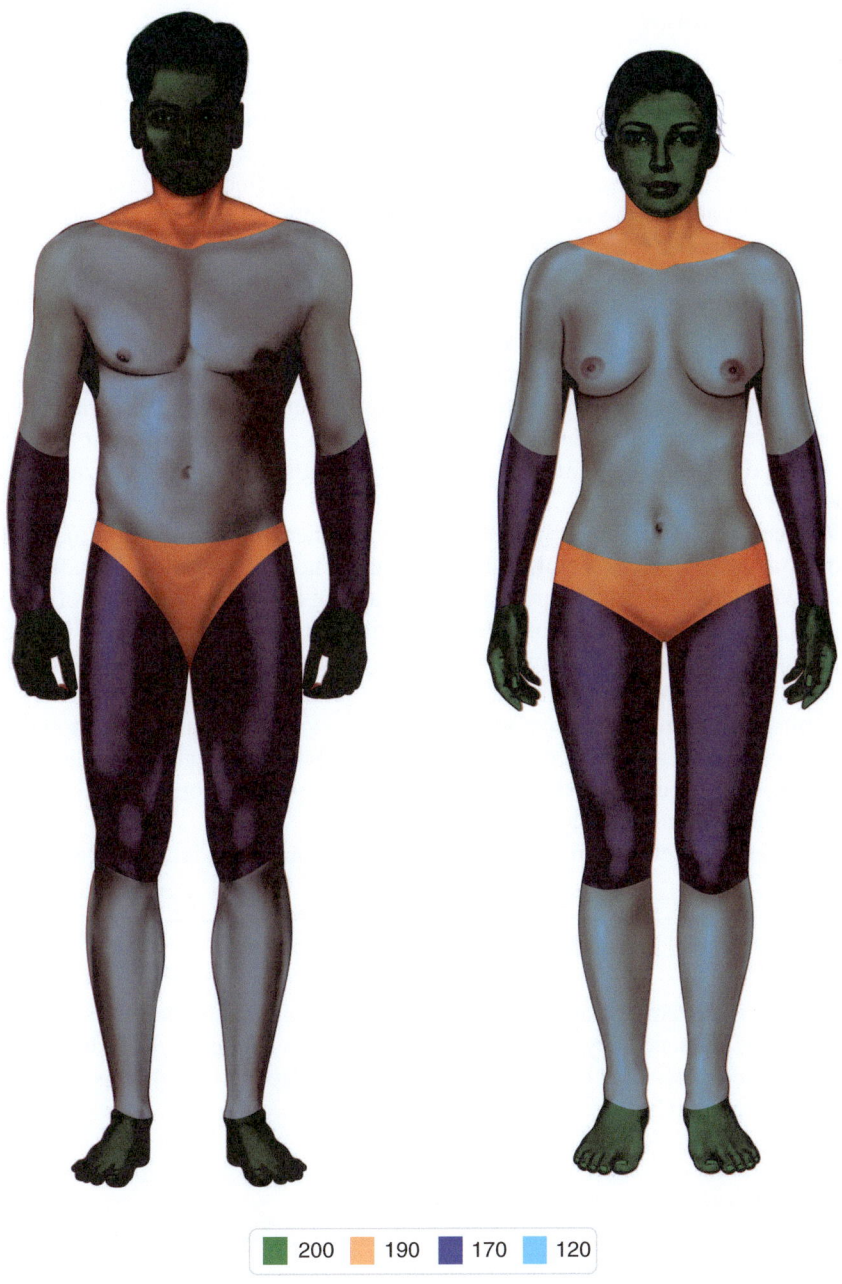

Fig. 13.1 Concentration of the eccrine glands according to the region of the skin considered

Apocrine Glands

The apocrine glands originate from the primary epithelial bud together with the sebaceous glands and hairs. They differ from the eccrine glands, not only by embryogenesis but also in function, distribution, size, and type of secretion.

While the eccrine glands are indispensable for thermoregulation, the apocrine glands have an odorous function, which is not important for humans but is important for sexual behavior in animals.

The apocrine glands are found in the armpits, mammary region, sternal, periumbilical, pubic and anogenital regions, and exceptionally in the trunk and scalp. The ceruminous glands of the auditory channels, the Moll glands of the eyelids, and the mammary glands are modified apocrine glands. They are located in the reticular dermis and are on average ten times larger than the eccrine glands. The excretory canal opens into the infundibulum, near the follicular orifice. In puberty, due to hormonal influence, the apocrine glands increase in size and initiate their secretion.

Innervation of the apocrine glands is sympathetic, with secretion induced by alpha and beta fibers being adrenergic and cholinergic. After stimulation, a yellowish-white viscous liquid containing varying amounts of cholesterol, triglycerides, fatty acids, cholesterol esters, and squalene is produced. Traces of ammonia, carbohydrates, and hormones such as dehydroepiandrosterone and androsterone can be found. The secretion, initially sterile and odorless, mainly occurs in the armpits. This secretion is decomposed by microorganisms, mainly Corynobacteria, which causes the appearance of odor. The odor is sui-generis and individually variable. It can be distinguished between continuous secretion from hormone or nervous/emotional stimulation.

Apocrine secretion diminishes with age, but it can persist into old age.

Eccrine Gland Disorders

Sweating is extremely variable from individual to individual, depends on age and race, and is influenced by endogenous and exogenous factors. Hyperhidrosis can be generalized or localized in some regions. Currently, neural hyperhidrosis is considered to be caused by:

- Stimuli of the cortex (cortical hyperhidrosis) due to the presence of hyperhidrosis.
- Stimuli that reach the hypothalamus (hypothalamic hyperhidrosis).
- Lesions in the central or peripheral nervous system, or from the sweat glands themselves and non-neural hyperhidroses.
- Hyperhidroses due to genetic alterations of the eccrine secretion.

Hyperhidroses of Neural or Non-neural Origin

Hyperhidrosis can be neural or non-neural in origin.

Hyperhidrosis of neural origin can be cortical, hypothalamic, gustatory, or caused by injuries to the spinal cord, trunk, and nerve fibers or reflexes. Non-neural hyperhidroses result from the action of heat on the skin, the action of drugs, altered bloodflow, or changes in the sweat glands themselves. Cortical or emotional hyperhidrosis is a more generalized hyperhidrosis in certain areas such as axillary, palmoplantar regions, and perineum-inguinal, and may eventually be a localized form.

It is frequently suggested that at least some cases of hyperhidrosis arise from autosomal dominant inheritance and therefore familial cases exist. The sweat glands are normal and there is no change in cholinesterase. It is assumed that specific nucleus impulses located in the cortex are processed by the hypothalamus from where they are led by the nerve pathways to the sympathetic fibers of the sweat glands, producing release of excessive amounts of acetylcholine with consequent increase in sweating. In fact, cortical hyperhidrosis improves during sleep, which would be explained by the diminution of the nerve impulses.

Generalized cortical hyperhidrosis occurs most often in the richer regions of the sweat glands, such as the scalp, forehead, groin, armpit, plantar region, and palms. In addition, it does not change in warmer environments, demonstrating no influence of thermally sensitive stimuli. When it occurs on the scalp and forehead it is unpleasant but usually does not bring secondary complications. In the groin area, it facilitates the installation of intertriginous eruptions, such as candidiasis or dermatophytosis (mycosis or tinea).

Axillary and palmo-plantar hyperhidrosis are the forms that cause major problems as they can alter the individual's quality of life, hamper work, and alter the psychosocial behavior of the individual. Plantar hyperhidrosis, usually of early onset, may facilitate the onset of fungal infections and a grooved plantar hyperkeratosis.

Axillary hyperhidrosis begins after puberty. There is a racial variation according to the development of the sweat glands. It is constant and naturally intensifies with emotional factors, heat, and exercise. Axillary hyperhidrosis may be the patient's main complaint, although 25% of cases also have discrete palmoplantar hyperhidrosis. Axillary hyperhidrosis, unlike palmoplantar hyperhidrosis, responds variably to thermal stimuli. It is to be noted that the apocrine glands are innervated by adrenergic fibers, unlike the eccrines, which are stimulated by cholinergic fibers.

Axillary hyperhidrosis may favor the appearance of pyogenic infections, erythrasma, candidiasis, and contact dermatitis caused by products used to reduce it.

Treatment

In cortical hyperhidrosis, the patient should be informed about the influence of emotional factors, possibly prescribing tranquilizers such as diazepines.

Anticholinergic drugs can be used to provide relief. For plantar hyperhidrosis, it is necessary to wear cotton socks whenever possible, and leather-soled shoes, preferably a sandal type. Closed shoes with no openings would worsen the problem because they prevent air circulation. The leather sole absorbs the moisture. When bacterial or fungal secondary infections occur, specific treatments are indicated.

Hypothalamic or Thermal Hyperhidrosis

Hypothalamic or thermal hyperhidrosis is caused by stimulation of the hypothalamic temperature-regulating centers that may possibly present an increased sensitivity. In this way, minimal stimulation can trigger intense hyperhidrosis. The main source of stimulation of the hypothalamus is an increase in temperature due to exogenous (heat) or endogenous causes: exercise and diseases that cause a temperature rise, infections, particularly tuberculosis, malaria, brucellosis, and lymphomas. In addition, a large number of conditions can cause hypothalamic hyperhidrosis, including metabolic changes (hyperpituitarism, hyperthyroidism), diabetes mellitus, gout, obesity, pregnancy, menopause, hypoglycemia, porphyrias, alcoholism. In diabetes, hyperhidrosis may occur in episodes of hypoglycemia.

Hypothalamic hyperhidrosis can be caused by the following drugs: antipyretics, non-hormonal anti-inflammatory drugs (acetylsalicylic acid, indomethacin, piroxicam, sulindac, naproxen), anticholinergics (acetylcholine, fisiostigmine, pilocarpine, methacholine), adrenergics (epinephrine, norepinephrine, dopamine, isoproterenol), drugs acting on the central nervous system (amitriptyline, amphetamine, caffeine, chlorpromazine, doxepin, phenothiazine, fluoxetine, haloperidol, yohimbine, nortriptyline), paroxic toxic substances for chronic arsenicism, and illicit drugs.

It should be noted that hypothalamic hyperhidrosis does not diminish during sleep and may become even more intense.

Treatment of hypothalamic hyperhidrosis is symptomatic or oriented towards correcting its cause.

Topical Treatment

It should be noted that while there is no definitive topical treatment, there are control treatments for hyperhidrosis, such as antiperspirants and deodorants that are widely used in the armpits for most of the population.

Antiperspirants are used to control sweating; they reduce sweating and therefore alter local bacterial growth.

Deodorants are made to fight the bad odor generated by the bacteria present in the microbiome. They basically contain antibacterial and fragrance aspects. Deodorants with potent antiperspirant properties can significantly improve the quality of life of millions of people worldwide.

Focal hyperhidrosis affects 2% of the population worldwide and only 40% of these people seek medical attention for treatment. The use of aluminum and its derivatives as an antiperspirant is already advised by the majority of dermatologists.

Aluminum chloride was the first antiperspirant active ingredient used with good efficacy. However, it has the drawback of causing skin irritation, blemishes, and tissue damage due to the pH of the aqueous solutions of this substance.

Aluminum hydrochloride has thus emerged to minimize the drawbacks of aluminum chloride. Their solutions have a pH closer to that of the skin and cause less damage to the tissues. The mechanism of action of the antiperspirants is the diffusion of the salt by the sweat duct which, after slow neutralization of the acidic solution of metallic salt, produces a gel or mucopolysaccharide complex. This obstruction prevents sweat from escaping and remains until the normal processes of cell renewal replace the affected keratin. There is no evidence of permanent damage to sweat glands, especially since normal sweating resumes immediately after discontinuation of the product.

Adverse Effects

Occasionally, the daily use of antiperspirants can irritate the skin, causing a burning sensation. The onset of irritation may occur immediately or after days or weeks of use. However, the cure begins to be observed within 3 days after the total withdrawal of the irritant.

Antiperspirants and Breast Cancer

Antiperspirants are products that inhibit or decrease perspiration. The difference between a deodorant and antiperspirant is that the former serves to remove the odor of the armpits, while the latter is responsible for reducing the amount of sweat produced. Most of the antiperspirants also work as deodorants, but most deodorants do not act as antiperspirants.

According to a technical opinion published by ANVISA (the Brazilian National Agency of Sanitary Surveillance), there no significant data in the scientific literature to date relating the aluminum salts present in antiperspirant formulae with the incidence of breast cancer.

Suggested Reading

Wolosker N, Fukuda JM. Editorial—current treatment of hyperhidrosis. J Vasc Bras. 2015;14(4): 279–81.

Axillary Hyperhidrosis and Bromhidrosis: The Dermatologist's Point of View

Roberta Vasconcelos and José Antonio Sanches Jr.

Axillary Hyperhidrosis

Introduction

Recent studies have shown that 2.8% of the US population has symptoms of hyperhidrosis, about 50.8% of whom have axillary hyperhidrosis. The mean age of patients with this condition is 40 years.

Physiopathology

Sweat is produced and excreted by the eccrine glands. There is no difference in the number or distribution of eccrine glands between patients with hyperhidrosis and normal individuals. However, patients with hyperhidrosis have a greater activity of the glands. There is probably deregulation involving the sympathetic and parasympathetic systems.

There is a genetic component in hyperhidrosis. Studies have shown that 65% of patients reported a family history of the disease. A genetic analysis showed that chromosome 14q is possibly associated with hyperhidrosis.

R. Vasconcelos
Department of Dermatology, São Paulo Cancer Institute—ICESP, São Paulo, SP, Brazil

J. A. Sanches Jr., MD, PhD (✉)
Department of Dermatology, School of Medicine, University of São Paulo, São Paulo, SP, Brazil

Clinical Presentation

The onset of hyperhidrosis usually occurs during puberty, after the inset of the axillary hairs. The affected area usually exceeds the haired area.

Sweating generally does not occur during sleep, and it worsens when the patient wakes up. Factors such as emotional stress, exercise, and high external temperature may worsen the condition, but are not necessary for it to occur.

The patient often reports impairment in quality of life and withdrawal from some activities that increase sweating. In addition, there may be a need to choose certain clothing colors and fabrics and several changes of clothing per day may be required to mask the condition.

To delimit the area with hyperhidrosis and verify the response after the treatments, a test with iodine and starch can be performed. After cleaning and drying the armpits, a layer of iodine (e.g., iodopovidone) is applied. After a few minutes, corn starch is sprinkled on the iodine. When there is moisture, in this case caused by sweat, the starch and the iodine are mixed and a bluish/purplish color is produced, delimiting the hyperhidrosis area (Fig. 14.1).

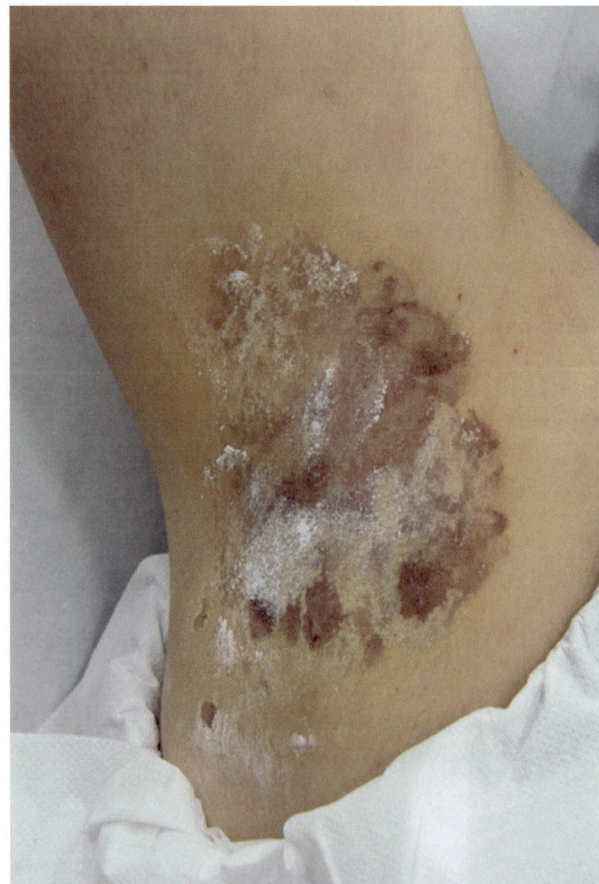

Fig. 14.1 Starch and iodine test. The purplish area is formed by the reaction of iodine with starch in a moist area, and delimits the hyperhidrosis in the axilla

Treatment

This chapter addresses the non-surgical treatment options for hyperhidrosis.

Classic Treatments

Topical Treatments
Antiperspirants with aluminum salts are considered the first line of treatment for hyperhidrosis. They occlude the distal ducts of the eccrine glands. Long-term blockade of the glands leads to functional and structural degeneration of the acini, reducing the production of sweat.

There are studies with aluminum chloride concentrations ranging from 12.5% to 30%, with satisfactory results. The formulation should be applied on dry skin at night. Common adverse effects include miliaria and local irritation.

Topical glycopyrrolate 2% is an anticholinergic drug that can be used locally to control axillary hyperhidrosis, although it is less effective for facial hyperhidrosis. It should be used twice a day.

Injectable Treatments
Botulinum toxin is an inhibitor of acetylcholine release. Two types of botulinum toxin were extensively tested for axillary hyperhidrosis: onabotulinumtoxin A (Botox®; Allergan) and abobotulinumtoxin A (Dysport®; Ipsen). There was no difference in efficacy between the two toxins if equipotent doses were used (3 U of abobotulinumtoxin A to 1 U of onabotulinumtoxin A).

The use of 50–100 U of onabotulinumtoxin A or equivalent in abobotulinumtoxin A is recommended in each axilla.

To minimize pain, anesthetic creams and local methods may be used, such as application of ice packs and vibration.

The application of botulinum toxin requires multiple injections, with 1–2 cm between them. The toxin vial is diluted in 2 mL of 0.9% saline solution and 2 U injected per point. To guide the area to be treated, the iodine and starch test, described previously, can be utilized.

The median duration of the antiperspirant effect of the toxin is 7.6 months. There is evidence that frequent applications increase the duration of effect between applications.

Complications associated with the procedure are rare. Tingling and pain on the treated area are the most frequent symptoms. There are reports of fatigue after the sessions and increased sweating in other areas.

Systemic Treatments
Oral anticholinergics are a potential treatment for hyperhidrosis. However, their use is restricted due to frequent adverse effects, which include dry mouth, dry eyes, and gastrointestinal symptoms.

Drugs that have more published studies relating to hyperhidrosis are glycopyrrolate and oxybutynin. Glycopyrrolate showed a response rate of 67% in adults and oxybutynin had a response rate of 70%. Bornaprine is another anticholinergic that has already been tested, but its use has been limited by its adverse effects in the central nervous system.

Other classes of medications have been used in axillary hyperhidrosis, such as β-blockers, benzodiazepines, and clonidine. However, efficacy data for these drugs are limited.

Emerging Therapies

Topical Treatments
The 3% oxybutynin gel is approved in the USA for treatment of overactive bladder. The effect of topical oxybutynin in the treatment of hyperhidrosis is currently being studied.

Botulinum toxin for transdermal application is being developed for the treatment of hyperhidrosis by the company Transdermalcorp. This formulation aims to eliminate the discomfort caused by toxin injections.

New Technologies
Microwave energy thermolysis can potentially reduce sweating permanently. In this procedure, eccrine and apocrine glands are destroyed by heat waves. The device currently marketed is MiraDry® (Miramar Labs, Inc., Sunnyvalle, CA, USA) and is approved by ANVISA (the Brazilian National Agency for Sanitary Surveillance) and the US Food and Drug Administration (FDA). In microwave energy thermolysis an injectable anesthetic is applied locally to decrease pain. Two applications are performed, with an interval of 3 months. The most common adverse effects are erythema, edema, pain, and ecchymosis, which can last for a few days after application. Sensitization may also occur in the treated area, lasting for up to 5 weeks. A rare complication is brachial plexus damage. Studies show a significant reduction of sweating for up to 2 years after treatment.

Radiofrequency applied with micro-needles in the dermis is a treatment that has demonstrated clinical reduction of sweating and histological decrease in the number of eccrine glands.

Dermatological lasers with different wavelengths have been tested in the treatment of hyperhidrosis: Nd-YAG (neodymium-doped yttrium aluminum garnet) 1064 nm, 1320 nm, 1440 nm, diode 924 nm, 975 nm, and 800 nm long pulse. Nd-YAG lasers have been tested in a limited number of cases, and the length of 1064 nm associated with surgical suction of the eccrine glands showed reduction of sweating in treated cases. For diode lasers, the combination of 924 and 975 nm lengths in the same session associated with surgical curettage showed a significant reduction in sweating. There was no significant effect for the 800 nm length.

Microfocused ultrasound has been investigated for the treatment of axillary hyperhidrosis. The equipment with the highest number of studies is called Ulthera® (Ulhtera Incorporated, Mesa, AZ, USA), and is already approved by the FDA and ANVISA for improvement of skin flaccidity. Ultrasound energy is applied to

4.5 mm of the skin surface in two treatments with a 30-day interval and clinical response was noted in about 50% of the treated patients.

Bromhidrosis

Introduction

Bromhidrosis is a clinical condition in which there is excessive and persistent nasty body odor. All sweat glands may be involved. The condition is more common in men after puberty, reflecting the maturation of the apocrine glands, but it can occur in any age group, including childhood.

Physiopathology

Bromhidrosis occurs as a result of increased secretion by the sweat glands associated with local bacterial proliferation. It is aggravated by poor hygiene and clinical situations that favor the proliferation of bacteria, such as diabetes mellitus, intertrigo, erythrasma, and obesity.

Several factors can affect the secretion of the eccrine glands, causing eccrine bromhidrosis, such as some types of food (garlic, onions, curry, and alcohol) and medications (penicillin, bromides). Some metabolic conditions, such as disorders in amino acid metabolism, isovaleric academia, and hypermethioninemia, can also cause this condition.

Clinical Presentation

Patients complain of a bad smell in the armpits in a permanent and intense way. On physical examination the bromhidrosis can be noticed or not.

Treatment

The patient should be advised about local hygiene, the use of antiseptic soap and antiperspirants based on aluminum salts. In cases of treatment failure, topical antibiotics such as clindamycin and erythromycin may be used.

Reducing local hair may reduce bacterial proliferation. For this purpose, laser epilation can be suggested. Another possible approach is to reduce local sweating by the same methods used for hyperhidrosis. The reduction of sweat would create a microenvironment less favorable to the proliferation of microorganisms.

Suggested Reading

Clerico C, Fernandez J, Camuzard O, Chignon-Sicard B, Ihrai T. Axillary hyperhidrosis, botulinium a toxin treatment: review. Ann Chir Plast Esthet. 2016;61(1):60–4.

Fujimoto T. Pathophysiology and treatment of hyperhidrosis. Curr Probl Dermatol. 2016;51:86–93.

Grabell DA, Hebert AA. Current and emerging medical therapies for primary hyperhidrosis. Dermatol Ther (Heidelb). 2017;7(1):25–36.

Kurta AO, Glaser DA. Emerging nonsurgical treatments for hyperhidrosis. Thorac Surg Clin. 2016;26(4):395–402.

Semkova K, Gergovska M, Kazandjieva J, Tsankov N. Hyperhidrosis, bromhidrosis, and chromhidrosis: fold (intertriginous) dermatoses. Clin Dermatol. 2015;33(4):483–91.

Botulinum Toxin for Axillary and Palmar Hyperhidrosis

Mônica Aribi, Gabriel Aribi, and Thalita Domingues Mendes

The History of Botulinum Toxin: From Poison to Medicine

Botulinum toxin (BTX) type A (BTX-A) is a neurotoxin derived from *Clostridium botulinum*, an aerobic bacterium. BTX temporarily chemodenervates the eccrine glands involved in hyperhidrosis by binding to the receptor located on the presynaptic membrane, blocking the release of acetylcholine from skeletal and autonomic cholinergic nerve terminals.

The first recorded case of food poisoning caused by the neurotoxin-producing bacterium *C. botulinum* (botulism) is believed to have been in 1735. In 1817, Dr. Justinus Christian Kerner (1782–1862) published a very precise description of the symptoms of patients suffering from botulism after eating uncooked, smoked sausages or ham.

During World War II, much research was conducted in the USA at Fort Detrick, Maryland, specially by Edward J. Schantz who was searching for an antidote to counteract BTX, which was thought to be a potential biological weapon ready to be used by several other countries. In 1949, Burgen showed that the block of acetylcholine release by BTX occurred in the presynaptic nerve endings and not, as previously believed, by postsynaptic blockage of receptors such as atropine. In the 1960s, Alan Scott, an ophthalmologist, was searching for a non-surgical alternative for the treatment of strabismus. His idea to weaken the extraocular muscles with BTX brought him in contact with Ed Schantz. After several trials on monkeys, BTX-A was approved in 1989 by the US Food and Drug Administration (FDA) for the treatment of strabismus, blepharospasm, and hemifacial spasm. Other fields of medicine

M. Aribi (✉) · G. Aribi · T. D. Mendes
Department of Dermatology, Ipiranga Hospital, São Paulo, SP, Brazil
e-mail: recepcao@monicaaribi.com.br

quickly became interested and BTX-A was used for a wide variety of indications, in particular for the treatment of hyperkinetic muscles. Bushara was the first to suggest a possible indication for BTX-A in the treatment of hyperhidrosis. Since 2002, BTX-A has been approved for the treatment of axillary hyperhidrosis in many countries and, most recently, in 2004, Botox® was approved in the USA by the FDA for axillary hyperhidrosis.

Commercially Available Botulinum Toxins

The seven serotypes of BTX that are produced by *C. botulinum* (A, B, C1, D, E, F, and G) affect the neural function, and there are many differences between each of them, such as size of the toxin complex, mechanism of action, formulation, and process of manufacture.

The first BTX available for clinical use was the BTX-A onabotulinumtoxin A, produced in the USA by Allergan Inc. under the name of BOTOX®/BOTOX_Cosmetic®. In Great Britain, Ipsen Limited manufactured another type of BTX-A, abobotulinumtoxin A, commercially called Dysport®. Dysport® has also been distributed by Medicis in the USA, Canada, and Japan under the name of Reloxin®.

Other preparations of BTX-A available in the world are Linurase® (Prollenium Medical Technologies Inc., Canada); the Chinese BTX-A (CBTX-A), commercially named Prosigne®/Lantox®/Redux® (Lanzhou Biological Products Institute, China); the BTX-A named Neuronox®/Meditoxin®/Botulift® (Medy-Tox Inc., South Korea), and the incobotulinumtoxin A known as Xeomin®/Bocouture® (Merz Pharmaceuticals, Germany).

The only other commercially available serotype is the BTX type B (BTX-B) manufactured by Solstice Neuroscience Inc., known as Myobloc® or Neuroblock® which has FDA approval to treat cervical dystonia. This preparation is also being used off-label to treat facial wrinkles (Table 15.1).

Patient Management and Considerations

Before treating patients with BTX a detailed patient history should be obtained, focusing particularly on clues regarding the presence of secondary hyperhidrosis, since the underlying primary disease must be addressed first. As with every other treatment, the potential adverse effects of the therapy, contraindications, and the alternative treatments should be explained to the patient. It is also recommended that the patient understands the mechanism of action of BTX, in particular the need for re-injection after 6–9 months. Patients should know not to be treated during pregnancy and lactation.

Table 15.1 Main commercial presentations of botulinum toxin A

	Onabotulinum-toxin A	Abobotulinum-toxin A	CBTX-A	BTX-A	Incobotu-linumtoxin A
Lab	Allergan, Inc.	Ipsen Inc./Medicis Inc.	Lanzhou	Medy-Tox Inc.	Merz Pharmaceuticals
Commercial names	Botox® Botox cosmetic® Vistabel® Vistabex®	Dysport® Reloxin® Azzalure®	Prosigne® Lantox® Redux®	Neuronox® Meditoxin® Botulift®	Xeomin® Bocouture®
Type—size	Type A—900 kDa	Type A—400–500 kDa	Type A—900 kDa	Type A—940 kDa	Type A—150 kDa
Mechanism	SNAP 25/SV2	SNAP 25/SV2	SNAP 25	SNAP 25	SNAP 25
Storage	2–8 °C	2–8 °C	2–8 °C	2–8 °C	Before diluting 25 °C After 2–8 °C

BoNT-A botulinum toxin serotype A, *CBTX-A* Chinese botulinum toxin A

Many practitioners have the patient sign a written consent form that becomes part of the patient's permanent record. Good follow-up procedures and prompt response to any complaints after treatment are important. The potential risks in treating patients for focal hyperhidrosis with BTX are comparatively small. However, clearly the treating physician must know the pharmacologic effect of the drug and the anatomic sites tov inject. It is necessary to participate in one or two training workshops to learn the injection technique prior to initiating treatment. Every practitioner must know in advance how to manage patients with unsatisfactory results. Successful treatments are predicated upon choosing the right patient for treatment, injecting them with the proper technique, and insisting on adequate follow-up visits in order to administer appropriate follow-up care.

Contraindications

BTX injections are not offered to patients who suffer from hyperhidrosis secondary to an underlying disease, who have undergone previous surgical debulking of sweat glands, or who have severe blood-clotting disorders.

Patients who have a concurrent infection at the injection site or systemic infection are asked to return the office after the infection has cleared. Treatment of patients who have an existing medical condition that may interfere with neuromuscular function, such as myasthenia gravis, Eaton-Lambert syndrome, or amyotrophic lateral sclerosis, should be avoided. Female patients who are pregnant or breastfeeding are also contraindicated.

Neutralizing Antibodies in the Treatment of Hyperhidrosis with Botulinum Toxin Type A (BTX-A)

BTX neurotoxins are bacterially derived, exogenous proteins that have the potential to elicit immune responses and antibody formation in humans. Neutralizing antibodies (NAbs) directed against the core neurotoxin can interfere with pharmacological activity, potentially leading to loss of clinical efficacy. Historically, the use of high doses of BTX-A at frequent injection intervals for the treatment of cervical dystonia was associated with the formation of NAbs in 4–10% of patients. However, studies across five different disorders show that NAb conversion was uncommon, occurring in only 11 of 240 subjects (0.5%) treated with BTX-A treatments.

The frequency and duration of treatment with BTX-A may also influence the rate of nAb formation. It is therefore good practice to administer doses that are sufficient to provide meaningful duration of clinical effect, but which are low enough to minimize the risk of seroconversion.

The present results suggest that NAbs are likely the cause of clinical non-responsiveness in only a small minority of patients.

Overall, the studies show strong evidence that BTX-A is associated with a low rate of NAb formation across multiple indications and suggests that other factors in addition to NAb serum conversion should be considered when subjects develop clinical non-responsiveness.

Technique

Minor Starch Test

The first step is to determine the exact area of the hyperhidrosis. This is most commonly achieved using the Minor Starch Test. First the hyperhidrotic area is completely dried and covered with an iodine solution, Lugol or Betadine® solution (Fig. 15.1), and it is then sprinkled with powdered starch (e.g., cornflower starch)

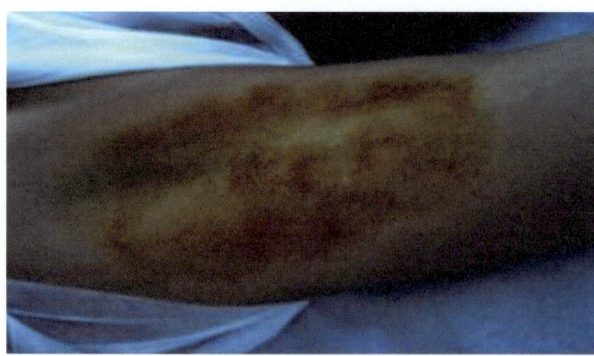

Fig. 15.1 Lugol solution applied to the hyperidrotic region

(Fig. 15.2). It is important that as little powder as possible is used to achieve a good colorimetric response. If too much powder is used, the powder will absorb the moisture of the sweat and the intensity of the patient's sweating may not be assessed correctly. After removing the excess purple color from the center of the outline, each injection site can be marked with gentian violet.

A semi-quantitative measurement of focal hyperhidrosis can be achieved using the Minor Starch Test, demonstrating the full extent of sweating in the affected area and, through the intensity of the purple coloration, the severity of sweating (Fig. 15.3).

Therefore, by performing a Minor Starch Test before each treatment, the physician can determine how many injection sites and how much BTX-A is needed prior to commencing therapy. It is important to take pictures of the result of the test prior to the treatment and during the follow-up visit, 15 days after the treatment, to assure the efficacy of the procedure.

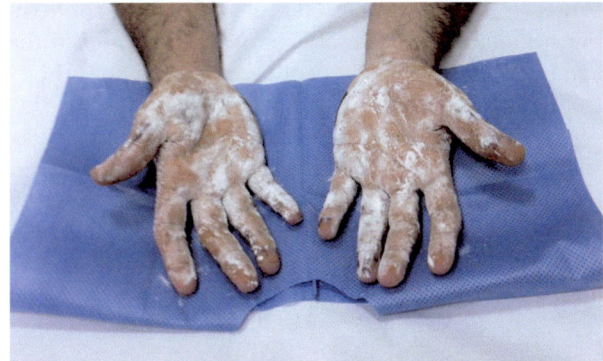

Fig. 15.2 Powder starch sprinkled to the same region

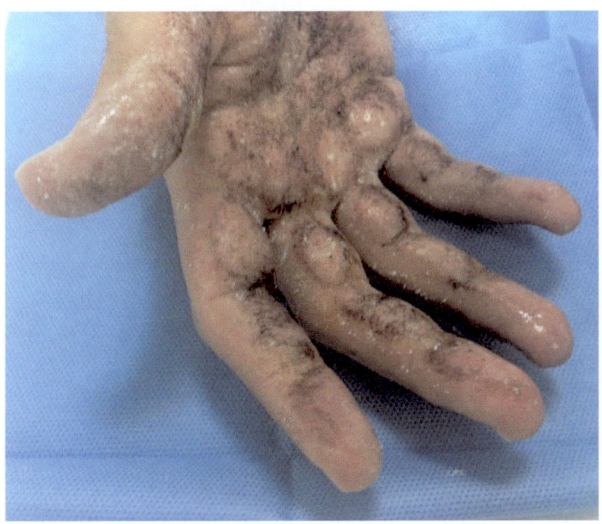

Fig. 15.3 Estimation of sweating areas allows to target the injection points

Therapy, Dilution, and Injection Technique

The volume of the dilution of the BTX-A depends on the option of the applicator. Once the vial of BTX-A is reconstituted without a preservative, it should be used in full within 4 h, due to the possibility the solution may not remain sterile for an extended period of time.

This issue is questioned by the studies, and we have learned that there are no adverse events or significant loss of potency resulting from the storage of reconstituted BTX-A for a few days and even a few weeks. After the dilution, the solution must be stored in a refrigerator (2–8 °C).

Some studies show that the volume of diluent used to reconstitute the product could increase the diffusion capacity of BTX-A [1], and thus some doctors prefer to increase this volume in order to have better results. Therefore, this author prefers to reconstitute a 100 U vial of onabotulinumtoxin A in 4.0 mL of sterile saline.

The injection of BTX-A should be with a 30-gauge needle or insulin syringe (Fig. 15.4). A needle is inserted at a 45 ° angle, approximately 2 mm into the dermis. For beginners, a very useful tip is to cut the lid of the syringe to be sure that the application is at the right depth level (2–2.5 mm) (Fig. 15.5).

The number of injection sites, and consequently the total dose of injected BTX-A, should no longer be defined as a total recommended dose for a given anatomic site, but instead by the number of units used per injection site. The minimum dose for each injection is from 2.0 to 2.5 U, but this also depends on the size of the colorimetric response exhibited by the Minor Starch Test. Since the diffusion capacity of BTX-A is about 1.0–1.5 cm in diameter, the injected points should be this distance apart (Fig. 15.6).

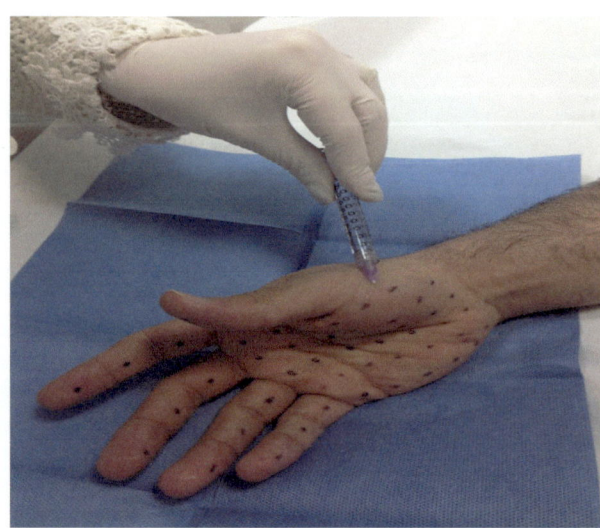

Fig. 15.4 Injection of BTX-A at the selected points

Fig. 15.5 The tip of cutting the lid of the syringe to avoid deeper injections

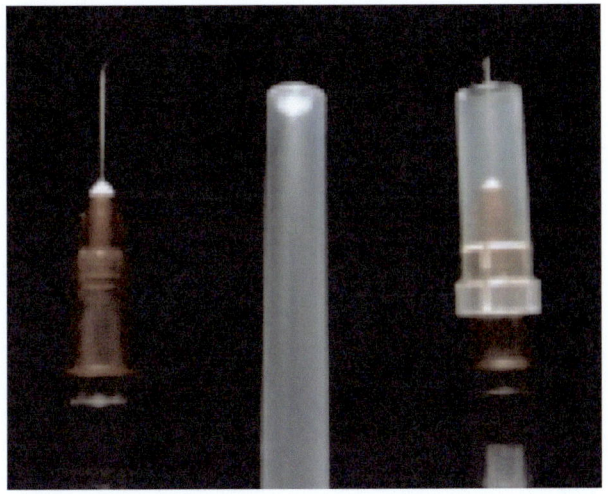

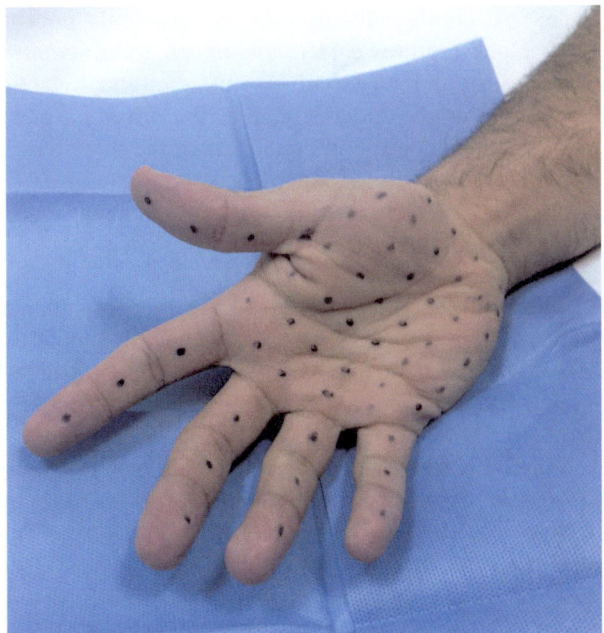

Fig. 15.6 Injection point distant 1.5 cm one to another

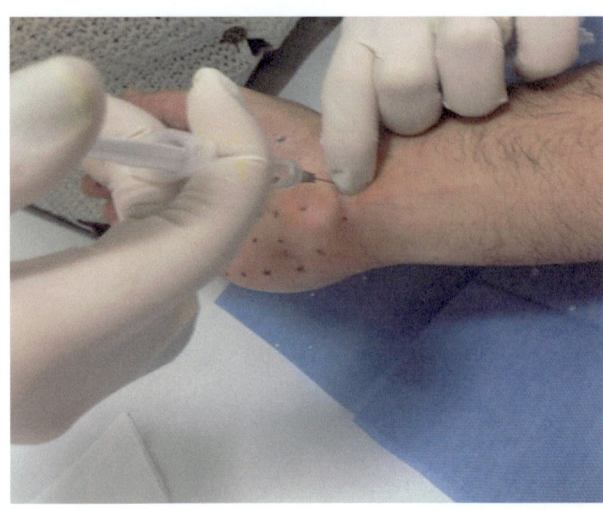

Fig. 15.7 Nerve block anesthesia for radial nerve

Anesthesia

Many trials of regional anesthesia have been reported, with differing results. For axillary hyperhidrosis the treatment can be performed using lidocaine cream or EMLA® 30 min before the treatment.

However, for treatment of the palm or in very sensitive patients the nerve block is the best choice, although this is commonly poorly accepted by patients. The nerve block requires careful and expert training and can be painful. The risk of nerve injury and severe adverse effects (anaphylactic shock, cardiac problems) also should not be underestimated. The different injection points of a nerve block of the hand can be found on the site of the three tendons (Fig. 15.7): for an ulnar nerve block the site of injection is over the *flexor carpi ulnaris*. For a median nerve block the site is on the tendon of *flexor carpi radialis*, and for the radial nerve the injection site is over the tendon of *extensor carpi radialis* and medial of the radial artery.

The needle should be inserted 0.5–1 cm perpendicular to the skin until firm resistance is felt and the deep fascia is pierced. It should then be retracted about 2 mm before 2 mL of lidocaine 2.0% without vasoconstrictor is injected.

Full anesthesia is achieved after 15–30 min in the palm and back of the hand (Figs. 15.8 and 15.9).

Finally, another type of anesthesia is cryotherapy used on the sites of injections (15 s spray) (Fig. 15.10), combined or not with iontophoresis with 2% lidocaine for 15 min per side. The collateral effect of this type of anesthesia is the formation of blisters in the day after.

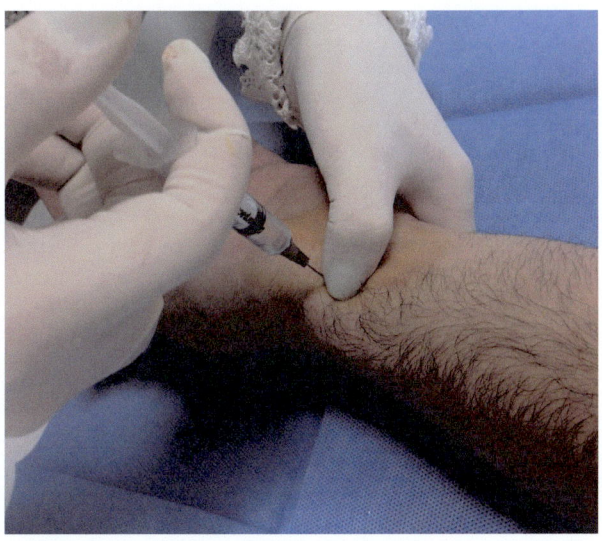

Fig. 15.8 Nerve block anesthesia for medial nerve

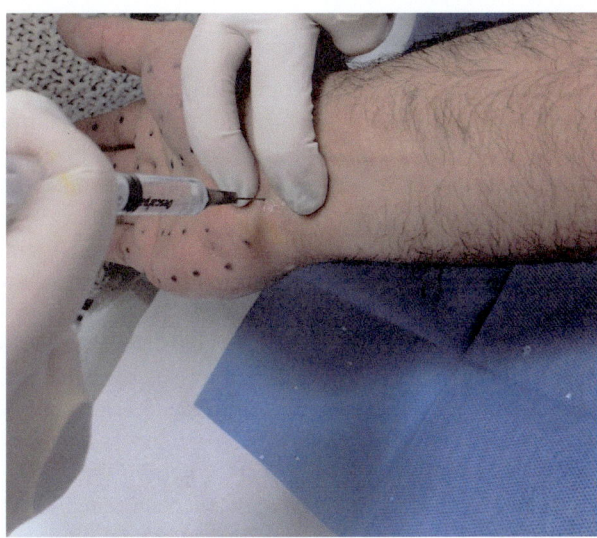

Fig. 15.9 Nerve block anesthesia for ulnar nerve

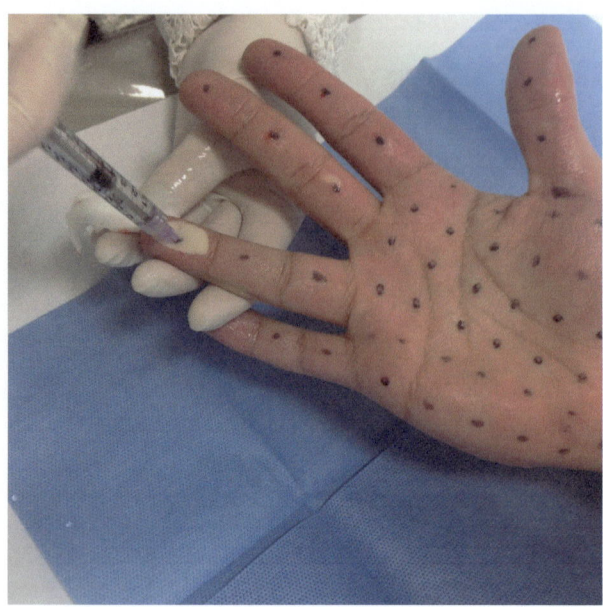

Fig. 15.10 Cryotherapy anesthesia just before BTX-A application

Advantages of BTX-A as Hyperhidrosis Treatment

Updated therapeutic algorithms are proposed for each commonly affected anatomic site, with practical procedural guidelines. For axillary hyperhidrosis, BTX injections are recommended as second-line treatment, oral medications as third-line treatment, local surgery as fourth-line treatment, and endoscopic thoracic sympathectomy as fifth-line treatment. For axillary and palmoplantar hyperhidrosis, topical treatment is recommended as first-line treatment.

Treatments with topical agents such as antiperspirant, mainly aluminum Chloridrate, have shown low efficacy. The anticholinergics, such as oxybutynin, show good results in palm, sole, axillary, and facial hyperhidrosis. The most common adverse effect is dry mouth, but it remains well-controlled at a dose of 10 mg/day.

Surgical resection of the sweat glands could be less sensible due to its collateral effects of scars, fibrosis, and hyperhidrosis recurrence. Sympathectomy surgery has shown to have compensatory hyperhidrosis as a collateral effect. The micro-needling radiofrequency could result in fibrosis and scars. Iontophoresis is considered the third-line therapy for palmar-plantar hyperhidrosis; its efficacy is high, but so are the initial levels of cost and inconvenience related to it [2].

Treatment with BTX-A is safe and efficient, and it has been approved by the FDA and EMA (European Medicines Agency). It is easily administered and recommended as second-line therapy in axillary hyperhidrosis. The lasting results provide great patient satisfaction and avoid the risks of a surgery procedure. In addition, recent studies have shown that repeated applications could improve the efficacy and the duration of the effect [3]. Patients reported the duration of symptom relief to be from 4 to 12 months, with a mean of 5.68 months [4]. We have observed some results in palmar hyperhidrosis to last from 6 to 10 months.

Conclusion
It is important that each case be evaluated individually, and the treatment must be the most convenient to the patient in all respects—social, economic, and physical.

References

1. Hsu TS, Dover JS, Amdt KA. Effect of volume and concentration on the diffusion of botulinum exotoxin A. Arch Dermatol. 2004;140(11):1351–4.
2. Walling HW, Swick BL. Treatment options for primary hyperhidrosis. Am J Clin Dermatol. 2011;12(5):285–95.
3. Lecouflet M, et al. Duration of efficacy increases with the repletion of botulinum toxin A injections in primary palmar hyperhidrosis; a study of 28 patients. J Am Acad Dermatol. 2014;70(6):1083–7.
4. DÉpiro S, Macaluso L, Salvi M, Luci C, Mattozzi C, Marzocca F, Salvo V, Scarnó M, Calvieri S, Richetta AG. Safety and prolonged efficacy of botulinum toxin A in primary hyperhidrosis. Clin Ter. 2014;165(6):e395–400.

Axillary Hyperhidrosis: Local Surgical Treatment with Aspiratory Curettage

16

Ronaldo Golcman, Murillo Francisco Pires Fraga, and Benjamin Golcman

Introduction

Because of the high density of sweat glands, armpits are a frequent location of hyperhidrosis. Eccrine glands, responsible for sweat production, are more numerous than the apocrine, odor-producing glands. Sweating with intense odor is called bromhidrosis. There is no direct relation between axillary hyperhidrosis and bromhidrosis.

Excessive sweating frequently stains clothes, exposing users to embarrassment, interfering in their social life and even employment situations, and becomes worse when associated with bromhidrosis.

Some of the following characteristics are considered desirable by patients when choosing the therapy to undertake:

- Single treatment, without periodic repetition
- Low risk
- Low-cost day clinic

R. Golcman
University of São Paulo, São Paulo, SP, Brazil

Brazilian Society of Plastic Surgery, São Paulo, SP, Brazil

Hospital Israelita Albert Einstein, São Paulo, SP, Brazil
e-mail: ronaldo@golcman.com.br

M. F. P. Fraga (✉)
Brazilian Society of Plastic Surgery, São Paulo, SP, Brazil

Faculty of Medical Sciences of Santa Casa of São Paulo, São Paulo, SP, Brazil
e-mail: murifraga@ig.com.br

B. Golcman
University of São Paulo, São Paulo, SP, Brazil

Brazilian Society of Plastic Surgery, São Paulo, SP, Brazil

- Local anesthesia
- Discreet scar tissue
- No compensatory sweating
- Quick recovery
- Minimum absence from work.

Considering these demands by the patient, aspiratory curettage is increasingly being indicated to treat axillary hyperhidrosis, with long-lasting results.

Shenaq et al. [1] proposed this procedure in 1987, which has subsequently been successfully used because it represents a low morbidity, low cost, and highly effective treatment in the long term.

In 2007 Bechara et al. observed that curettage with greater caliber (4–6 mm) and more aggressive cannulas offered further reduction of hyperhidrosis in comparison with lesser caliber (<3 mm) cannulas.

Considering factors such as fewer absences from work, quick return to normal life, and definitive and low-risk treatment, surgical treatment of hyperhidrosis by aspiratory curettage is increasingly taking a greater place in modern therapeutics.

Operating Techniques

Surgical Positioning and Preoperative Demarcation

The patient should be in a dorsal decubitus position, with arms at 90 ° and hands near the head.

Demarcation of the axillary hairy area must have a 1 cm peripheral border because we know there is a close relationship between axillary hair and density of eccrine and apocrine glands. Patients with long hair may need trichotomy after demarcation.

Anesthesia

Local anesthesia with sedation, or local anesthesia alone, should be administered.

Anesthesia starts with venous sedation at the anesthesiologist's discretion. Local infiltrative anesthesia is composed of a 200 mg lidocaine solution plus 100 mg bupivacaine, 140 mL saline solution, and 0,5 mL adrenaline. The procedure starts with an anesthetic button being introduced before an incision is made (4 mm) to allow introduction of the aspiration curettage cannula. Once the incision is ready, infiltration is completed through the incision with a Klein needle (subcutaneous superficial plan). The total infiltration volume varies from 40 to 80 mL per armpit, taking into consideration the extent of the patient's hairy area and weight. Ten minutes after infiltration, vasoconstriction and intra- and post-surgical sedation occur, thus ensuring a less traumatic and tumescent aspiratory curettage (Figs. 16.1, 16.2, and 16.3).

16 Axillary Hyperhidrosis: Local Surgical Treatment with Aspiratory Curettage

Fig. 16.1 Demarcated area for curettage, Klein infiltration cannula, and curettage (blunt) cannula

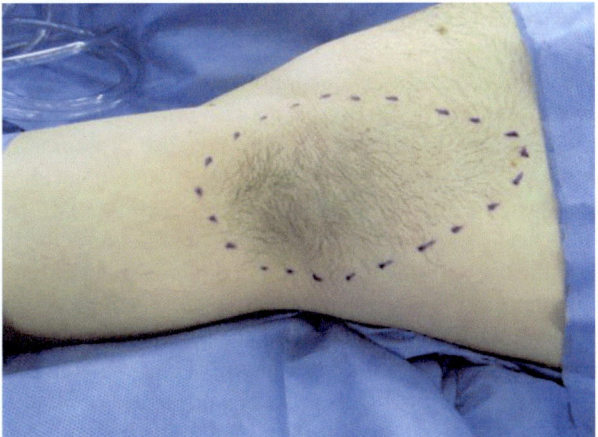

Fig. 16.2 Demarcated area for curettage, Klein infiltration cannula, and curettage (blunt) cannula

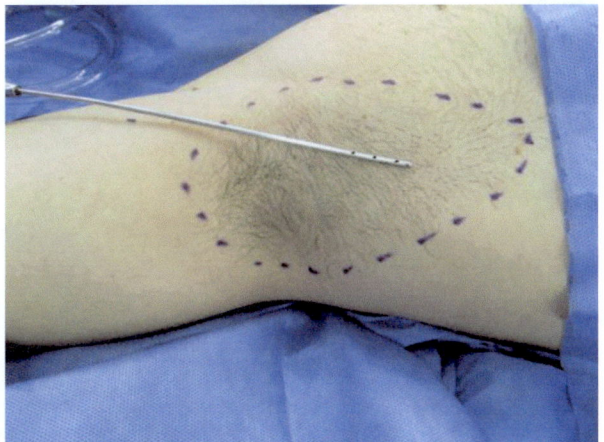

Fig. 16.3 Demarcated area for curettage, Klein infiltration cannula, and curettage (blunt) cannula

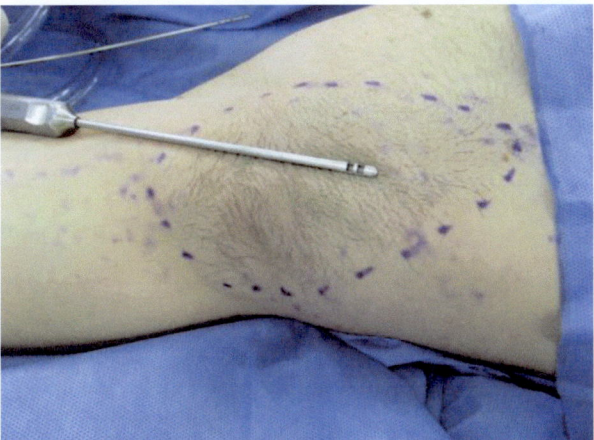

Surgical Technique

An aspiratory curettage cannula is introduced through a 4 mm incision in the interior of the arm (bicipital fold), 1–1,5 cm distant from the previously marked area.

Tunneling is initiated, without negative pressure, in the previously marked area with a 3,7 or 4 mm flat-blunt cannula (duckbill), with one or two holes (rectangular or square) with moderated cutting edges (Fig. 16.4).

After tunneling is completed, and maintaining the connections between the skin and the deeper plans due to vascular elements and fibrous beams, the vacuum sucker is connected, charged with a 60 cmHg negative pressure, and the cannula hole is turned towards the skin. This is the beginning of the aspiratory curettage.

Aspiratory curettage evaluation and intra-operative control are performed by evaluating the bi-digital skin fold, as well as the cannula contour (initially unapparent, though perfectly defined at the end of the procedure) (Figs. 16.5, 16.6, 16.7, and 16.8).

Aspiratory curettage begins with the smaller caliber cannulas (3.7–4 mm) and progressively uses the 5 mm ones.

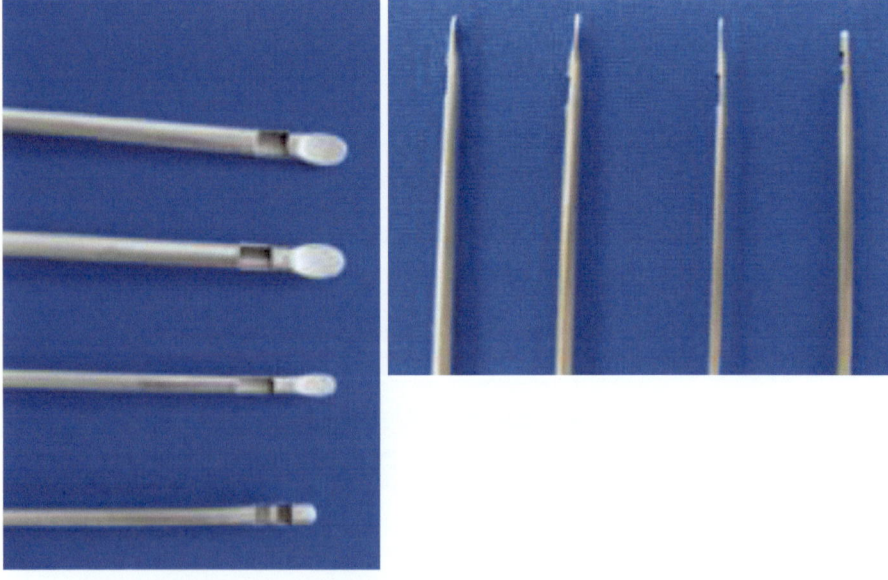

Fig. 16.4 Blunt cannulas (front and profile)

Fig. 16.5 Cannula relief in the beginning and end of procedure

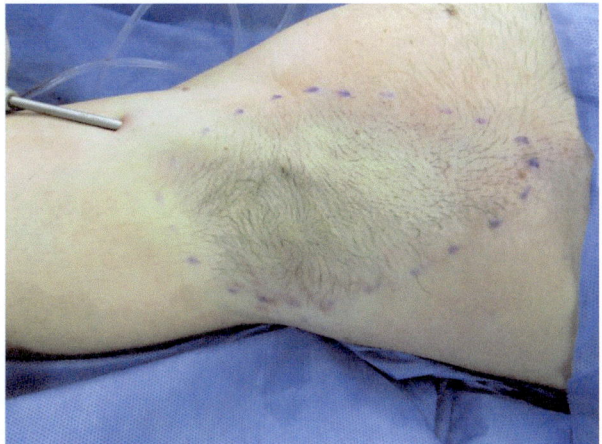

Fig. 16.6 Cannula relief in the beginning and end of procedure

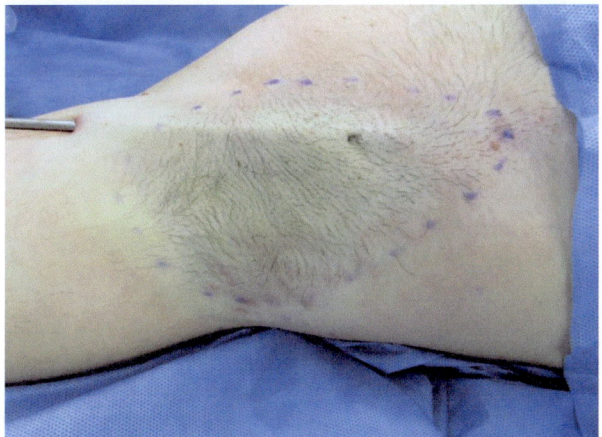

Fig. 16.7 Thickness of skin flap in the beginning and end of procedure

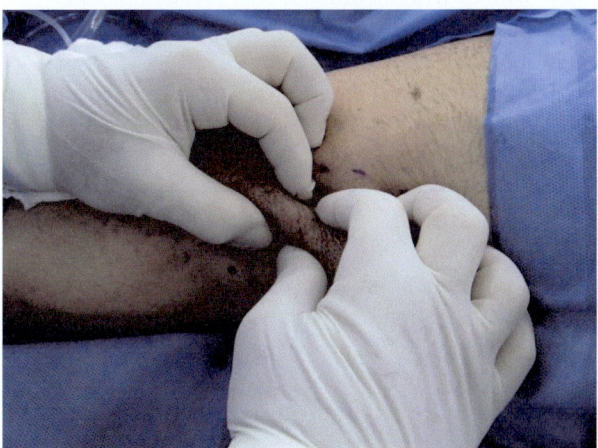

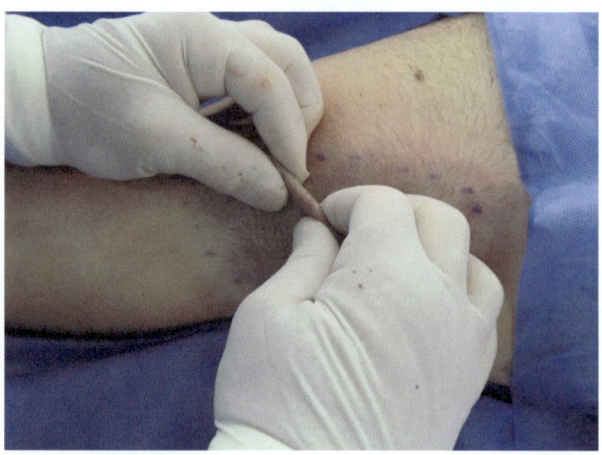

Fig. 16.8 Thickness of skin flap in the beginning and end of procedure

Intradermal suture takes place at the end of the procedure with one or two stitches of poliglecaprona 5-0 (absorbable), followed by *steril strip*® and *opsite*®. Cotton balls are placed in the axillary cavus so that the weight of the patient's arm produces the necessary compression upon the wound. The patient should be observed for a period of approximately 30 min if he received local anesthesia and 6 h following anesthetic sedation. At the end of this period he can go home.

Postoperative Care

Compression is temporarily removed when taking a shower and permanently after 24 h. Limitation of arm movements is restricted for 3 days after the operation and arm friction should be avoided for 10 days. During this period armpit skin should be kept slightly oily using a skin protector and a lubricant (DERSANI®). Later on, if the area looks stiff or if the skin is contracted, hand massaging and lymphatic drainage—with or without ultrasound—is recommended twice a day. Several times a day the arm should be gradually exposed to slow hyperextension so as to speed up mobility recovery and skin elasticity.

Pain killers and antibiotics (second-generation cephalosporins) are recommended for a 5- to 7-day period.

Complications

Most complications are local and the majority can be solved quickly. These complications are most commonly seromas or bruises and can be treated by drainage through needle puncture. When an expansive hematoma (Fig. 16.9) appears immediately after the surgery, urgent drainage is required, followed by 48 h of compression. Late seromas should be treated through serial puncture, every other day, until total remission. Epitheliolysis or segmental necrosis of the skin may occur when curettage is too intense, to the detriment of skin tissue vascularization (Figs. 16.10 and 16.11).

Fig. 16.9 Expansive hematoma in the immediate period post-surgery

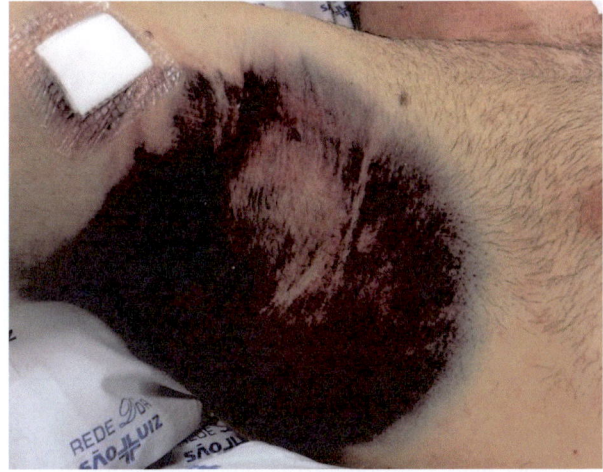

Fig. 16.10 Epitheliolysis and segmental necrosis 7 days postoperative. Resolution with clinical treatment. Transient hyperchromia may occur

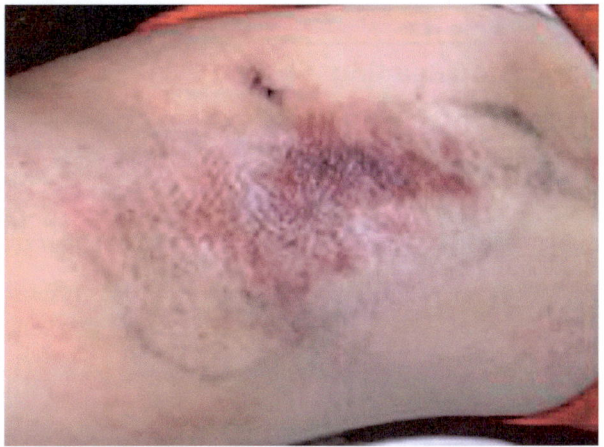

Fig. 16.11 Epitheliolysis and segmental necrosis 7 days postoperative. Resolution with clinical treatment. Transient hyperchromia may occur

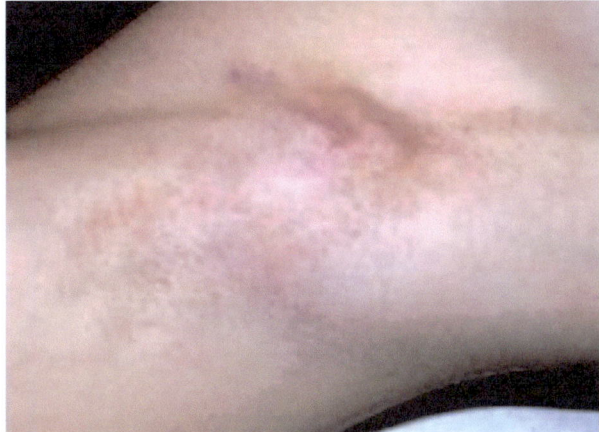

Treatment is restricted to chemical debridement ointment (collagenase) in association with antibiotics.

It is possible that a more conservative aspiratory curettage may only be partially successful. In those cases the procedure has to be repeated in order to achieve the final goal.

Ecchymosis occurs in 100% of surgeries, being a normal feature in this sort of procedure, as also occurs in postoperative liposuction.

Skin dyschromia (hypo- or hyperchromia) may be observed in some patients and healing, in most cases, is spontaneous. Hyperchromia can be treated with creams containing hydroquinone to accelerate the process. Permanent dyschromia may also occur, but is less frequent.

Conclusion

Vacuum curettage improves the quality of life in patients with axillary hyperhidrosis and/or bromhidrosis and can be the first option regarding a surgical approach.

Suggested Reading

Golcman R. Axillay hyperidrosis – surgical treatment using vacuum curettage. Procedimentos Estéticos Minimamente Invasivos, Livraria Santos Editora LTDA, c. 36. p 293–299, São Paulo 2006.

Golcman R, Golcman B, Fraga MFP. Axillay hyperidrosis – surgical treatment using vacuum curettage (Hiperidrose axilar – tratamento cirúrgico através da curetagem aspirativa). Einstein. 2005;3(4):271–4.

Lee MR, Ryman W. Liposuction for axillary hyperhidrosis. Australas J Dermatol. 2005;46(2):76–9.

Shenaq SM, Spira M. Treatment of bilateral axillary hyperhidrosis by suction assisted lipolysis technique. Ann Plast Surg. 1987;19(6):548–51.

Wu WH, Ma S, Lin JT, Tang YW, Fang RH. Surgical treatment of axillary osmidrosis: an analysis of 343 cases. Plast Reconstr Surg. 1994;94:288.

Part III

Sympathectomies for Hyperhidrosis

Anatomy of the Sympathetic Nervous System in Relation to Surgical Hyperhidrosis Treatment

17

André Felix Gentil and Arthur W. Poetscher

Introduction

The autonomic nervous system (ANS) is the efferent portion of the visceral nervous system, responsible for control of the body's vegetative functions. It is divided into sympathetic (ANSs) and parasympathetic (ANSp) systems. Among its various functions, the ANSs controls the secretion of the sweat glands. Normally, in situations of stress or exercise there is an increase in the production of sweat. In some people, the ANSs do not properly regulate this production. This unbalance of ANSs is one of the causes of hyperhidrosis, a disease in which patients perspire in an exaggerated manner, often for no apparent reason. The hyperactivity of the sweat glands is most striking where they are most concentrated: on the palms of the hands, armpits, and the soles of the feet. These regions are constantly wet, with important impairment of the quality of life of these individuals.

There are several treatments for hyperhidrosis. Surgical treatment, in particular, of this condition has undergone major modifications in the last 50 years. The sympathetic chain, the target of the interventions, is located deep inside the thoracic cavity and complex surgeries were necessary to access it. The delay in postoperative recovery and the morbimortality associated with the operation meant indication of the procedure is restricted to a few cases. In the last 15 years, however, with the development of video-assisted surgery, the technique to access the sympathetic chain has become safe and effective. The procedures became minimally invasive

---

A. F. Gentil (✉)
Neurosurgeon of the Hospital Israelita Albert Einstein in São Paulo, São Paulo, SP, Brazil

School of Medicine, University of São Paulo, São Paulo, SP, Brazil

A. W. Poetscher
Neurosurgeon of the Hospital Israelita Albert Einstein, São Paulo, SP, Brazil

School of Medicine, University of São Paulo, São Paulo, SP, Brazil

Albert Einstein Institute for Teaching and Research, São Paulo, SP, Brazil

and with low operative risk. Endoscopic thoracic sympathectomy (ETS) has become the procedure of choice for the surgical treatment of hyperhidrosis. The procedure has been refined and the extent of the sympathectomy has been minimized in order to treat only the structures of the thoracic sympathetic chain responsible for excessive sweating in a particular site of the body, minimizing the possible adverse effects. Several methods have been developed to interrupt the segments of the sympathetic chain, among them excision, electrocauterization, ultrasonic destruction, and clipping. The technical simplicity and success rates between 95% and 99% meant indication of the procedure has had an exponential growth.

Knowledge of the anatomy of ANS, especially ANSs, as well as their variations, has become essential for the surgeon who intends to perform ETS. There is still great debate about which are the ideal targets among the segments of the thoracic sympathetic chain for the effective treatment of hyperhidrosis and in what way very frequent anatomical variations can influence the results of the operations.

In this chapter, a description is given of the anatomy and physiological aspects of the ANS, with emphasis on its sympathetic division and its implications in the treatment of hyperhidrosis.

The Autonomic Nervous System (ANS)

As already mentioned, the ANS is generally responsible for maintaining the constancy of the internal environment of the organism, or homeostasis, a term introduced by Cannon. ANS regulates vital functions such as breathing, circulation, digestion, temperature adjustment, and part of metabolism. It allows the organism to adapt to internal and external changes through processes that occur almost automatically, with little or no volitional influence.

ANS is extremely complex at the biochemical–functional level. The classical view of this system has been modified since the 1970s, but it is still didactic and facilitates the basic understanding of its functioning. We discuss here only the main concepts currently accepted.

Central Control

The central control of ANS occurs through fibers originating from five areas of the central nervous system (CNS): the limbic system, prefrontal area, hypothalamus, brainstem nuclei, and spinal cord. Among these, the hypothalamus exerts the greatest influence, being subject to the interferences of the other centers and also of endocrine origin. Fibers originating in the hypothalamus descend through the reticular formation of the brainstem and into the spinal cord. Changes in internal and external environments, as well as emotional oscillations, modify the hypothalamic activity and influence the ANS activity. There is evidence that the activity of the anterior portion of the cingulate gyrus, an emotion-related cerebral cortical structure, is partly responsible for the abnormal secretion of sweat in patients with hyperhidrosis. There is other evidence that ANS activity on the heart would be modulated in part by the cerebellum.

Some conscious knowledge of ANS activity may occur through ascending afferent fibers. In fact, there are some people who can change their heart rate, temperature, and aspects of metabolism.

ANS Basic Functions

As already mentioned, the SNA is divided into sympathetic and parasympathetic. The functions of ANSp are not as well-defined as those of ANSs. The parasympathetic activity on the pupils, salivary glands, heart, lungs, gastrointestinal tract, bladder, reproductive organs, and metabolism aim to conserve and resupply body energy, acting mainly during rest. Some of the structures innervated by ANSp are directly influenced by voluntary motor control. In some cases, as in the control of the bladder and rectus muscles, the movements of the striated muscle fibers, controlled by the motor cortex, are closely related to the movements of the smooth muscle fibers under parasympathetic modulation.

ANSs has more clearly defined functions. Its fibers are distributed throughout the body, promoting catabolic actions and increasing the rate of metabolism. The ANSs innervates the iris and ciliary muscle of the eye, salivary, lacrimal and sweat glands, mucous membranes of the nose and palate, erector muscles of the hairs, blood vessels, heart, larynx, trachea and bronchi, gastrointestinal tract organs (including the esophagus, stomach, small intestine, liver, biliary system, and large intestine), adrenal gland, kidney, bladder, and reproductive organs.

The effects of ANS activity are most evident in situations of high emotional arousal, such as stress or fear, and are classically referred to as fight or flight responses. The sympathetic system prepares the organism to fight or escape through various actions: it increases the heart rate, increases the force of contraction of the ventricles (dilating coronary vessels), contracts the arterioles of the skin and the intestine and dilates those of the skeletal muscles (allowing more activity), dilates the pupils, relaxes the smooth muscles of the bronchi (increasing the airflow of the lungs), relaxes the smooth muscles of the intestines and bladder (stimulating the sphincters), stimulates erecting muscles of the hairs, and increases sweating (allowing greater heat loss). There are also metabolic changes such as increased blood glucose and the release of adrenaline from the marrow of the adrenal gland.

Anatomy of the ANS

The ANS is composed of brain–spinal nuclei and nerves, forming a network of ganglia and plexuses that innervate various target organs such as viscera, smooth muscles, and secretory glands. Each of the sympathetic and parasympathetic divisions of the ANS have distinct central origins. The ANSs arise from segments of the spinal cord in the thoracolumbar region, whereas the fibers of the ANSp originate in the craniosacral region.

The connection of the ANS to the target organs is done through an anatomical organization comprising four main structures: preganglionic fibers, peripheral ganglia, postganglionic fibers, and neuro-effector junctions.

The main anatomical difference between the sympathetic and parasympathetic ANS is the location of the peripheral ganglion in relation to the target organs. In the ANSs the ganglia are close to the medulla and distant from the target organ, usually determining short preganglionic fibers and long postganglionic fibers. In the ANSp the ganglia are located far from the marrow, near or even within the target organs, determining long preganglionic fibers and short postganglionic fibers.

Most of the target organs receive innervation of the two systems, which, in general, act in an antagonistic and reciprocal way, producing different physiological effects. However, in some cases, the actions of the two systems are synergistic. In fact, at the target organ level, the sympathetic and parasympathetic systems are not independent. Neuro-effector junctions of the two systems are found side by side in most organs.

Preganglionic Fibers

The preganglionic fibers of the ANSs originate in the thoracolumbar region of the spinal cord. The cellular body of the neurons of these fibers are located in the intermediate zone of the gray portion of the marrow and is disposed face-caudally between the T1 and L2 segments. There are anatomical variations and sometimes there is collaboration of neurons of the segments of C8 and L3.

The preganglionic fibers exit the medulla by the ventral root of the spinal nerves and enter the white communicating branch, so called because most of its fibers are myelinated; they go to the ganglia of the paravertebral sympathetic chain where they synapse with the cellular body of the postganglionic neuron; the preganglionic axon can synapse with several postganglionic cells, going up or down to other levels of the chain. A portion of the sympathetic preganglionic fibers do not synapse within the paravertebral sympathetic chain, following directly through the splanchnic nerves to the pre-vertebral sympathetic chain; another small portion of fibers follows directly into the adrenal gland, where it makes a synapse in the adrenal medulla.

Because preganglionic fibers can synapse with more than one ganglion, CNS-derived impulses can diffuse through peripheral ANS. Modulation of these impulses also occurs through inhibitory synapses originating from internuclear neurons present between the ganglia, collateral branches of the postganglionic fibers, or visceral afferent fibers. The presence of dopamine, a classically inhibitory neurotransmitter, has been demonstrated in sympathetic ganglia, proving the existence of inhibitory synapses.

Postganglionic Fibers, Ganglia, and Plexus

The axons of the postganglionic fibers leave the sympathetic chain ganglia through the gray communicating branch, so called because their fibers are amyelinic, returning to the peripheral nerve and following it to different target organs.

Most of these fibers accompany the peripheral nerves of the chest wall, distributing between the vessels and the skin of the thorax. Postganglionic fibers present vesicles at their extremities, where neurotransmitters are stored for use in synapses with target organs.

The sympathetic ganglia are located in the paravertebral region, forming the paravertebral sympathetic chain or, in the pre-vertebral region, supplied by the splanchnic nerves. The paravertebral sympathetic chain consists of two elongated plexuses, each composed of a series of ganglia usually organized in a segmental fashion and joined by ascending and descending fibers. Each of the chains has 22–24 ganglia: three cervical, 10–12 thoracic, four lumbar, and four to five sacral. Merges between the ganglia are frequent, especially in the thoracic and lumbar regions. The chains extend from the level of the second cervical vertebra to the coccyx.

Cervical Sympathetic Chain

The cervical sympathetic trunk is composed of the superior, middle, and inferior cervical ganglia, which receive ascending preganglionic fibers from the thoracic levels of T1 to T5. Its postganglionic fibers innervate structures of the head, neck, upper limbs, and part of the thorax.

The superior cervical ganglion is the largest and is located laterally to the second and third thoracic vertebrae, behind the internal carotid artery and between the carotid sheath and the pre-vertebral fascia. The preganglionic fibers that make a synapse in this ganglion originate mainly from the first four thoracic spinal segments. The internal carotid nerve is an extension of this ganglion that penetrates the skull and provides sympathetic innervation to the internal carotid artery. Other fibers originating from this ganglion form nerve plexuses around the internal and external carotid artery, maxillary artery, cavernous sinus, and middle meninges artery. From these plexuses depart fibers that will participate in the innervation of the ciliary, sphenopalatine, optic, and submaxillary ganglia. The fibers of the gray communicating branches of the spinal nerves of C2 to C4 control the piloerection, sweating, and vasomotricity of the head and neck. There are also connections between the superior cervical ganglion and cranial nerves, pharyngeal plexus, carotid body and bulb (with vasomotor function), heart, and superior cardiac nerves.

The middle cervical ganglion, the smallest of the three cervical ganglia, is located at the level of the seventh cervical vertebra, receiving fibers from the medullary segments T2 and T3. Eventually it may be double or absent. It provides postganglionic fibers to the fifth and sixth cervical nerves that participate in the formation of the middle cardiac nerve and other branches that will innervate the thyroid gland.

The lower cervical ganglion is also located at the level of the seventh cervical vertebra. All of its preganglionic fibers originate from the first thoracic ganglion. It supplies fibers to the sixth, seventh, and eighth cervical nerves, which in turn provide branches to the lower cardiac nerve and to other large blood vessels, including the vertebral and basilar arteries.

In most cases, the lower cervical ganglion fuses with the first thoracic ganglion, forming the star-shaped ganglion (or cervicothoracic ganglion). It has a variable shape and can sometimes also include the middle cervical ganglion or the second thoracic ganglion. The stellate ganglion often supplies fibers to the sixth, seventh, and eighth cervical nerves, the first and second thoracic nerves, and to the vertebral artery.

The trunk between the mid and lower cervical ganglia can be double, including the subclavian artery. The more superficial cord may form a loop that sends branches to the sympathetic innervation of the artery, called the subclavian loop.

Thoracolumbar Sympathetic Chain

There is a change of direction of the paravertebral sympathetic chain at the transition between its cervical and thoracic portion. The cervical portion of the chain is located ventral to the transverse processes and to the vertebral bodies, due to the presence of the long neck muscle. When it enters the thorax, the chain goes backwards, circumvents the transverse process of the seventh cervical vertebra, and happens to be located on the lap of the ribs.

The thoracolumbar sympathetic trunk receives preganglionic fibers from every intermediate column of the medulla (T1 to L2, eventually collaborations from C8 and T3). It is covered by the costal portion of the parietal pleura and the interganglion fibers are between the pleura and the intercostal vessels. The fibers T1 to T5 enter the thoracolumbar trunk, but do not synapse, going directly to the cervical ganglia. Some of the T6 to T12 fibers form gray communicating branches and synapse in the paravertebral sympathetic chain giving rise to postganglionic fibers that will go to the skin to exert control over piloerection, sweat secretion, and vasomotricity. Another part of these fibers does not synapse in the thoracolumbar trunk and will form the splanchnic nerves. The L1 to L2 (or L3) fibers descend into the lumbosacral trunk to innervate the pelvis and genitals, as is studied below.

The postganglionic fibers of the T2, T3, and T4 thoracic ganglia are responsible for innervation of the face, axillary region, and hands. The second thoracic ganglion is usually located in the second intercostal space at the level of the cervical vertebrae of C2 and C3. Fusion may occur between the first and second thoracic ganglia and between the star ganglion and the second ganglion, as already mentioned. The first five thoracic ganglia provide branches to the cardiac, pulmonary, esophageal, and aortic plexuses.

Branches of the seven lower thoracic ganglia join to form three thoracic splanchnic nerves, which cross the diaphragm and provide sympathetic innervation to the abdominal organs. These nerves are composed mostly of preganglionic fibers that did not synapse in the sympathetic chain and will innervate neurons present in the glands of the pre-vertebral chain.

The major splanchnic nerve is formed by fibers from T5 to T9. In the thorax, it participates in the innervation of the esophagus, thoracic aorta, and thoracic duct. Its fibers then cross the diaphragm and terminate in the celiac ganglion, at the level of the first lumbar vertebra, behind the stomach and the small omentum, in front of the crura of the diaphragm and the abdominal aorta, between the adrenal glands. Celiac ganglion synapses in it give rise to postganglionic fibers that will innervate the pancreas, gallbladder, and stomach. Another group of fibers does not synapse and goes directly to form the adrenal plexus. The preganglionic fibers that innervate the adrenal gland, as already mentioned, synapse directly with the chromaffin stem cells. These cells have the same embryological origin as the postganglionic neurons, both developing from the neural crest. They secrete catecholamines into the bloodstream, especially epinephrine (adrenaline).

The smaller splanchnic nerve is formed by branches of T10 and T11 and travels along with the larger splanchnic nerve until it crosses the diaphragm. Its fibers terminate in the aorticorenal ganglion, located at the origin of the renal artery and responsible for the sympathetic innervation of the kidneys and part of the aorta. One part of the fibers collaborates to form the superior mesenteric ganglion, which will innervate the pancreas and small intestine.

The inferior splanchnic nerve is formed by fibers of T12 or possibly by fibers of the minor splanchnic nerve. It also crosses the diaphragm with the other two splanchnic nerves and participates in the formation of the renal plexus.

Lumbo-Sacral Sympathetic Chain

The abdominal portion of the sympathetic chain is located in the anterolateral region of the vertebral column, accompanying the medial border of the psoas major muscle. The lumbar and sacral paravertebral sympathetic chain receives preganglionic fibers descended from the T10 to L3 segments. There are cross-communications between the two chains below L5.

The preganglionic fibers of L1 to L2 (or L3) contribute to the formation of two or three lumbar splanchnic nerves, which descend in front of the aorta and bifurcate upon reaching the pelvis. These nerves provide fibers to the lower mesenteric ganglion, which participates in the innervation of the colon and is part of the upper hypogastric plexus and hypogastric nerves, which accompany the ureters and participate in the formation of the lower hypogastric plexus within the pelvis. The hypogastric plexuses are located in front of the fifth lumbar vertebra, between the two common iliac arteries. Fibers from these plexuses innervate the rectum, vas deferens, bladder, ureters, and prostate.

The sacrococcygeal trunk, composed of five sacral ganglia and one odd coccygeal ganglion, receives fibers originating from T12 and L1. These structures are located in front of the sacrum, medial to the anterior sacral foramen. These ganglia, together with fibers originating in the lower hypogastric plexus, form the pelvic plexus, responsible for the sympathetic innervation of part of the bladder and prostate, the male and female reproductive organs, and the vasomotricity of the lower limbs.

Neuroeffective Junctions and Neurotransmitters

When they reach the target organs, the postganglionic fibers exhibit small dilatations, from which neurotransmitters are released.

In the classical model, all the pre-ganglionic fibers of the ANS and the postganglionic parasympathetics have acetylcholine as the only neurotransmitter, and norepinephrine would be the only neurotransmitter of the sympathetic postganglionic fibers. Knowledge about neurotransmitters has evolved a lot in recent decades. The existence of several other neurotransmitters is known today, in particular in the parasympathetic intestinal nervous system. Most are peptides and coexist with classic neurotransmitters. Several modulatory substances influence the action of neurotransmitters, mainly at the level of the target organs. Such substances may act by modifying the release of neurotransmitters or their efficacy. Tissue metabolites and hormones are part of this class of substances.

Much of what is known today about the physiology of ANS is due to observation of the actions of different pharmacological substances on individual portions of the system. Receptors for acetylcholine in ANS are classically of two types: nicotinic in autonomic ganglia (so-called because they can be activated by nicotine) and muscarinic in target organs (activated by muscarine). Initially, only two types of receptors for norepinephrine were believed to exist and they were classified as alpha or beta. Alpha receptors are found in smooth muscles and also in some secretory glands, while beta receptors are located in the heart, promoting increased heart rate and the strength of contractions.

Skin- and Vessel-Specific Aspects

Sympathetic innervation of the skin presents particularities. Stimulation of the ANSs promotes hair erection, vasoconstriction, and increased secretion of sweat, promoting loss of body heat. ANSp does not participate in the innervation of sweat glands and hair.

The sweat glands of the skin are innervated by postganglionic sympathetic cholinergic fibers in their majority (unlike the classic model). These fibers act on sweat glands that cover the whole body, stimulating muscarinic receptors and promoting the release of sweat. Other substances are released together with acetylcholine, such as bradykinin and vasoactive intestinal peptide, promoting vasodilation around these glands.

The secretion of odorous glands from sweat of the axilla, areolar region, and pubic region is controlled by sympathetic adrenergic postganglionic fibers, which promote the contraction of arterioles and secretion of these glands.

Autonomic control over the different blood vessels in the body is not fully understood. Most arterioles, capillaries, and veins are innervated by sympathetic fibers. The density of nerve endings varies according to the caliber of the vessel, being greater in vessels of smaller caliber. Most receptors are alpha-1, promoting vasoconstriction, but there are some beta receptors, which promote vasodilation. Thus, the same adrenergic stimulus may promote vasoconstriction in some vascular territories and vasodilation in others (e.g., in the coronary arteries). The sympathetic effects on these vessels are more evident in the splanchnic region, in the skin, and in the muscles.

Sympathetic stimulation promotes paleness in the skin and decreased circulation in the mucous membranes. Injection of epinephrine or other sympathomimetic drugs promotes vasoconstriction and increased blood pressure. The action of the SNAp on the caliber of the vessels seems to be of less importance than the sympathetic action.

Communicating Branches

As already described, shortly after exiting the medial portion of the marrow, the sympathetic fibers pass through a mixed nerve and enter the paravertebral sympathetic chain through a white communicating branch. The fibers that leave the sympathetic chain return to the intercostal nerve through the gray communicating branch. Normally, each segment of the sympathetic chain supplies fibers to the intercostal nerve at the same level, and vice versa. However, microscopic studies have shown that there is a wide variability in the nerve connections between the spinal cord, the sympathetic chain, and the sympathetic nerves. A network of nerve fibers of various sizes interconnects these structures. In fact, studies on corpses and intraoperative findings have shown that there is great anatomical variation between the communicating branches of the uppermost part of the thoracic chain. There are ascending branches, which communicate a ganglion to an intercostal nerve of a higher level, and descending branches. It is believed that this anatomical variation may contribute to some cases of recurrence or even failure of the sympathectomy, since even after the apparently adequate denervation of one or more levels of the thoracic sympathetic chain, alternative pathways through these branches can maintain innervation in the area affected by hyperhidrosis. There are authors who argue that the interruption of these inconstant sympathetic pathways may contribute to a decrease in the rare cases of failure of the operation.

A sympathetic ganglion may give rise to more than one communicating branch. In most cases, there are at least two branches to the second thoracic ganglion, which is the one with the greatest anatomical variation among the thoracic sympathetic ganglia. In only 15% of the individuals studied, the anatomy of the communicating branches was similar.

Kuntz Nerve

One of the types of communication that deserves special attention is the intrathoracic branch (or Kuntz nerve), which communicates the ventral branch of the first thoracic nerve to the second intercostal nerve.

In clinical studies, the incidence of the Kuntz nerve is approximately 60%. Studies on corpses have demonstrated that the presence in the Kuntz nerve occurs in up to 68% of the cases, being bilateral in 48%. In only 7.6% of the cases studied, their presence or the existence of ascending communicating branches were not observed starting from the second thoracic nerve. In the same study, the presence of the star ganglion was observed in 84% of the patients and the fusion between the star ganglion and the second thoracic ganglion occurred in 9.1% of the cases, forming a single large ganglion. The second thoracic ganglion generally (50%) was located in the second intercostal space.

Some authors argue that resection of the Kuntz nerve, when it exists, is essential for the success of the surgery. However, when the clipping technique for the sympathetic blockade of the second thoracic ganglion (above and below the ganglion) is used, the Kuntz nerve fibers are preserved, but this does not cause an increase in the failure rate of the surgery. Thus, there are still doubts about the role of the Kuntz nerve in STE surgery.

Suggested Reading

Cho HM, Lee DY, Sung SW. Anatomical variations of rami communicantes in the upper thoracic sympathetic trunk. Eur J Cardiothorac Surg. 2005;27(2):320–4.

Chung IH, Oh CS, Koh KS, Kim HJ, Paik HC, Lee DY. Anatomic variations of the T2 nerve root (including the nerve of Kuntz) and their implications for sympathectomy. J Thorac Cardiovasc Surg. 2002;123(3):498–501.

Goetz CG. Textbook of clinical neurology. 2nd ed. Philadelphia: W.B. Saunders Company; 2003.

Kloot ER, Drukker J, Lemmens HA, Greep JM. The high thoracic sympathetic nerve system – its anatomic variability. J Surg Res. 1986;40(2):112–9.

Lin CC, Wu HH. Kuntz's fiber: the scapegoat of surgical failure in sympathetic surgery. Ann Chir Gynaecol. 2001;90(3):170–1.

Loewy AD, Spyer M. Central regulation of autonomic functions. Oxford: Oxford University Press; 1990.

Singh B, Ramsaroop L, Partab P, Moodley J, Satyapal KS. Anatomical variations of the second thoracic ganglion. Surg Radiol Anat. 2005;27(2):119–22.

Wolosker N, Kauffman P. Upper extremity sympathectomy. In: Rutherford's vascular surgery, vol. II, cap 124. 8th ed. Philadelphia: Elsevier; 2014. p. 1923–35.

Criteria for Surgical Patient Selection

18

Sérgio Kuzniec and Paulo Kauffman

Until the last decade of the twentieth century, the surgical treatment of primary hyperhidrosis consisted of open sympathectomy. Access options involved explorations of the supraclavicular fossa, cervicotomies, thoracotomies, or retroperitoneal explorations by the flanks, depending on the portion of the sympathetic chain to be excised. The aggressiveness of this approach brought high morbidity, restricting the surgical indication to more severe and selected cases.

In the 1990s this aspect changed. The technological development of videosurgery made it possible to approach the sympathetic chain through small incisions, with minimal surgical trauma. These mini incisions became sufficient for the introduction of operative equipment and visibility of the procedure with safety. In this way, sympathectomy has been offered as an effective treatment of hyperhidrosis to more and more patients. The operation has become more secure, standardized, and effective. Several publications showed nuances and technical variations, mainly related to thoracic sympathectomy, directed at the treatment of palmar, axillary, or craniofacial hyperhidrosis, and to facial flushing.

However, negative repercussions of sympathectomy emerged, mainly related to compensatory sweating. Although the vast majority of operated patients were satisfied with the result obtained, even with the constant occurrence of increased sweating in other areas of the body, some definitely regretted having undergone the operation, sometimes with severe psychological or social repercussions.

S. Kuzniec (✉)
Hospital Israelita Albert Einstein, São Paulo, SP, Brazil

P. Kauffman
Department of Vascular and Endovascular Surgery, University of São Paulo School of Medicine, São Paulo, SP, Brazil

Sympathectomy should be considered as definitive. Once performed, methods of reversing the operation are controversial, just as drug treatment of compensatory sweating is not fully effective.

The major problem, therefore, ceased to be operative aggressiveness and became selection of patients who would benefit most from the reduction of hyperhidrosis with less possibility of regret.

The diagnosis of hyperhidrosis is made by clinical criteria, based on personal history and clinical examination. There is no specific laboratory or imaging test for confirmation. It should be ruled out whether it is secondary to another condition (secondary hyperhidrosis, e.g., in neuropathies or hormonal disorders). Clinical criteria are the presence of visible focal sweating for at least 6 months, with no other obvious causes, aligned with at least two of the following criteria: bilateral and symmetrical, affecting daily activities, occurring more than once a week, had started before the age of 25, a family history of hyperhidrosis, and absence of night sweats. Sweating is clearly influenced by emotional status and stress situations.

There are devices to measure sweating volume but they are not practical for clinical use, only as research equipment.

Primary hyperhidrosis is a disease that affects quality of life. Excessive sweating can become intolerable and interfere intensively with daily activities. It does not cause damage to the body, but it restricts, on a variable scale, social, affective, professional, and functional aspects. Thus, when we offer therapeutic options, mainly surgical, risks and adverse effects should be well understood, emphasizing compensatory sweating in the case of sympathectomy and local effects in the excision operations of axillary glands.

Those who have hyperhidrosis, but do not feel restrictions or do not have the quality of life impaired by it, should not be operated. More objectively, evaluation of quality of life is performed with a specific questionnaire that scores several areas, such as professional, affective, and functional. For all patients, this questionnaire should be answered at the first evaluation, since the option of surgery will only be offered to those who present poor scores in this questionnaire, indicating poor or very poor quality of life, in aspects related to hyperhidrosis. The worse the quality of life before treatment, the greater the improvement obtained after the procedure.

Initial treatment of primary hyperhidrosis is conservative. If the patient gains relief from their symptoms without limiting adverse effects, it avoids invasive treatment. Initially, topical therapy is offered, but this may be effective only in milder cases. Iontophoresis may result in temporary improvement of palmar and plantar hyperhidrosis, but it has a low adherence because it takes time to achieve results and because of its temporary nature.

Injection of botulinum toxin also solves hyperhidrosis with temporary results. It is a high-cost treatment with an average durability of less than 1 year and can satisfy patients prone to repeat injections. However, some patients who experience the hyperhidrosis-free period offered by temporary localized treatments will seek something more definitive.

Systemic anticholinergic drugs are effective in reducing sweating at the expense of frequent adverse effects with mucosal thinning. However, it has been observed that with doses lower than those recommended for these drugs when used for other purposes, such as urinary incontinence, hyperhidrosis can be relieved without undesirable effects, or at least to a lesser extent and with tolerance. The standardization of the use of oxybutynin for the different types of hyperhidrosis allowed a greater acceptance and, therefore, reduction of the need for operative treatment for many patients who were did not respond to topical treatments.

The operation is offered to patients who have already undergone conservative treatment and who either have not had success or opted for definitive treatment. Because hyperhidrosis is neither lethal nor does it produce relevant organic morbidity, patients should not be operated without belief in their acceptance of possible undesirable effects, and nor should they be operated on if there is any risk or clinical limitation.

Most hyperhidrosis patients are healthy young adults. The basic preoperative evaluation is sufficient to eliminate or adjust any eventual clinical problem. Excess weight is a predictor of more compensatory sweating in the postoperative period. The higher the body mass index (BMI), the greater the degree of compensatory sweating, but this does not always cause regret after the operation. In any case, it is suggested to restrict surgical treatment to those with a BMI below 25. If possible, stimulate weight loss as a preparation for the operation in order for it to be safer and more effective.

Videothoracoscopic sympathectomy is performed via the virtual cavity between the visceral and parietal pleurae, which spontaneously move away with the entrance of air (or other gas or liquid). Previous pulmonary diseases, such as recurrent bronchopneumonias, tuberculosis, empyema, pneumothorax, rib fracture trauma, thoracic operations, and other possible conditions that cause pleural adhesion predict difficulty or even the impossibility of performing the operation safely. Pre-operative radiography or other imaging tests can sometimes inform the degree and difficulty to be found in the operation. The clinical history of the patient is the best predictor of adherence.

Individual psychological factors may predispose to failure. Anxiety is a common trait in these patients, and waiting for a perfect result may frustrate them when an adverse effect occurs as a result of the operation, even if discreet. Prior psychological analysis selects patients with this risk, and this is discussed in Chap. 7.

Suggested Reading

Cameron AE. Selecting the right patient for surgical treatment of hyperhidrosis. Thorac Surg Clin. 2016;26(4):403–6.
De Campos JR, Wolosker N, Takeda FR, et al. The body mass index and level of resection: predictive factors for compensatory sweating after sympathectomy. Clin Auton Res. 2005;15(2):116–20.
Hoorens I, Ongenae K. Primary focal hyperhidrosis: current treatment options and a step-by-step approach. J Eur Acad Dermatol Venereol. 2012;26(1):1–8.
Wolosker N, Kauffman P. Upper extremity sympathectomy. In: Rutherford's vascular surgery, vol. vol II, cap 124. 8th ed. Philadelphia: Elsevier; 2014. p. 1923–35.
Wolosker N, Yazbek G, de Campos JR, et al. Quality of life before surgery is a predictive factor for satisfaction among patients undergoing sympathectomy to treat hyperhidrosis. J Vasc Surg. 2010;51(5):1190–4.

Surgical Techniques for the Realization of Thoracic Sympathectomy

19

Eduardo de Campos Werebe, Carlos Levischi, and Rodrigo Sabbion

Introduction

Primary hyperhidrosis does not have a well-established cause. Anatomically, we know that there is a sudomotor efferent pathway that originates in the cerebral cortex and makes connections in the hypothalamus and medulla, crosses before the bridge, descends through the lateral horn of the spinal tract, connects to the sympathetic ganglion, and reaches the sweat glands by fibers postganglionic. The neurotransmitter is acetylcholine, which binds to the muscarinic receptors of the sweat glands [1]. This activation is part of an atavistic neural response that prepares the individual to run or fight and is mediated by the sympathetic autonomic nervous system [2–8].

The fight–flight reaction involves a complex model involving the central nervous system (CNS), adrenal system, and autonomic nervous system in target organs [9].

In the CNS, the stimulus of fear can occur in two ways. The first involves the cortex, and the second involves the amygdala and is very rapid [10].

The more proximal the pathway, the more intense the stimulus. In the case of the fight–flight response, the pathway is proximal with intense stimulus.

Basically, there are two ways in which the fear stimulus can travel—the high road and the low road:

- The high pathway involves the adrenocortical system.
- The lower lane involves the amygdala and the sympathetic system.

The autonomic nervous system is divided into sympathetic and parasympathetic. In the case of the low path in the fight–flight response, only the sympathetic is activated. Several actions of the autonomic nervous system occur in the various target

---

E. de Campos Werebe (✉) · C. Levischi · R. Sabbion
Hospital Israelita Albert Einstein, São Paulo, SP, Brazil

© Springer International Publishing AG, part of Springer Nature 2018
M. P. Loureiro et al. (eds.), *Hyperhidrosis*,
https://doi.org/10.1007/978-3-319-89527-7_19

organs. In the skin, the sympathetic response involves bruising, vasodilation, and sweating.

The effector stimulus leaves the marrow through the anterior branch, meets the spinal nerve, and through its anterior branch travels the communicating branches to the ganglion in the sympathetic chain.

In the case of the sweat glands, the sympathetic preganglionic branch is short and the postganglionic branch is long. The neurotransmitter is acetylcholine, which binds to the muscarinic receptors. In the anatomy of the skin we can observe the existence of sweat glands, eccrines, and apocrines. Those responsible for hyperhidrosis are the eccrine glands. They have no association with the hair follicle and can produce the equivalent of 10 L of sweat per day, if an individual would sweat all day long. We must remember that the pathways assume anatomical variations that may affect the final response to an intervention in the sympathetic system.

Typical primary hyperhidrosis is diagnosed clinically. There are no commercially available tests to quantify it effectively and, in addition, they would not be able to stablish a differential diagnosis to secondary hyperhidrosis. The typical clinical findings are exaggerated sweating that is localized, has occurred since childhood, with a family history, linked to emotion, and does not occur during sleep.

Scientists from Newcastle in England have shown that wrinkled hands and feet increase the adhesion of these surfaces, improving performance when moist [3]. This fact may be related to the fight–flight response, increasing grip in the hands and feet and explaining why 90% of primary hyperhidrosis occurs in these regions. A US publication has studied these effects in primates in depth [11]. They compared this phenomenon with flat or furrowed tires and speculate that in wet conditions this phenomenon would increase the grip of the primates.

The main differential diagnoses are panic syndrome and secondary hyperhidrosis. Both have a major impact on the outcome of surgical treatment of hyperhidrosis.

Panic syndrome typically begins suddenly, during adolescence or young adulthood. Sweating is usually widespread and can occur during sleep. Hyperhidrosis is not usually the predominant symptom, occurring simultaneously with tachycardia, chest pain, dry mouth, perception of death, depersonalization, suffocation, tingling, and tremors.

Secondary hyperhidrosis occurs through several different stimuli, unrelated to fear, has a later onset, may occur during sleep, and is not localized. Sympathectomy often triggers or worsens its manifestation. As there are no examinations to differentiate it from primary hyperhidrosis, and definitive treatment may worsen it, the therapeutic choice must be made with great care.

The treatments can be divided into palliative or definitive, and the palliative effect is dependent on its use. Among the several forms of palliation, we highlight the use of anticholinergic drugs.

On the other hand, the universally validated definitive treatment is sympathectomy. Among the surgical forms, we believe that sympathectomy with ganglion ablation will provide two complementary effects for the control of typical primary hyperhidrosis. Effect A involves the anterior effector branch of the sympathetic system and has the effect of abolishing the eccrine sweat action at that treated level. Effect B involves the exchange of afferent and efferent information between the limbic system and the sympathetic system, improving the effect of the fight–flight response. In this sense, secondary hyperhidrosis in untreated body regions may appear or worsen. Surgery is indicated only in cases of typical primary hyperhidrosis, in order to avoid the onset and/or worsening of secondary hyperhidrosis.

Thoracic Sympathectomy Surgical Techniques

Introduction

In order to offer the best treatment for patients with primary palmar hyperhidrosis, improving their psychological symptoms, social, and occupational challenges, we have to keep in mind some important concepts. Conservative treatment is not always effective, and sometimes patients are not compliant to use medication indefinitely. When this occurs and other forms of treatment are not accepted, surgery becomes the best option for definitive treatment [12].

Surgical techniques that open through the posterior, transaxillary, or supraclavicular spinal muscles are currently avoided for a variety of reasons, among them a very high morbidity for the disease in question associated with an aesthetic result that is currently unacceptable. Due to all of the reasons given earlier, minimally invasive surgery is the gold standard for the treatment of hyperhidrosis. While minimally invasive surgery is understood as the use of the videothoracoscope, this is now being extended to other techniques such as endoscope use, as discussed later in this chapter.

With the advent of video and advancement in endoscopic video-assisted techniques, the thoracoscopic approach, first described by Kux in 1951, has undergone rapid progression and is now widely accepted as the approach of choice [13]. Further discussion has upraised regarding the technique to be used: although the video-assisted approach has been accepted as the approach of choice with minimal postoperative morbidity and near perfect success rate [14–16], the optimal technique remains controversial. Many aspects have to be reviewd such as method of interrupting the sympathetic chain, level of intervention and thoracic approach.

The optimal procedure, or the best option, such as sympathicotomy or sympathectomy (excision), remains also controversial. What is the best form of sympathetic chain ablation: use of electrocautery or other forms of energy?

In this chapter we will discuss all of the questions raised here and describe the techniques employed, the numerous variants available, combinations of techniques, patient positioning and/or trocars, materials used, sympathetic operated levels, and the section method used. Each of these is discussed in detail, including a description of the technique used and the results achieved.

Chain Approach and Patient Positioning

Anterior Approach

In the anterior approach [12], general anesthesia is induced and intubation is performed with a double lumen endotracheal tube to allow monopulmonary ventilation most of the time. This type of intubation is not mandatory; intubation can be performed with a simple tube and using apnea during the introduction of trocars and ablation of the sympathetic chain. In this method, the patient is placed in a semi-seated position, with an angle of 75 °, and the arms abducted 90 ° on the shoulder. The operating table is also inclined to 15 °. With this placement, the lung on the operated side falls toward the diaphragm.

After initiation of monopulmonary ventilation or apnea (in the case of intubation with single tube), a 5 or 10 mm trocar is inserted anteriorly into the pleural cavity generally in the fourth intercostal space. In this approach (the most commonly used) there are various incision sites that can be used, among them:

- the line of the mammary sulcus (in women), at the bisector of the external quadrant of the breast;
- the line of the pectoralis major (in men), in the bisector of the external quadrant of the muscle;
- fourth or fifth intercostal spaces in the anterior axilla line;
- incision infra-areolar, in the external quadrant of the areola (in men).

The first incision is used to place the 5 or 10 mm optics (camera) and guide the second trocar. The second incision is made in the third intercostal space in the median axillary line, 5 mm, for introduction of the working instrument.

After visual confirmation of the head of the second, third and forth ribs, the section of the sympathetic chain is made using the working instrument (scissors, electrocautery, or harmonic scalpel) through the 5 mm trocar of the third intercostal space.

Finally, the pleural cavity is evacuated through the lateral line, trough a cannula placement, and the trocars are removed under the application of continuous positive airway pressure. Usually muscle and skin are closed, and there is no need for thoracic drainage maintenance.

Posterior Approach

The use of the posterior approach [17] is justified by its authors due to the fact that in the lateral approach, the lung moves to the medial-ventral side and in the anterior approach, the lung moves caudally, partially obscuring the view of the sympathetic chain, which sometimes forces us to take the lungs out of the operative field using a work tool and this can cause injury leading to unwanted fistulas. In addition to these advantages, monopulmonary ventilation is unnecessary, thus using the simple endotracheal tube, which theoretically is less traumatic than a double lumen tube and may result in lower morbidity [18]. The tidal volume should be reduced by 30%; this reduction is compensated by a higher frequency of ventilation under capnographic control.

With the posterior approach, the lung moves to the ventral side of the thorax. Remarkably, after introduction of the videoendoscope, the sympathetic chain immediately appears, without the need for manipulation of the lung. This approach offers better visibility—according to its proponents—and, like the previous approach, bilateral treatment is possible in a single session without changing the patient's position (in contrast, repositioning is mandatory in the lateral approach). Better visibility and exposure of the sympathetic chain in relation to the other approaches is described as occurring with this technique.

The patient is placed in a jackknife position, with ventral decubitus and greater flexion in the hips, to obtain a thoracic kyphosis and to open the intercostal spaces as much as possible. The arms are bent 90 ° at the elbows, and the shoulders are maximally abducted. The forearms are immobilized with arm supports to lateralize the scapulae.

For the sympathetic chain approach by the posterior wall, a Verres needle is inserted into the pleural cavity through the sixth intercostal space, distally to the lower angle of the scapula. Pneumothorax is created by infusing 1000 mL of carbon dioxide with a maximum pressure of 4 mmHg. The Verres needle is then replaced by a 10 mm trocar suitable for the thoracoscope.

Two operative trocars are inserted medially into the scapula in the second and fourth intercostal spaces. One of these trocars is also suitable for a stapler device. The force of gravity moves the lungs to the ventral side of the thorax. This gives excellent visual exposure of the sympathetic chain without the need for pulmonary collapse or the use of a pulmonary valve. After locating the second to fifth ribs, the parietal pleura medial to the sympathetic chain is incised with an electrosurgical hook. The T2 to T4 thoracic ganglia and their interconnecting fibers are resected by electrocoagulation.

The sympathetic chain distal to the star ganglion is resected by scissors without the use of electrocoagulation to avoid damage to this ganglion. In the case of face hyperhidrosis or flushing, resection of the distal third of the starved ganglion with scissors is described.

After the sympathectomy, a chest drain is placed through a trocar and suction drainage of 10 cm H_2O is applied, and the lung is inflated under direct camera vision. The procedure is repeated on the other side during the same operation without the need to change the patient's position.

All patients in the described series were treated postoperatively with chest drainage for at least 24 h. Although recent literature shows that routine thoracic drainage is unnecessary, some authors emphasize that postoperative pneumothorax can be a cause of serious complications.

Lateral Approach

In the lateral approach [19], the patient is positioned in the lateral decubitus position, with cushions placed in the tip of the scapula. The legs are positioned so that the ipsilateral leg is flexioned, and the contralateral extended, with protection between them. The ipsilateral arm to the decubitus is extended, while the arm above is positioned with a 90 ° angle between the shoulder and the middle axillary line and also the elbow. The intubation is selective.

After the patient is positioned, the operative side is collapsed and the pleural cavity is accessed by two trocars. The incisions are made in the second or third intercostal space in the mid axillary line (trocarter of 5 mm), and in the fifth intercostal space in the posterior axillary line (5 or 10 mm). Generally the patient should be rotated to allow gravity to retract the lung away from the surface of the spine.

After these steps, all the chain and the chain section itself should be identified. In the series described, surgery was terminated by the introduction of a single thoracic tube number 16F connected to the active suction of −20 cm H_2O, for 24 hours and withdrawn in the immediate postoperative period or first PO - postoperative day.

The great disadvantage of this technique, besides the mandatory use of selective intubation, is that the patient must be repositioned and the same surgical procedure must be performed on the opposite side.

Chain Section Methods: Sympathectomy Versus Sympathicotomy, Clipping, or Ramicotomy

Among the various nuances that have emerged over the course of the use of the thoracoscopic technique, a constant concern is the possibility of neural regeneration with recurrence of symptoms when the trunk is only cauterized (sympathicotomy) or there is no resection (as regularly in sympathectomy).

In the studies conducted to compare the two thoracoscopic procedures of sympathicotomy and sympathectomy for hyperhidrosis [15, 16, 20], Collin [15] reported recurrence in four of 54 patients treated by sympathectomy with scissors in the second rib within 9–12 months after the procedure; Kuda et al. [20] reported that there was no difference in recurrence between sympathicothomy and sympathectomy. In 2001, Bo-Young King et al., using what they called a "sympatheticotomy", but which can be interpreted as a "mixed technique", did not observe recurrence during the follow-up period after sympatheticotomy: "We think that reinnervation with recurrence of symptoms [does not is] a problem of the procedure itself but a matter of technique and can be prevented by cephalic cauterization of the chain and cauterization of the caudal sympathetic chain after separation".

To alleviate any doubt, Aydemir et al. [21] published a study in 2015, the objective of which was to evaluate and compare thoracoscopic sympathectomy and sympatheticotomy in the third level of ganglia (T3) for the treatment of primary palmar hyperhidrosis. In terms of initial surgical results, in relation to complications and satisfaction, the patient was followed up for 6 months postoperatively using a detailed interview and scored on a 1–3 scale (1 = very satisfied, 2 = satisfied and 3 = unsatisfied). In their results, no therapeutic failures occurred. The mean time of operation was 50 min for the sympathectomy group and 36 min for the sympatheticotomy group. Compensatory sweating occurred in 40 patients (89% for the sympathectomy group and 85.11% for the sympatheticotomy group). The satisfaction rate was 91.11% for the sympathectomy group and 93.61% for the sympatheticotomy group. Thus, there was no significant difference between thoracoscopic sympathectomy and sympatheticotomy of the third ganglion (T3) in the treatment of primary palmar hyperhidrosis in terms of initial surgical results, complications, and patient satisfaction.

To clarify whether sympatheticotomy is sufficient, Lin et al. in 2015 [22] carried out a prospective, randomized study with 200 patients. In this study, two groups of thoracic sympathectomy (R3) and thoracic sympatheticotomy were randomized plus racemic at the same level (R3+) ($n = 100$ each). Clinical observations were recorded over a 3-year follow-up period. The results showed that the curative rates of palmar and axillary hyperhidrosis were 100% for two groups. There was no statistically significant difference between the groups in the increase in left hand temperature after thoracic sympathetic nerve transection (3.6 ± 1.4 °C vs. 3.5 ± 1.3 °C), right hand increase (40% vs. 44%), recurrence rate (1% vs. 2%), and postoperative satisfaction rate (92% vs. 90%). However, the pain scores of the R3 group were significantly lower than those of the R3+group (3.0 ± 1.9 vs. 3.6 ± 1.9, $p < 0.05$).

Simple transection of the thoracic sympathetic chain is sufficient in the treatment of palmar hyperhidrosis, and there is no need for the ramicotomy.

The idea of the use of the ramicotomy only arose because of the possibility of denervation in a smaller area and, consequently, a lower rate of compensatory sweating. However, the study by Lee et al. [23] showed that although the rate of compensatory sweating with the use of the isolated ramicotomy is actually lower than in other methods, the patient satisfaction index is much worse with the use of isolated ramicotomy (around 67% vs. 90% with other methods). On the basis of these data the technique has practically been abandoned.

Another imagined form of sympatheticotomy is the use of chain clipping. Theoretically, this technique would be less invasive, have less postoperative pain, and provide the future possibility of reversion if the interruption of compensatory hyperhidrosis became a major factor.

The study conducted in 2015 by Hida et al. [24] compared the effects of sympatheticotomy by cutting or clamping on T3 in two outcomes—postoperative palmar transpiration and compensatory sweating—and also evaluated postoperative patient satisfaction.

They studied 289 patients undergoing sympathetic interruption bilaterally in T3 level for palmar hyperhidrosis. These patients were sent questionnaires by mail to assess the reported degree of postoperative palmar sweating and compensatory sweating, as well as their level of satisfaction. Of the 92 patients who responded to the questionnaire, 54 had been submitted to cut sympatheticotomy (cut group) and 38 by clamping (clipping group).

Sympathicotomy by T3 clamping was less effective in reducing the primary symptom of postoperative palmar sweating, but induced less compensatory sweating than cut sympathicotomy in T3. However, both methods were similar in relation to patient satisfaction. The degree of postoperative palmar sweating and the severity of compensatory sweating were inversely correlated with the degree of satisfaction of the patient.

Sympathic Chain Section Level

From the literature, we can observe some inferiority, when comparing sympathectomy without the need of ramicotomy. The use of the clipping was not as effective as the section of the chain, and the comparative postoperative between the two techniques is equivalent in terms of results.

With this in mind, the next question would be what level of the chain is most indicated to be sectioned, and to have an expected better outcome with lower indexes of compensatory sweating? Classically used levels were T2 and T3, or between these. The first study using the T4 level was performed by Lin in 2001 [25], with experience in 165 patients:

> Compensatory hyperhidrosis is one of the complications that surgeons strive to avoid. We have found that the preservation of the sympathetic chain to the head is the main influent factor to avoid reflex sweating in sympathicotomies; and with the sympathetic lower ganglion blocked, the sympathetic tonus for the head is preserved. T4 sympathetic block is an ideal procedure that can treat palmar and/or axillary hyperhidrosis and preserve most of the sympathetic tone to the head. We used sympathetic-T4 block in the treatment of 165 cases of palmar hyperhidrosis and axillary and we obtained excellent operative results without reflex sweating, from August 1, 2000 to February 28, 2001. We conclude that sympatheticotomy at the T4 level is the method that can treat the hand and axillary hyperhidrosis without inducing reflex sweating.

Following this line of reasoning, several other studies have been published with the same objective, and the vast majority of them corroborated Lin et al.'s conclusions, both in patient satisfaction index and in related complications: occurrence of compensatory hyperhidrosis is lower than following the use of higher chains, and even when present it is classified as "extremely uncomfortable" by only 3.2%. The satisfaction index for the surgery reaches an average of 94% and, incredibly (perhaps because of the compensatory hyperhidrosis being smaller), the remaining 6% who were not satisfied did not regret the operation [26].

Uniportal Versus Multiportal

Currently the most commonly used surgical technique for the sympathetic chain section is the anterior approach, with the patient sitting. Because it is a minimally invasive surgery and a non-malignant disease, the desire for favorable results, reduction of morbidity (mainly postoperative pain), and patient satisfaction became an obsession. In addition to these requirements, and since the vast majority of patients are young, aesthetic concerns are also a point of great interest.

Uniportal techniques (either with a single portal in the mammary furrow or in the third axillary space) have gained ground, and the choice varies depending on surgeon experience and patient preference. But would there be any gain with this technique?

Ibrahim and Allam [27] conducted a study comparing the two techniques (uniportal and multiportal) with 71 patients, of whom 35 were submitted to a multiportal technique and 36 to a uniportal technique. Preoperative, intraoperative, and postoperative variables were compared: morbidity, recurrence, and mortality.

The final results showed that the procedure was successful in 100% of patients; none presented recurrence of palmar hyperhidrosis, Horner's syndrome (oculomatous paralysis), severe postoperative complications, or death. There was no need for conversion to an open procedure.

In the postoperative period, with a multiportal technique, there was residual minimal pneumothorax in two patients (5.7%), while in the other group there was only one (2.8%). A minimum hemothorax occurred in one patient (2.9%) in the multiportal group and three patients (8.3%) in the uniportal group. Compensatory hyperhidrosis occurred in seven patients (20%) in the multiportal group and eight patients (22.2%) in the uniportal group.

With these results, the authors' conclusion was that no difference was found between the multi- and uniportal methods. Both are minimally invasive, effective, and safe procedures that permanently improve quality of life in patients with palmar hyperhidrosis.

Types of Energy

With the advent of technology applied to minimally invasive procedures, other forms of energy for tissue dissection and sectioning emerged with promises of lower postoperative pain, increased safety due to less heat dissipation in tissues, less neuromuscular stimulation, and less smoke in the operative field. These new forms of energy also entered our milieu and became a real option for procedures, among them sympathicotomy. But would the use of these new forms of energy make any difference in practice?

The 2015 Th2–Th4 study by Kuhajda et al. [28] was performed in 79 patients with palmar, axillary, or craniofacial hyperhidrosis. All patients were approached laterally, with 2 5 mm portals: the first in the medial axillary line, third space, and the second in the fifth space, posterior axillary line. The chain was sectioned on two, three, and four ribs bilaterally and ablated laterally the chain by 4–5 cm to section possible accessory branches. In the first 39 patients, section of the chain was performed with an electric scalpel and in the next 40 patients the harmonic scalpel was used.

In this study, no significant differences were found between the electric or harmonic scalpel. There was no significant difference between complications and severity of pain, with a slightly higher intensity of pain using harmonic scalpel ($p < 0.05$). Both provided adequate treatment for primary hyperhidrosis, although the electric scalpel had lower costs.

Besides the harmonic scalpel, there is another option for energy: ultrasonic. Divisi et al. [29] compared ultrasound scalpel section (ligature) and radiofrequency in terms of complications and effectiveness. A total of 130 sympathectomies were performed in 65 patients: electrocoagulation was performed in 20 procedures (15%), ultrasonic scalpel in 54 (42%), and radiofrequency dissection in 56 (43%).

Twelve complications (9%) were observed: thoracic pain in six patients (four with electrocoagulation, one with ultrasonic scalpel, and one with radiofrequency dissector); paresthesias in three patients with electrocoagulation; bradycardia in one ultrasound patient, normalized at the fourth postoperative hour; and unilateral relapse in two patients with electrocoagulation. Assessment of quality-adjusted life-years and quality of life revealed a statistically significant improvement ($p = 0.02$) in excessive sweating and general satisfaction after surgery, with Ultracision® and LigaSure™ showing better findings than electrocoagulation.

This study concluded that the latest-generation devices offered greater effectiveness in the treatment of hyperhidrosis, minimizing complications and facilitating the resumption of normal work and social activity of patients; however, they did not take into account that the satisfaction rates with the use of electrocoagulation are comparable to the new devices, as well as a lower cost with the former.

It is up to each surgeon to make a decision regarding device use, taking into account evidence-based medicine, patient satisfaction, and their own self-assurance with the use of these new devices.

Other Techniques Described

Transareolar Uniportal Thoracic Sympathectomy Under Intravenous Anesthesia Without Intubation

The transareolar uniportal thoracic sympathectomy under intravenous anesthesia without intubation technique was described by Chen et al. [30] in a randomized controlled trial, with the objective of evaluating its viability and safety. Endocópio was used in the pleural cavity, the insertion of which was made by an infrareolar incision of 2 mm and the patient was anesthetized and using laryngeal masks.

A total of 168 male patients underwent endoscopic uniportal thoracic sympathectomy, divided into groups A or B. Group A patients underwent a non-intubated transareolar technique (with laryngeal mask) with an endoscope and a 2 mm needle, and the patients in group B underwent intubated transaxillary sympathectomy with a 5 mm thoracoscope.

According to the results of this study, all procedures were performed without intercurrences, and the palms of all patients became dry and warm immediately after surgery. The mean recovery time was significantly lower in non-intubated patients. Postoperative sore throat occurred in four patients in group A and 32 patients in group B ($p < 0.01$). The mean length of the incision was significantly shorter in group A than in group B and the mean postoperative pain scores were markedly higher in group B than in group A. The mean cost of anesthesia was considerably lower in non-intubated than intubated patients and the mean cosmetic scores were higher in group A than in group B ($p < 0.01$).

Transumbilical Thoracic Sympathectomy

The transumbilical thoracic sympathectomy technique was described in a single-center trial of 148 cases with up to 4 years of follow-up [31]. In the reports of this transumbilical thoracic sympathectomy technique , an ultrafine flexible endoscope inserted into the umbilical region was used. After a 5 mm umbilical incision, the muscular region of the diaphragmatic dome was incised and the bronchoscope positioned in the thoracic cavity. The sympathetic chain was identified at the desired thoracic level and sectioned with electrocautery with the biopsy forceps.

This is the newest and largest study to date, and used a prospective database in the retrospective analysis of 148 patients (61 males, 87 females, mean age 21.3 years) operated on by the same surgeon in a single institution from April 2010 to March 2014. All procedures were performed under general anesthesia with intubation with double lumen endotracheal tube. The demographic, postoperative, and long-term data of the patients were recorded and statistical analyses were performed. All patients were followed up for at least 6 months after the procedure through clinical visits or telephone/e-mail interviews.

The procedure was successfully performed in 148 of 150 patients. Two patients had to be converted to a conventional thoracoscopic procedure because of severe pleural adhesions. The mean operative time was 43 min (range 39–107 min) and the mean postoperative time was 1 day (range 1–4 days). All patients were interviewed 6–48 months after surgery and no diaphragmatic hernia or syndrome was observed. The resolution rate of hyperhidrosis and axillary hyperhidrosis was 98% and 74.6%, respectively. Compensatory sweating was reported in 22.3% of patients. Almost all patients were satisfied with the surgical results and the cosmetic result of the incision.

It is suggested that this technique could avoid chronic pain and chest wall paresthesia associated with the thoracic incision, besides providing cosmetic benefits.

Subxiphoid Thoracic Sympathectomy

Subxiphoid thoracic access was reported by Chen et al. [32] in a single patient of 34 years old who underwent bilateral sympathectomy at the T3 level.

The patient was positioned in proclive (reverse "Trendelemburg"), anesthetized, and ventilated with selective intubation. Using a 2 cm incision in the subxiphoid region, the surgeon manually dissected a subcostal tunnel and, with his finger, entered the pleural cavity. An on-site Alexis and 10 mm optics were inserted.

After the strand was severed, the pneumothorax was removed with the probe and the patient did not need a drain. The operative time described was 60 min.

The author discusses whether this technique is better in relation to the transumbilical because the transumbilical needs a very long trocarter to reach the thoracic cavity, bringing risks to the patient. According to the author, the subxiphoid technique also does not cause intercostal pain to the patient postoperatively.

Unilateral Sympathectomy for Hyperhidrosis

According to the various authors who have published on the unilateral sympathectomy approach, among them Ravari and Rajabnejad [33], one of the first to publish the technique with a considerable number (52) of patients, videothoracoscopic surgery with sympathectomy on the "dominant" side of the patients' symptoms would resolve bilateral hyperhidrosis.

In their series [33], from July 2010 to June 2013, 52 patients with primary palmar hyperhidrosis were submitted to unilateral video-assisted thoracoscopic sympathectomy for the dominant hand. Results were analyzed regarding the resolution of symptoms, occurrence of complications, rate of recurrence and compensatory hyperhidrosis, and need for surgery to the opposite side.

According to the authors, all patients were followed for 6–42 months. Palmar hyperhidrosis was completely relieved and absolute dryness was achieved in all patients in the same hand after the operation. Palmar hyperhidrosis in the opposite hand was cured until complete dryness in 24 (46.15%) patients. In 22 (42.3%) patients, there was no change in the opposite hand, but there was an increase in six (11.53%) patients. Only seven (13.46%) patients had to undergo contralateral sympathectomy. Compensatory hyperhidrosis occurred in 13 patients (25%) after unilateral sympathectomy. Five other patients (in total 18 [34.6%]) had compensatory hyperhidrosis after contralateral sympathectomy. It was mainly in the trunk in all 18 patients.

According to these authors, these numbers indicate that only a small number of patients will eventually need a contralateral sympathectomy in the non-dominant hand.

Prior Technical Design: Two Incisions

Anesthetic Induction
Patient will undergo general anesthesia with intubation oro-tracheally. The use of an oro-tracheal double lumen (broncocath) tube is optional; however, we see it as an advantage in most cases. If the single-track tube is chosen, the use of inhalation gases as a single anesthetic technique should be avoided, since the use of periods of apnea may lead to insufficient anesthesia.

Positioning
The patient is maintained in supine position until the end of anesthetic induction; having the anesthesiologist permission, the arms are positioned abductively—forming an angle of just over 90° relative to the trunk. The forearms are slightly flexed to avoid joint stress. Care should be taken at this time to avoid any distension to the brachial plexus structures. We also place a pillow under the patient's knees. After the positioning, the trunk is raised to a semi-seated position.

Incisions
We usually start the procedure on the left side, since we believe that after the left sympathectomy there may be a reduction in the heart rate, which is safer to evaluate soon after the beginning of the procedure—in the vast majority of cases, bradycardia is transient. We perform the first incision in the infra-mammary sulcus in females and in the areolar transition line in males. It is an incision approximately 6/7 mm to admit a 5 mm plastic disposable trocar. The subcutaneous tissue and musculature are crossed by blunt dissection using a pair of "Kelly" haemostatics or "Metzenbaum" scissors —. On the moment of entering into the pleural space, it is ideal to have the lung collapsed by bolcking it or just putting the patient is in apnea. The trocar is then introduced through the previously dissected course. Via this trocar a 4 or 5 mm camera with 30° viewing angle is introduced.

The next incision, which is between 5 and 6 mm, is performed in the axilla, in the middle axillary line, inferior to the region of the local ones. A permanent 5 mm trocar will be introduced; it enters the pleural cavity under direct vision. The instrument of dissection is positioned in this trocar, usually by use of the harmonic scalpel or a hook coupled to the electrocautery.

Sympathectomy

We first perform the opening of the parietal pleura on both sides of the sympathetic chain, at the fourth and fifth rib height, following the pleural opening throughout the medial and lateral portion of the chain. After the pleural opening we are able to clearly visualize the sympathetic chain. We begin with the complete section of the upper portion of the chain, and then proceed with the section of the lower portion, which is carried out in the medial portion of the rib to avoid the vascular-nervous bundle. With the chain released, we start the fulguration—it must retract completely freely; if this does not happen, probably some branches were not completely released.

Pulmonary Expansion and Aspiration of the Residual Air

With the end of the sympathectomy, a nasogastric tube is introduced via the axillary trocar as a drain. The anterior trocar is withdrawn through the camera, holding it in position to observe complete lung expansion. The anesthetist re-inflates the lung, and the probe is connected to a vacuum system. The camera is removed after confirmation that the lung is lying against the chest wall. The anterior incision is closed with 4.0 monocryl wire at continuous points. After closing it is necessary to check if there is aerial fistula; this is done by introducing the probe/drain into a vat filled with water or saline. The anesthesiologist ventilates the lung and checks for bubbles; if there is no vent after the maneuver, the catheter is removed and the incision is closed as above.

References

1. Lakraj A-AD, Moghimi N, Jabbari B. Hyperhidrosis: anatomy, pathophysiology and treatment with emphasis on the role of botulinum toxins. Toxins (Basel). 2013;5:821–40. http://www.mdpi.com/journal/toxins
2. Sheski FD, Mathur PN, Finlay G, editors. Therapeutic uses of medical thoracoscopy therapeutic uses of medical thoracoscopy Page 2 of 5. Alphen aan den Rijn: UptoDate; 2013. p. 1–5.
3. Changizi M, Weber R, Kotecha R, Palazzo J. Are wet-induced wrinkled fingers primate rain treads? Brain Behav Evol. 2011;77(4):286–90.
4. Vretzakis G, Simeoforidou M, Stamoulis K, Bareka M. Supraventricular arrhythmias after thoracotomy: is there a role for autonomic imbalance? Anesthesiol Res Pract. 2013;2013:413985.
5. Cerfolio RJ, De Campos JRM, Bryant AS, Connery CP, Miller DL, DeCamp MM, et al. The society of thoracic surgeons expert consensus for the surgical treatment of hyperhidrosis. Ann Thorac Surg. 2011;91(5):1642–8. https://doi.org/10.1016/j.athoracsur.2011.01.105.
6. Ribas Milanez de Campos J, Kauffman P, Wolosker N, Munia MA, de Campos Werebe E, Andrade Filho LO, et al. Axillary hyperhidrosis: T3/T4 versus T4 thoracic sympathectomy in a series of 276 cases. J Laparoendosc Adv Surg Tech A. 2006;16(6):598–603. http://www.ncbi.nlm.nih.gov/pubmed/17243877

7. Licht PB, Pilegaard HK, Ladegaard L. Sympathicotomy for isolated facial blushing: a randomized clinical trial. Ann Thorac Surg. 2012;94(2):401–5. http://www.ncbi.nlm.nih.gov/pubmed/22633477
8. Weng W, Liu Y, Zhou J, Li H, Yang F, Jiang G, et al. Thoracoscopic indocyanine green near-infrared fluorescence for thoracic sympathetic ganglions. Ann Thorac Surg. 2016;101(6):2394. http://linkinghub.elsevier.com/retrieve/pii/S0003497516002149
9. Janszky I, Szedmák S, Istók R, Kopp M. Possible role of sweating in the pathophysiology of panic attacks. Int J Psychophysiol. 1997;27(3):249–52.
10. Méndez-Bértolo C, Moratti S, Toledano R, Lopez-Sosa F, Martínez-Alvarez R, Mah YH, et al. A fast pathway for fear in human amygdala. Nat Neurosci. 2016;19(8):1041–9. https://doi.org/10.1038/nn.4324
11. Wilder-Smith EPV. Water immersion wrinkling: physiology and use as an indicator of sympathetic function. Clin Auton Res. 2004;14(2):125–31.
12. Kim BY, Oh BS, Park YK, Jang WC, Suh HJ, Im YH. Microinvasive video-assisted thoracoscopic sympathicotomy for primary palmar hyperhidrosis. Am J Surg. 2001;181(6):540–2. /das/journal/view/36919996-2/N/12595072?ja=301839&PAGE=1.html&ANCHOR=top&source=
13. Kux M. Thoracic endoscopic sympathicotomy in palmar and axillary hyperhidrosis. Arch Surg. 1978;113:264–6.
14. Adar R, Kurchin A, Zweig A, et al. Palmar hyperhidrosis and its surgical treatment: a report of 100 cases. Ann Surg. 1977;186:34–41.
15. Collin J. Treating hyperhidrosis surgery and botulinum toxin are treatments of choice in severe cases. BMJ. 2000;320:1221–2.
16. Johannes Z, Martin I, Erik RH, et al. Video assistance reduces complication rate of thoracoscopic sympathicotomy for hyperhidrosis. Ann Thorac Surg. 1999;68:1177–81.
17. Haan J, Mckaay AJ, Cuesta M, Rauwerda J. Posterior approach for the simultaneous, bilateral thoracoscopic sympathectomy. J Am Coll Surg. 2001;192(3):418–20. /das/journal/view/36919996-3/N/11742608?ja=318620&PAGE=1.html&ANCHOR=top&source=MI
18. Fredman B, Olsfanger D, Jedeikin R. Thoracoscopic sympathectomy in the treatment of palmar hyperhidrosis anaesthetic implications. Br J Anaesth. 1997;79:113–9.
19. Kuhajda I, et al. Semi-Fowler vs. lateral decubitus position for thoracoscopic sympathectomy in treatment of primary focal hyperhidrosis. J Thorac Dis. 2015;7(S1):S5–S11.
20. Kuda T, Oshiro J, Nagamine N, et al. Comparison of thoracoscopic sympathectomy and sympathicotomy for primary palmar hyperhidrosis. Chest. 1998;114(suppl 4):S391–2.
21. Aydemir B, Imamoglu O, Ok T, Celik M. Sympathectomy versus sympathicotomy in palmar hyperhidrosis comparing T3 ablation. Thorac Cardiovasc Surg. 2015;63(8):715–9.
22. Lin M, Tu Y, Chen J, Li X, Lai F, Lin J. Efficacy comparison of two methods of r3 sympathicotomy for palmar hyperhidrosis. Zhonghua Yi Xue Za Zhi. 2014;94(47):3745–7.
23. Lee DY, Paik HC, Kim fazem H, Kim HW. Comparative analysis of T3 selective division of rami communicantes (ramicotomy) to T3 sympathetic clipping in treatment of palmar hyperhidrosis. Clin Auton Res. 2003;1:I45–7.
24. Hida K, Sakai T, Hayashi M, Tamagawa T, Abe Y. Sympathotomy para hiperhidrose palmar: os métodos de corte versus clamping. Clin Auton Res. 2015;25(5):271–6. https://doi.org/10.1007/s10286-015-0293-y. Epub 2015 14 de maio
25. Lin CC, Wu HH. T4-sympathetic endoscopic locking by clamping (ESB4) in the treatment of hyperhidrosis palmaris et axillaris - experiences of 165 cases. Ann Chir Gynaecol. 2001;90(3):167–9.
26. Choi BC, Lee YC. Sim SB. Treatment of palmar hyperhidrosis by endoscopic cut of the upper part of the sympathetic ganglion T4. Preliminary results. Clin Auton Res. 2003;Suppl 1:I48–51.
27. M I, Allam A. Comparing two methods of thoracoscopic sympathectomy for palmar hyperidrosis. JAAPA. 2014;27(9):1–4.
28. Kuhajda I, Durie D, Koledin M, Ilic M. e cols. Electric vs. harmonic scalpel in treatment of primary focal hyperhidrosis with thoracoscopic sympathectomy. Ann Transl Med. 2015;3(15):211.

29. Divisi D, Di Leonardo G, De Vico A, Crisci R. Electrocautery versus Ultracision versus LigaSure in surgical management of hyperhidrosis. Thorac Cardiovasc Surg. 2015;63(8):729–34.
30. J C, Q D, M L, J L, X L, F L, Y T. Transareolar single port acute thoracic sympathectomy under intravenous anesthesia without intubation: a randomized controlled trial. J Laparoendosc Adv Surg Tech A. 2016;26(12):958–64.
31. Zhu LH, Chen W, Chen L, Yang S, Lu ZT. Transumbilical thoracic sympathectomy: a single-center trial of 148 cases with up to 4 years of follow-up. Eur J Cardiothorac Surg. 2016;49(Suppl 1):i79–83.
32. Chen JT, Liao CP, Chiang H, Wang B. Subxiphoid single-incision thoracoscopic bilateral ablative sympathectomy for hyperhidrosis. Interact Cardiovasc Thorac Surg. 2015;21:119–20.
33. H R, A R. Unilateral sympathectomy for primary palmar hyperhidrosis. Thorac Cardiovasc Surg. 2015;63(8):723–6.

Bilateral Thoracic Sympathectomy: How I Do It?

20

Davi Wen Wei Kang, Benoit Jacques Bibas, and Mauro Federico Luis Tamagno

Surgical Indications

The main indications for thoracic sympathectomy are primary or essential hyperhidrosis, facial flushing, ischemic pathologies of the hands, post-traumatic pain syndromes, long QT syndrome, thoracic angina, and Raynaud's phenomenon.

Primary hyperhidrosis can be palmar, plantar, axillary, or craniofacial, leading the patient to have psychosocial embarrassment, and creating problems in the educational, social, professional, and affective spheres (Figs. 20.1, 20.2, 20.3, 20.4).

The ischemic pathologies of the hands occur by arteritis leading to thrombophlebitis and distal arterial obstructions. Patients present digital ischemic lesions and intense pain of difficult control, as in the thromboangiitis obliterans. Thoracic sympathectomy promotes vasodilation, decreasing pain and delimiting distal tissue necrosis more quickly.

Post-traumatic pain syndromes, better known as causalgia or reflex sympathetic dystrophy, refer to burning pains, diffuse, with cutaneous hyperesthesia, vasomotor and sudomotor instability, and eventually edema. These phenomena occur due to injury to local nerves. Thoracic sympathectomy is useful for pain relief of the affected upper limb.

Long QT syndrome is an idiopathic, congenital arrhythmia with a broad QT interval on the electrocardiogram, which can lead to tachyarrhythmias, syncope, and sudden death. Thoracic sympathectomy (most often associated with continuous

---

D. W. W. Kang (✉)
Thoracic Surgeon at Hospital Israelita Albert Einstein, São Paulo, SP, Brazil

B. J. Bibas, MD
Department of Thoracic Surgery, University of São Paulo, São Paulo, SP, Brazil
e-mail: benoit.bibas@hc.fm.usp.br

M. F. L. Tamagno, MD
Thoracic Surgeon, São Paulo, SP, Brazil

© Springer International Publishing AG, part of Springer Nature 2018
M. P. Loureiro et al. (eds.), *Hyperhidrosis*,
https://doi.org/10.1007/978-3-319-89527-7_20

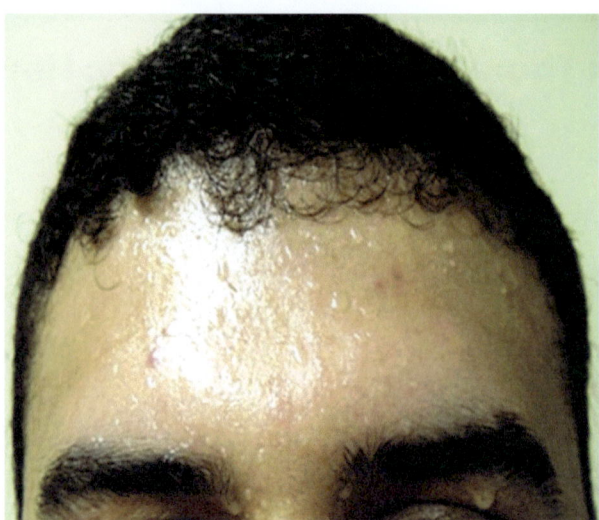

Fig. 20.1 Craniofacial hyperhidrosis

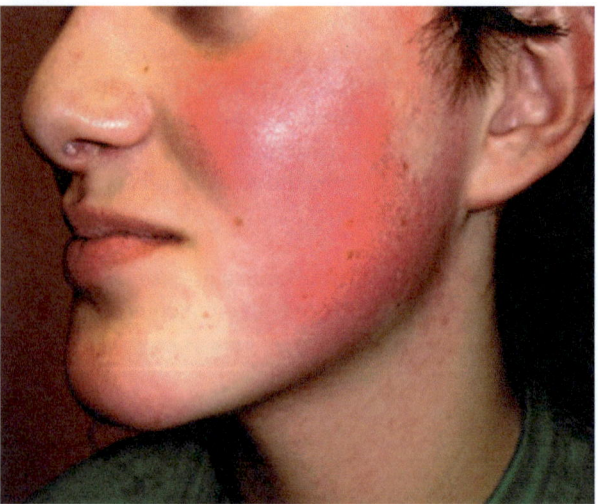

Fig. 20.2 Facial flushing

use of β-blockers) reduces the release of sympathetic mediators in the ventricles, decreasing the incidence of serious cardiac events or syncope.

In intractable thoracic angina with diffuse or microangiopathic coronary disease (no indication for angioplasty or revascularization) or in patients already revascularized but without clinical–surgical conditions for a new operation, thoracic sympathectomy may promote a direct anesthetic effect and reduce the heart's demand for oxygen (by decreasing heart rate and systolic pressure).

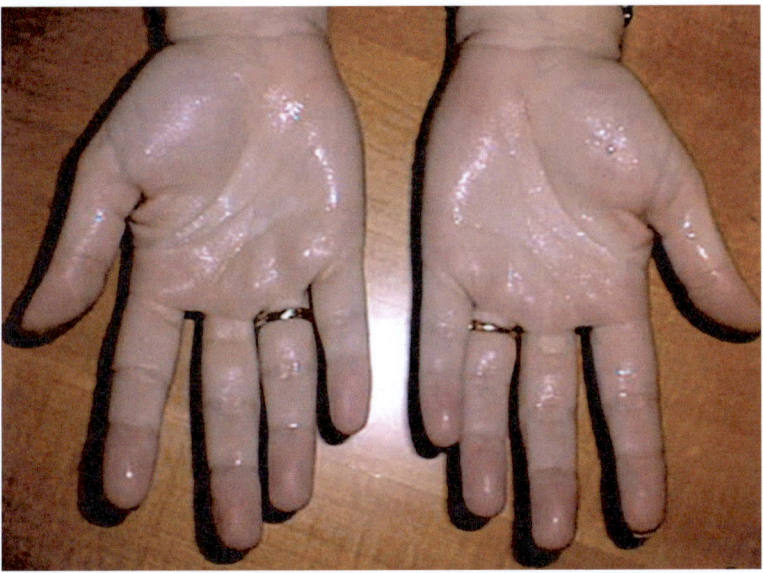

Fig. 20.3 Palmar hyperhidrosis

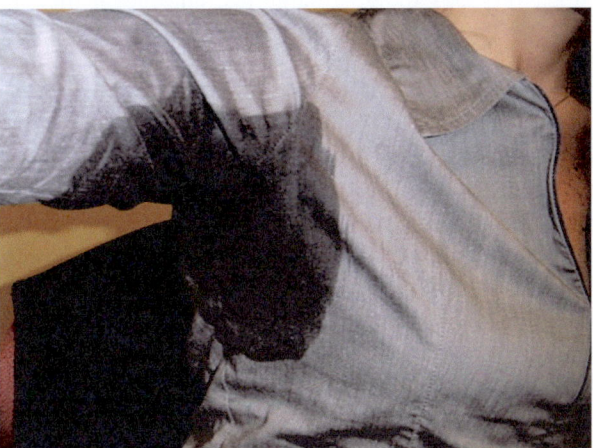

Fig. 20.4 Axillary hyperhidrosis

Raynaud's phenomenon is characterized by episodes of vasospasm in distal arterioles, with a clinical sequence of pallor, cyanosis, and flushing of the extremities. In the crisis, there is pain, hypothermia, paresthesias and, depending on the severity, ischemic phenomena may occur. This phenomenon can be primary (Raynaud's disease) or secondary (to diseases of collagen, hemopathies, neurological diseases, ischemic pathologies and traumas). Thoracic sympathectomy is rarely employed, and has an effect similar to that indicated in upper-limb ischemic pathologies [1].

Since 1995, we have gathered the experience of the Thoracic Surgery Department of the Hospital das Clínicas of the Medical School of the University of São Paulo with that of the private clinic. In our series, less than 2.5% of the patients had a diagnosis other than essential hyperhidrosis (such as causalgia, thromboagitis obliterans, and long QT syndrome). All in all other cases, the surgical indication was primary hyperhidrosis [2].

In primary hyperhidrosis, 61% of the patients were female and 39% were male. Age ranged from 7 to 70 years (mean of 25.6 years). The main indications were palmoplantar hyperhidrosis (38%), palmoplantar and axillary hyperhidrosis (33%), pure axillary hyperhidrosis (23%), and craniofacial hyperhidrosis (6%) [3].

Surgical Technique

In bilateral thoracic sympathectomy, we used the following standardized surgical technique:

1. Patient is submitted to general anesthesia, usually with prophylactic antibiotic therapy for induction of anesthesia and use of simple orotracheal intubation. If there are preoperative indications that the patient may have pleuropulmonary adhesions (e.g., previous thoracic surgeries, antecedent pleural effusion), we indicate the use of a selective intubation with the use of an endotracheal double-lumen catheter that allows ventilation to be stopped on the side that is being operated and keep the other side ventilating. The selective tube chosen is on the left side, to facilitate its positioning (avoiding atelectasis of the right upper lobe when the right side tube is used). The positioning is done with the aid of the pulmonary auscultation to verify if the blockade is correct, but in case of doubts or difficulties of positioning, radioscopy and/or bronchoscopy should be used.
2. The patient is placed in the supine position, in a semi-seated position (trunk raised to 45 °), and with the arms in abduction at 90 °, supported on the arches of the surgical table. Thin pillows are placed behind each shoulder that extend through the trunk on each side, providing better armpit exposure. Another larger pillow is placed under the knees and the patient is taped to the operating table at the hip.
3. Axillary trichotomy is performed in the nipple and peri-mammillary region, followed by asepsis and antisepsis and placement of the surgical drapes.
4. The video monitor is placed behind one of the patient's abducted arms with the monitor angled so that both the surgeon and the assistants can see it (Fig. 20.5).
5. We start the surgery with a 6 mm incision in the anterolateral region of the thorax in the anterior axillary line (in men: in the transition between the skin and the nipple; in women: in the submammary sulcus), where a trocar of 5.5mm diameter is placed between the fourth or fifth intercostal space, after blunt dissection of the pathway between the skin and the parietal pleura. The dissection of the intercostal space and introduction of the trocar through the parietal pleural is done with the patient in a short period of apnea and with the ventilation system open to avoid inadvertent lesion of the visceral pleura. We introduce through this trocar the video optics of 4 or 5 mm with 30 ° angulation.

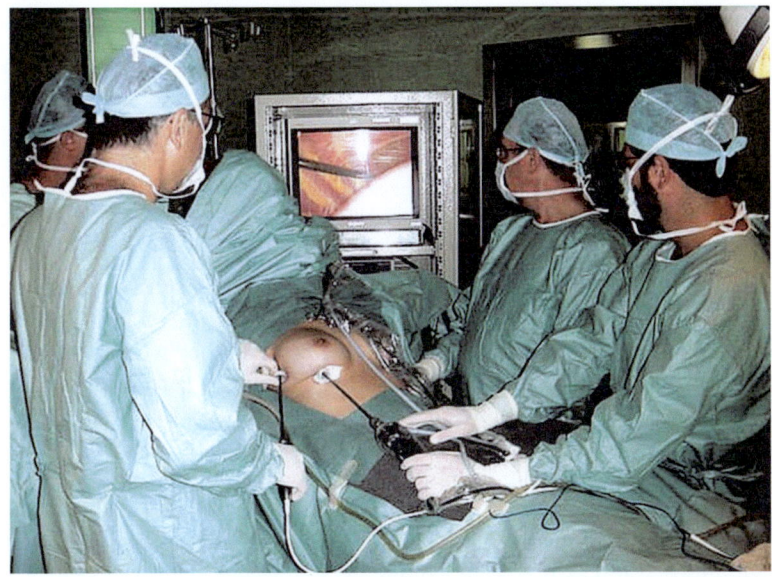

Fig. 20.5 Positioning of the surgical team and the video monitor

6. Once the optic is positioned in the pleural space, we place the second trocar 5.5 mm in the mid axillary region at the second intercostal space, under direct vision. The parameter we commonly use to locate this incision is where the axillary hair ends.
7. Through this second trocar a hook (electrocautery) is introduced, and in a second short period of apnea, the lung is collapsed allowing the sympathectomy to be performed.
8. We identify the sympathetic chain through the mediastinal pleura as a longitudinal, whitish cord, protruding in the region corresponding to the heads of the ribs when they articulate with the thoracic vertebrae. The hook can be used to palpate and make sure the sympathetic chain is present.
9. To identify the level of the ganglions for thermoablation, we use the ribs as an anatomical parameter. The first rib visible at the top of the thoracic cavity is the second rib and the sympathetic ganglion T2 starts from it and extends to the third rib where T3 begins; and so on. See the resection levels recommended in Table 20.1.
10. The mediastinal pleural is opened with the hook (electrocautery) around the sympathetic chain over the corresponding rib and the complete section of the chain is performed at this level. The same is done in the rib below, followed by complete cauterization of the sympathetic chain that was isolated between these two ribs. At this time (during cauterization), we observe the retraction of the isolated sympathetic chain, ensuring the term-ablation of this sympathetic ganglion.
11. After the hemostasis has been reviewed, a nasopharyngeal tube 16 Fr is inserted through the axillary trocar and we connect this tube to a vacuum. At the same

Table 20.1 Levels of sympathectomy currently recommended

Facial hyperhidrosis	Bilateral	Ganglion	T2
Palmar hyperhidrosis	Bilateral	Ganglion	T3
Palmar–axilar hyperhidrosis	Bilateral	Ganglion	T4
Axilar hyperhidrosis	Bilateral	Ganglion	T4
Vascular patologies	Unilateral	Ganglion	T2, T3, T4 + stellate ganglion
Long QT syndrome	Left	Ganglion	T2, T3, T4, lower third of the stellate ganglion

time, we ask the anesthesiologist to inflate the lungs to full expansion under direct vision, and then remove the video optics.

12. After the suture of the inferior incision, we perform the "we perform a simple maneuver to check for pneumothorax or air fistula", where we disconnect the pleural tube from the vacuum and insert the distal end of the pleural tube into a bowl with saline solution. The anesthesiologist manually ventilates the patient through the endotracheal tube until the airflow (bubbling) of the tube immersed in the saline solution ceases. The pleural tube is removed using a Valsalva maneuver and then this incision is sutured. If there is persistent air fistula, the pleural tube is left as if it were a drain and connected to a water seal system or replaced by a pigtail drain connected to a Heimlich valve.
13. Occlusive dressings are performed on the incisions and a chest X-ray is performed in the patient's room with the patient seated to confirm the full expansion of the lungs.
14. The patient is discharged the next day for outpatient return. If the patient has a drain, they are discharged after removal of the chest drain [4].

Results and Complications

After a follow-up period of 3–96 months (mean of 49 months), we observed the results listed here.

About 95.9% of the patients had no complications and were discharged the day after the operation or on the same day; 3.9% after 48 h and only 0.2% were hospitalized for 72 h.

Therapeutic success was achieved in 93.3% of cases of hyperhidrosis, with 6.6% recurrence [5].

The most common and severe technical difficulty during the procedure was pleural adhesion in 6.7%; azygos lobes were observed in 0.4% and apical blebs in 0.2% of patients. The most frequent immediate postoperative complication was postoperative pain in 97.4% patients (with spontaneous regression in 2 weeks using analgesics); pneumothorax requiring thoracic drainage occurred in 3.5%, neurological disorders involving upper limbs in 2.1%, Horner syndrome in 0.9%, significant bleeding in 0.4%, and one patient had extensive subcutaneous emphysema. The most frequent late complication was compensatory sweating, which occurred in 88.4% of the cases. Although 27.2% of the patients reported compensatory hyperhidrosis (severe compensatory sweating), only 2.5% expressed regret at having undergone surgery. Gustatory sweating occurred in 19.3% [6].

In patients with organic diseases, all had improved pain or scarring of ischemic lesions (thromboangiitis obliterans), relief of symptoms (causalgia), and stabilization of the cardiac condition (long QT syndrome). No conversion to open surgery or death occurred in our series.

References

1. Kauffman P, Milanez de Campos JR. Simpatectomia cervicotoracica por videotoracoscopia. In: de Andrade Filho LO, editor. Cirurgia Torácica Diagnóstico e Tratamento. 1ª ed. Rio de Janeiro: Cultura Médica; 2007. p. 391–414.
2. Kauffman P, JRC M, Jatene F, et al. Simpatectomia cervicotorácica por vídeotoracoscopia: experiência inicial. Rev Colégio Bras Cirurgiões. 1998;25:235.
3. Kauffman P, Milanez de Campos JR, Wolosker N, et al. Simpatectomia cervicotorácica videotoracoscópica: experiência de 8 anos. J Vasc Bras. 2003;2:98–104.
4. Milanez de Campos JR, Kauffman P, Kang DWW. Simpatectomia torácica no tratamento da Hiperidrose primária. In: Moraes IN, editor. Tratado de Clínica Cirúrgica. 1st ed. São Paulo: Editora Roca Ltda; 2005. p. 1015–9.
5. De Campos JRM, Kauffman P, Werebe EC, Wolosker N, et al. Quality of life, before and after thoracic sympathectomy: report on 378 operated patients. Ann Thorac Surg. 2003;76:886–91.
6. de Andrade Filho LO, Kuzniec S, Wolosker N, Yazbek G, Kauffman P, Milanez de Campos JR. Technical difficulties and complications of sympathectomy in the treatment of hyperhidrosis: an analysis of 1731 cases. Ann Vasc Surg. 2013;27(4):447–53.

Endoscopic Thoracic Sympathectomy for Primary Palmar Hyperhidrosis

21

Alan E. P. Cameron

Introduction

Sweaty palms are a terrible handicap. Perhaps 1% of the population suffer from the condition, but many of these are not treated. Many feel that the condition is not bad enough to seek help, or that it is too embarrassing or too trivial to bother the physician; many others are referred to dermatologists (physicians who treat skin diseases) and are not referred on to surgeons because the dermatologists seem prejudiced against surgery. Many articles about hyperhidrosis written by dermatologists never mention surgery—perhaps this is because surgery offers the only permanent cure! This chapter outlines the options for treatment, focusing on surgical interventions.

Symptoms

Perhaps the best description of sweaty hands comes in Charles Dickens' book *David Copperfield* published in 1850. Uriah Heep is an evil swindler and Dickens gives him horribly sweaty hands to add to his nastiness. David says "what a clammy hand his was. I rubbed mine afterwards to warm it and rub his off" and later on he sees Heep's "lank forefinger leaving snail-like tracks upon the page". This accurately describes the unpleasantness of shaking hands with a hyperhidrosis sufferer, but overlooks the effect on the person with the awful hands. Somebody with palmar hyperhidrosis becomes shy, insecure, and anxious.

A. E. P. Cameron
Surgical Department, Ipswich Hospital, Ipswich, UK
e-mail: alan.cameron@ipswichhospital.nhs.uk

At this point I should mention that sweating and anxiety go together; we talk about a "sweaty situation" or conversely that something straightforward was "no sweat". Sweating, palpitations, and so on are part of the "fight or flight" primitive responses mediated by the sympathetic nervous system so it is not surprising that sweating and anxiety are connected. People with hyperhidrosis are undoubtedly anxious, but maybe it is the sweating which comes first; they worry about sweating, which then exacerbates the wetness, which then reinforces the anxiety into a depressive downward spiral. So they are anxious *because* they sweat and not vice versa.

Diagnosis

The diagnosis of primary palmar hyperhidrosis is straightforward. The condition can start in childhood. Small children can be very cruel and a child with sweaty hands will be teased unmercifully. Other children will refuse to hold hands; having wet fingers makes holding pens and pencils difficult so teachers may criticize them for untidy writing; drawings and writings may be smudged and messy. More commonly the symptoms arise around puberty; the reason for this is unknown. Many sufferers are told they will "grow out of it", but this is not true; adolescence can be bad enough without the added agony of sweaty hands. Going on a "date" must be a nightmare.

Although the specific gene has not yet been identified, there is a strong familial element to primary hyperhidrosis: there is a family history in up to 40% of cases. Interestingly, parents who have had successful treatment for sweating will often recognize the symptoms in their young children. From their own experience they know that the condition will not improve so they may bring the children early on to avoid distress during adolescence.

Palm sweating can be very variable; for example, it can be affected by emotion or by ambient temperature. Characteristically, sweating does not occur at night. In the very worst cases sweat will drip off the hands onto the floor. In addition to social effects, palm sweating can affect peoples' occupation; many will consciously avoid a job which involves contact with clients. People who wear gloves for work, such a doctors and dentists, may find that the gloves fill with liquid. Keyboards may be damaged; manipulation of tools may be hazardous if the fingers are slippery. One of my cases was a car delivery driver who had a crash because his hand slipped on the steering wheel.

There are validated assessments which can be used to try to quantify the distress being caused. The Dermatology Quality of Life Index and the Hyperhidrosis Disease Severity Scale are two examples. These are rarely employed in routine clinical practice but very helpful for research studies.

The essential feature is that the sweating *upsets the patient* and is reducing their quality of life. There is no absolute criterion for making the diagnosis.

Examination

There is often very little to find on examination of the hands. When talking to their physician the patient should be relaxed and open and therefore in such circumstances—provided the doctor is also relaxed and compassionate—there will be no anxiety and therefore no excessive sweating. While it may be reassuring to the surgeon to observe the dripping hands, usually the diagnosis and treatment depends solely on the sufferer's story.

Although there are some objective tests for measuring the amount of sweat produced, these are really only research tools and are not useful in clinical practice. Gravimetric measurement involves putting the patient into a temperature-controlled environment and then weighing swabs placed on the hands or armpits. The difficulty here is not only that the results are very unreliable, but also that there is no actual quantifiable amount of sweat which can be labelled as "excessive". More sophisticated laboratory tests may include sudometry where gas is passed over the hands and the moisture released is measured or measurement of sweat production after electrical stimulation of the nerves. These are of no practical value in assessing the individual case.

Other Tests

There are of course other causes of sweating; it is a feature of all infectious diseases and of some cancers (the Pel-Ebstein fever of Hodgkin's lymphoma being the most memorable). But in these cases the underlying disease is usually entirely obvious and patients are never referred because of the sweat.

Hyperhidrosis is said to occur secondary to some other conditions; however, these must be very rare because I have never seen a case! Generalized secondary hyperhidrosis can be secondary to some endocrine-secreting tumors; it can be caused by certain drugs, especially the newer antidepressants which can therefore cause confusion in an anxious/depressed sweaty patient. Menopausal hot flushing can be associated with sweating. Some patients with diabetes or thyrotoxicosis do have generalized sweating.

The characteristic of these conditions is that the sweating is all over the body and occurs at night. Primary hyperhidrosis by contract is focal on the hands, armpits, feet, or head and does not occur at night.

It is also stated that focal hyperhidrosis can be caused by rarities such as tumors or traumatic injury of the sympathetic nervous system. Again, I have never seen or even heard of such a case.

Thus, the diagnosis is clinically based on the sufferer's history and no investigation is necessary.

Non-Surgical Options

Unlike in the armpit, where non-surgical options may be preferable, the available treatments for the hands are unsatisfactory.

Topical treatment with zirconium or aluminum compounds would be ineffective and too irritant.

Oral systemic treatment with anticholinergic drugs such as oxybutynin or glycopyrronium bromide is not possible. To control the severe focal sweating on the hands would require such high doses that the adverse effects would be absolutely intolerable.

Equally, topical ointment preparations containing anticholinergic drugs would be too greasy and thus unsuitable for the hands.

Injection of Botox® does control palm sweating. I have no personal experience of this but I have seen a few cases who had one such set of injections. The treatment was so painful that it was unendurable and they refused a repeat so came for surgery! It is possible to limit the pain of the multiple injections by giving a nerve block at the wrist but the effect of the Botox® is temporary and many patients will seek a more permanent solution.

Local surgery such as subdermal curettage is clearly impossible in the palm. The relatively new miraDry® microwave device has promising results in the axilla. It is being assessed for use in the palm but no results are currently available.

The only non-surgical option for the hands is iontophoresis.

Iontophoresis

Iontophoresis was first described in the 1950s and is still useful even though the mechanism of action is obscure. Possibly there is some interference with the neurological transmission to the sweat glands; alternatively, the system may cause simple plugging of the orifice of the eccrine glands themselves. The technique uses a generated direct current of 15–20 mA which is passed through the skin by putting the hands (or feet) into a water bath; usually just tap water is employed but some benefit can be gained by adding anticholinergic drugs to the solution. Each treatment takes 30–40 min but does need to be repeated every week. In the UK, the initial course of treatment is provided in hospital by physiotherapists. If successful then patients may buy their own machines for use at home. Adverse effects can include tingling and paresthesia and occasionally minor burns.

Iontophoresis is, of course, not a permanent cure and many patients become disenchanted with the need for repeated treatments. However, I think it has two main applications before proceeding to endoscopic thoracic sympathectomy (ETS) surgery.

Firstly, in the occasional pediatric case the treatment may give symptom control while the child is growing; children need to be a reasonable size, and have reasonable understanding, before ETS surgery can be performed.

Secondly, in adults it may be helpful to try iontophoresis prior to surgery so that the patient knows that all conservative options have been exhausted; this cautious approach may also help overcome the reluctance of our dermatology colleagues who think we are too aggressive!

Axillary Sweating

It has been known for many years that the results of ETS for sweating confined to the armpit are not as good as for the hands. Furthermore, there are other options for the treatment of such sweating apart from ETS.

However, if the patient has combined palm and armpit sweating then ETS is a good option, with a slight extension of the denervation as discussed BELOW in Adverse Effects.

Incidentally, the secretion of the eccrine glands is salty water and does not smell; beware patients who complain of malodorous armpits—they are not candidates for ETS.

Patient Information

In *Henry IV*, Shakespeare wrote that "Falstaff sweats to death", but this is not true as nobody has ever died from sweating. All surgery must carry some risk, and while we all accept that it is good practice to inform patients undergoing any operation of the risks and benefits, this is even more essential when dealing with a benign non-fatal condition. In fact, ETS is a very safe operation with very low reported mortality but there can be unpleasant adverse effects so it is important to have a frank discussion. It is also important to document the full discussion with the patient and very helpful to give them a written fact sheet.

The adverse effects are discussed in the section below "Complications and Adverse Effects".

Preoperative Assessment

The majority of patients are fit young adults so there are very few contraindications to ETS. One paradoxical contraindication is the "super fit" athlete. There is evidence that ETS can reduce maximal heart rate and maximal exercise output. The vast majority of sportsmen might not notice this, but it might just slightly impair the performance of the very highest-level athletes, so I would be wary of offering the procedure to them.

The operation does depend on creating a space above the lung so a history of pneumothorax might be important, and a history of surgical pleurodesis would be worrying. Apical tuberculosis would be equally difficult to overcome. Heavy smokers or those with a history of pneumonia may have developed adhesions at the apex of the lung but these can usually be overcome by careful dissection.

The decision on when to operate on a child is usually a simple question of size; the operation can be performed as soon as the child is large enough for the instrument to pass fairly easily between the ribs—and the child is aware enough to understand, of course.

A preoperative chest X-ray is unhelpful because apical adhesions do not show. The presence of an azygos lobe can cause confusion inside the chest but it is rarely picked up on preoperative radiology. I never request one.

As the cases are fit and healthy, preoperative blood tests are not essential but may be dictated by anaesthetic protocols.

Evolution of My Technique

I performed my first ETS a long time ago; although the principle of destroying part of the sympathetic chain has remained the same, there have been some changes in technique. Many different types of ETS have been described, ablation, resection, clipping, harmonic scalpel, and so on, but I have made little change!

My initial operations were in 1984, in the days before video-endoscopy became available. So I operated by peering through a direct-vision gynecological laparoscope (which meant that nobody else could see what was going on as there was no television monitor!). We used a double-lumen tube with 3-L pneumothorax to collapse the operated side and initially did one side at a time. This quickly changed to a synchronous bilateral procedure. I initially used one port in the axilla for the telescope and a port in the second interspace anteriorally for the electrode but soon changed to two axillary ports. All cases of palmar sweating had electrocoagulation of the sympathetic chain at four levels, T2–5 inclusive. All cases had a chest X-ray in the recovery room and all were kept in hospital for a day or so.

Gradually the technique changed to simple endotracheal intubation, single-port operating thoracoscope in the mid-axillary line, limited coagulation, and day-case surgery.

In the UK many ETS operations are performed by vascular surgeons such as myself. One of the things that has not changed since I started is that I always have a set of chest instruments and chest drainage equipment immediately available. As a non-thoracic practitioner I certainly hope never to use these instruments but my policy is to "prepare for the worst but expect the best".

Current Technique

We operate under general anesthesia: either endotracheal intubation or laryngeal mask. Only a single intravenous line is inserted and no invasive monitoring is needed. Pneumatic calf compression devices are applied; this not only helps prevent venous thrombosis but also helps venous return in the semi-upright position. The table is adjusted to raise the patient into the "beach chair" position. The arms are abducted to 90 °, being careful to avoid overstretch. I use a 7 or 8 mm operating thoracoscope which has a 3 mm operating channel for the electrode or scissors so only one puncture is necessary.

Bupivacaine 0.5% is injected into the chest wall in the second or third interspace in the mid-axillary line and a small incision is made. The anesthetist then disconnects the ventilator and a trocar is passed into the pleural space. To avoid damage, this trocar should be blunt. The thoracoscope is inserted and ventilation restarted. In the semi-upright position the lung usually falls away from the apex of the chest cavity and there is usually a good view. Occasionally adhesions to the apex prevent the lung from falling away; filmy adhesions can be divided by micro-scissors down the operating channel but large vascular adhesions are best circumvented if possible. If the lung needs to be depressed further then CO_2 is insufflated as required; the anesthetist can stop ventilating as well if necessary.

For palmar sweating I destroy the chain at the level of the third and fourth ribs by pressing an electrode firmly against the mid-point of the rib and applying a diathermy current. In cases of concomitant axillary sweating I would go down to T5 as well.

After adequate destruction of the chain the thorascope is passed up to the apex of the chest and low-pressure suction applied to evacuate any gas (high pressure may suck lung tissue into the instrument). The anesthetist applies positive pressure ventilation as the instrument is removed. The skin is sutured and the procedure performed on the other side. This technique is simple and speedy. No chest drain is required.

Many cases experience chest heaviness or tightness as they are waking up so it is worth mentioning this preoperatively. Routine postoperative chest X-ray is not required. We do request selective radiographs if the oxygen saturation is <92% on air, or if there is excessive shortness of breath, or there is excessive chest pain. In practice this is rare.

Most patients will go home the same day.

There is often a little postoperative discomfort at the back of the chest, probably due to diathermy of the ribs, but this is controlled by simple analgesia. Quite a few patients get a "rebound" of sweating on the third postoperative day and may think the operation has failed. They can be reassured that this passes after 24 h; the cause is unknown.

Complications and Adverse Effects

As already mentioned, in experienced hands ETS is a safe operation and very few deaths or major complications have occurred. There have been a few instances of damage to major thoracic vessels, but these have tended to be where the surgeon was not sufficiently trained. Other immediate problems are also rare; sometimes residual air in the chest may need a temporary chest drain, for example.

The vast majority of patients are very satisfied and have a greatly improved quality of life. However, the long-term effects of ETS are important.

In 1933 Ross wrote that "some of our patients have stated emphatically that the secretion of sweat has been considerably more profuse in the areas not affected by the operation [open thoracic sympathectomy]. The remark has been so frequently made … that the possibility of compensatory hypersecretion cannot be excluded". Compensatory sweating remains the chief unwanted side effect of ETS. It is reduced by limiting the extent of the sympathectomy (see the American Thoracic Society guidelines for a fuller discussion). As with primary hyperhidrosis, compensatory sweating is a subjective sensation observed by the patient. It is therefore difficult to quantify. Most patients get it to some degree, but only a few are really bothered by it if a more focused ETS has been done. Compensatory sweating seems to be a more severe and intractable problem where the highest level of T2 has been divided. This level is necessary for treatment of craniofacial symptoms, which is why such cases need very careful discussion before offering ETS and why surgeons are increasingly reluctant to treat such symptoms.

Management of compensatory hyperhidrosis is difficult; generalized sweating may be helped by oral anticholinergic drugs; localized areas may respond to Botox®.

Paradoxically, the hands may become too dry and cracked after ETS; some moisture is necessary to for grip and cosmetic creams may help.

Gustatory sweating on the upper lip after hot or spicy food may occur after ETS, again less commonly after the more limited ablations.

Horner's syndrome of the small pupil and drooping of the eyelids is an occasional complication of ETS, but again is only really seen after the higher-level ablations.

Minor changes in cardiac output and thus in exercise capacity may occur, but the vast majority of cases will not notice these.

The "post-ETS syndrome" is a worrying constellation of symptoms occasionally occurring but widely disseminated via the internet. Indeed, a cohort of such dissatisfied patients has called for ETS to be banned. The syndrome includes severe compensatory sweating but also other complaints such as a feeling of temperature deregulation, dislike of bright lights or loud noise, lethargy, depression, loss of libido, and so on. These are hard to explain so it is tempting to dismiss them as purely psychological but they do follow ETS, so whatever the mechanism they are a consequence of the surgery. Again, however, they seem to be more common after extensive denervation.

Conclusion

Palmar sweating has a very debilitating effect on the sufferer. Many studies have shown that ETS offers a dramatic and durable long-term cure. Careful attention to detail can reduce many of the unwanted side effects.

The bottom line is to make sure the right patient gets the right operation performed by the right surgeon.

Suggested Reading

Cerfolio RJ, de Campos JR, Bryant AS, et al. The Society of Thoracic Surgeons expert consensus for the treatment of hyperhidrosis. Ann Thorac Surg. 2011;91(5):1642–8.

de Campos JR, Kauffman P, Werebe EC, et al. Quality of life before and after thoracic sympathectomy; report on 378 operated patients. Ann Thorac Surg. 2003;76:886–91.

Dickens C. The personal history, adventures, experience and observation of David Copperfield the younger of Blunderstone Rookery. London: Bradbury and Evans; 1850.

Herbst F, Plas EG, Fugger R, et al. Endoscopic thoracic sympathectomy for primary hyperhidrosis of the upper limbs. A critical analysis and long term results of 480 operations. Ann Surg. 1994;1:86–90.

Ross JP. Sympathectomy as an experiment in human physiology. Br J Surg. 1933;21:5–19.

Smidfelt K, Drott C. Late results of endoscopic thoracic sympathectomy for hyperhidrosis and facial blushing. Br J Surg. 2011;98(12):1719–22.

Evolution of Surgical Methods and Difficulties Relating to Endoscopic Thoracic Sympathectomy

22

Paulo Kauffman

Introduction

Until the 1980s, thoracic sympathectomy to treat palmar hyperhidrosis was conducted via open access and the technique used was the supraclavicular access as it offers advantages over other open access: it is extrapleural, heals easily leaving an almost invisible scar, allows the bilateral procedure to be performed in a single surgery, recovery is rapid, reducing the period of hospitalization, and complications are infrequent in the hands of experienced surgeons. It is a slightly aggressive surgery, which involves manipulation of nerve trunks of the brachial plexus and the subclavian artery and has an inconvenient approach via the stellate ganglion to identify the sympathetic chain, which determines appearance of Horner syndrome. Its most feared manifestation, eyelid droop, has an only an aesthetic impact, but is unacceptable to the majority of patients, even though it is transient in most cases, mainly in women, who constitute the majority of patients that seek treatment.

Currently, the open technique is indicated only when endoscopic thoracic sympathectomy cannot be performed for technical reasons and where it is associated with open procedures, such as neurovascular decompression of the thoracic outlet.

Until the 1980s, the following axiom was in force: "great surgeons, great incisions". However, since medicine is not an exact science, its concepts and behaviors are not immutable, evolving with the progressive knowledge gained from research and improvement of medical technology, and thus this axiom is no longer true following the practical introduction of minimally invasive endoscopic techniques that have obvious advantages over conventional open-access routes because they are less aggressive, easier to perform, better accepted, and promote faster patient recovery.

With the recent advances in the optical, video, and instrumental systems for endoscopic surgical procedures, thoracic sympathectomy has been made possible

---

P. Kauffman
Department of Vascular and Endovascular Surgery, University of São Paulo School of Medicine, São Paulo, SP, Brazil

using a videothoracoscopic technique, a procedure that has been used by our team for more than 20 years. The experience gained with this technique and the results obtained in many studies carried out at the Hyperhidrosis Outpatient Clinic of the Hospital das Clínicas of São Paulo constitute the basis of all the considerations that are discussed in this chapter.

Surgical Tactics

- *Anesthesia*: general anesthesia is used, and a simple intubation or double-lumen catheter can be used, the latter also being called selective intubation as it allows lung ventilation to be blocked on the operated side, collapsing it and facilitating the visualization of the chain. To verify proper positioning of the probe, a bronchoscope may be used. At the beginning of our experience with this surgery, we routinely used a double-lumen probe, which is still preferred when acting on the fourth ganglion (G4) of the thoracic sympathetic chain and also in patients with a history of lung infections in whom there is a greater probability of pleural adhesions. When thermoablation is performed in higher ganglia, as in the third (G3) and possibly in the second (G2), a simple probe with adequate pulmonary ventilation control is enough to perform the surgical intervention and has become our routine technique.
- *Position on the surgical table*: the patient was initially positioned with the trunk elevated at 30 ° and the arms raised and fixed in an arch on the table, which in some cases resulted in complaints of paresthesia and even transitory paresis in the upper limbs by distension of the brachial plexus nerves (Fig. 22.1a); to avoid these complications, the patient was placed in a seated position, with the trunk elevated at approximately 45 °, the arms supported on the armbands of the table and with two cushions under the shoulders that, besides reducing the distension of the brachial plexus, aim to facilitate the movement of surgical instruments (Fig. 22.1b). Also to avoid distension of the lumbar plexus, we use a cushion

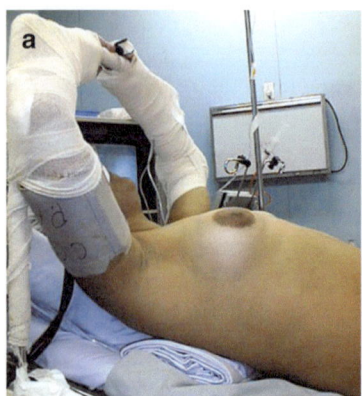
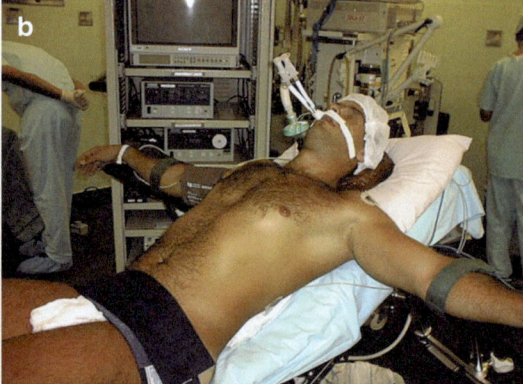

Fig. 22.1 Position on the surgical table: (**a**) previous position; and (**b**) current position

under the knees to keep them semi-flexed. The patient has a band placed at the hip, to prevent their movement when performing lateral rotation on the table.
- *Tactic*: the level of the sympathetic chain targeted varies according to the affected body segment.
- *Palmar hyperhidrosis*: at the beginning of our experience we performed thermoablation of the segment of the thoracic chain located between the first, second, and third costal arcs, including G2 and G3. Due to the denervation of a very extensive area of the organism (cranial–facial segment, neck, and upper limbs), this resulted in important compensatory hyperhidrosis, which made us limit the thermoablation to only G2; however, this did not reduce the intensity of the compensatory hyperhidrosis, notably in the trunk, which continued to manifest in a significant number of patients (64%), causing 4% of patients to regret the intervention. In order to overcome this inconvenience, we conducted a study comparing results of the sympathectomy performed at two levels (G2 and G3) in patients with palmar hyperhidrosis. Palmar anhidrosis was observed after the intervention in both groups, but the intensity of compensatory hyperhidrosis was significantly higher in the group submitted to G2 thermoablation. We then proceeded to routinely perform G3 thermoablation in the treatment of palmar hyperhidrosis, with a tendency in some patients to lower the level of the procedure even further by performing G4 thermoablation, which was effective in reducing the intensity of palmar hyperhidrosis, without, however, resulting in anhidrosis in a significant number of them; the advantage of lowering the level of sympathectomy was the reduction in the intensity of compensatory hyperhidrosis, a proven observation using a sweat gauge, an objective method of measuring sweating. Thus, in patients duly informed about the advantages and disadvantages of G4 thermoablation in the treatment of palmar hyperhidrosis, such a technique may be adopted, particularly in those who already experience a high level of sweating in other regions of the body and are therefore at greater risk of intense compensatory sweating after the procedure.
- *Axillary hyperhidrosis*: in the early days of its use, the sympathectomy was extensive, including G2, G3, and G4 ganglia, with the drawback of compensatory hyperhidrosis, as previously reported. From the observations made in our outpatient clinic, we stopped working on the G2 in patients with pure axillary hyperhidrosis, performing instead G3 and G4 thermoablation, and later, new observations showed similar results in terms of axillary anhidrosis when we performed thermoablation of G3–G4 and G4 only in these patients, with the advantage of less marked compensatory hyperhidrosis and a higher degree of satisfaction in the G4 group. Since then, we have adopted the conduct of G4-only thermoablation to treat pure axillary hyperhidrosis.
- *Craniofacial hyperhidrosis and/or facial flushing*: thermoablation of the G2 is the most appropriate procedure to obtain sympathetic denervation of the cephalic segment in cases of craniofacial hyperhidrosis and/or facial flushing, although there are authors who report good results with the sympathetic blockade of G3 in patients with craniofacial hyperhidrosis, acting only on G2 when there is facial flushing.

Contraindications

Some situations contraindicate the performance of videothoracoscopic thoracic sympathectomy, namely previous pulmonary infections that evolved with pleural effusions, requiring drainage or simply puncture, resulting in dense pleural adhesions, which also occurs in those who have had pulmonary diseases such as tuberculosis, previous thoracic surgeries, and radiotherapy in the thoracic region. Sinus bradycardia is also a contraindication to the sympathetic intervention. We have contraindicated thoracic sympathectomy in obese patients because, despite the high degree of satisfaction of these patients with the surgical procedure, the intensity of compensatory hyperhidrosis is usually greater than in patients with normal weight.

Difficulties

In obese patients, the identification of the sympathetic chain is usually more problematic, since it is covered by a greater amount of adipose tissue, making it difficult to visualize; its identification is made by "palpation" with the scalpel. This also occurs in some patients over 40 years old with some degree of overweight. In addition, in these patients, it may be difficult to correctly identify the level of the costal arches, a condition necessary to perform the thermoablation of the segment of the chain indicated in the case in question, since we use the costal arcs, not the ganglia that are usually between them, as parameters in the surgical intervention. The first costal arch is usually covered by the adipose layer located at the apex of the pleural cavity, so that, when we enter the pleural cavity, the second costal arch is the most easily visualized and used as a reference for counting other arches.

The most common technical difficulty is pleural adhesion, and was found in 116 (6.7%) of a total of 1731 patients in our series. From the literature we know that approximately 3–5% of patients undergoing endoscopic chest surgery have more or less dense pleural adhesions, which cannot be diagnosed by preoperative imaging (radiography or computed tomography of the chest). Its release, when loose, is easy, allowing sympathectomy to be performed normally, which was observed in 47.5% of our patients who had these adhesions during the surgical procedure (Fig. 22.2); however, when these adhesions are firm and extensive, with a more or less intense degree of vascularization, due to previous pleuropulmonary diseases, they may render the intervention via the endoscopic route unfeasible, leaving open surgery as the only alternative. In those patients where it is suspected that pleural adhesions may be found, based on the clinical history, the anesthesiologist may be required to use a double-lumen tracheal tube for the purpose of discontinuing the ventilation of the homolateral lung for the longer period of time necessary for the surgeon to undo the adhesions, identify the sympathetic chain, and promote its thermoablation. The conditions that favor the occurrence of these extensive and firm adhesions are pulmonary tuberculosis, pulmonary infections that occur with empyemas, requiring punctures and pleural drainage, and chest trauma with hemothorax formation.

Fig. 22.2 Appearance of a loose adesion

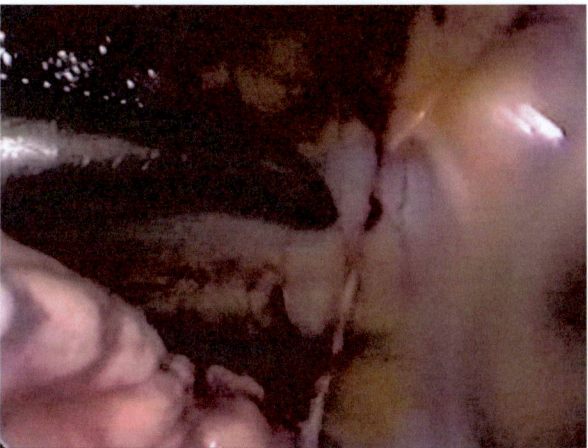

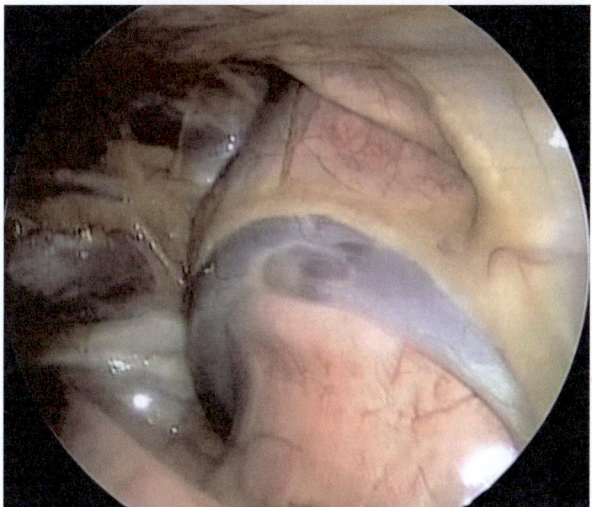

Fig. 22.3 Surgical aspect of the azygos lobe with the vein in front

The presence of an azygos lobe constitutes an uncommon anatomical variation, affecting about 1% of the population and identified in 0.4% of chest X-ray examinations, which, when present, makes it difficult or even impossible to perform video-assisted thoracoscopic surgery (VATS). The azygos lobe is an accessory lobe located at the apex of the right lung, which although clinically irrelevant, began to be surgically valued with the increasing use of videoendoscopic thoracic sympathectomy in the treatment of patients with hyperhidrosis. This is because it can determine important morphological alterations in the upper mediastinum and constitute an obstacle to the intervention, due to the difficulty of identifying the sympathetic chain at this level and also the possibility of injury to the vein itself, causing abundant hemorrhage that is difficult to control endoscopically (Fig. 22.3).

In our experience of 1876 operated patients, we found the azygos lobe in seven (0.35%), and in five of them the diagnosis was made preoperatively by chest radiography, which is capable of identifying this anatomical abnormality in most cases, thus allowing the surgeon to be alerted to the potential risk it poses. In case of doubt, chest tomography can be used.

In order for VATS to be successfully performed, it is necessary to have a broad and complete view of the structures located in the upper mediastinum and the sympathetic chain with their ganglia in relation to the heads of the ribs posteriorly, the subclavian artery superiorly, and, in the right hemithorax, the vena cava medially and the azygos vein below. In the presence of the azygos lobe, the sympathetic chain is partially or totally obscured by this congenital anomaly, making it difficult to achieve the surgical procedure. Some authors contraindicate the endoscopic operation in the presence of the azygos lobe, preferring, in this situation, the open thoracotomy. In order to obtain good visualization, intubation with a double-lumen probe is the most adequate, since it allows a greater reduction of lung volume, favoring the identification of anatomical variation, including the pleural reflex membrane, which is present most of the time and also facilitates the exposure of the sympathetic chain, especially the third and fourth ganglia that constitute the target ganglia of the surgical procedure (Fig. 22.4). Despite the difficulties encountered during the operation to perform the sympathetic chain thermoablation, the goal was achieved in the seven patients, with total success in relation to their initial complaints and without major complications.

It should be emphasized that at the end of the surgical procedure it is necessary to observe whether the azygos lobe returned to its place of origin (Fig. 22.5), because if it expands outside its place of origin, there is a possibility that it remains partially or totally collapsed, as happened in a patient in our series; this fact may favor the occurrence of pneumonia in the postoperative period.

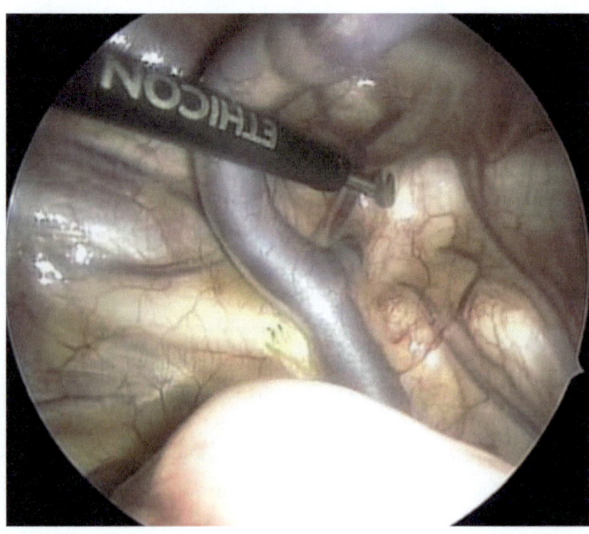

Fig. 22.4 Identification of the sympathetic chain after removing the azygos lobe from its original position

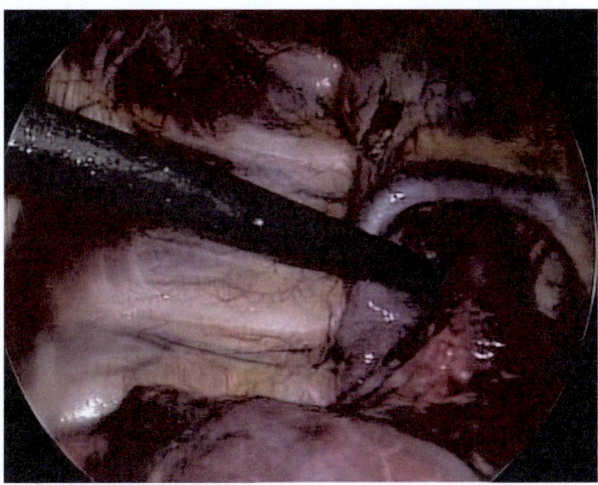

Fig. 22.5 Replacement of the azygos lobe in its original position at the end of the surgical procedure

Suggested Reading

Campos JRM, Kauffman P, Gomes O Jr, Wolosker N. Video-assisted thoracic sympathectomy for hyperhidrosis. Thorac Surg Clin. 2016;26:347–58.

de Andrade Filho LO, Kuzniec S, Wolosker N, Yazbek G, Kauffman P, Milanez de Campos JR. Technical difficulties and complications of sympathectomy in the treatment of hyperhidrosis: an analysis of 1731 cases. Ann Vasc Surg. 2013;27(4):447–53.

Kauffman P, Wolosker N, de Campos JR, Yazbek G, Jatene FB. Azygos lobe: a difficulty in video-assisted thoracic sympathectomy. Ann Thorac Surg. 2010;89:e57–9.

Wolosker N, Kauffman P. Upper extremity sympathectomy. In: Cronenwett J, Johnston KW, editors. Rutherford's vascular surgery. 8th ed. Philadelphia: Saunders; 2014. p. 1923–33.

Yazbek G, Wolosker N, Kauffman P, Campos JR, Puech-Leão P, Jatene FB. Twenty months of evolution following sympathectomy on patients with palmar hyperhidrosis: sympathectomy at the T3 level is better than at the T2 level. Clinics (Sao Paulo). 2009;64:743–9.

Is the Clipping Method for Sympathetic Nerve Surgery a Reversible Procedure?

Javier Pérez Vélez and Carlos Martinez-Barenys

Introduction

Hyperhidrosis is a dysfunction of the autonomic sympathetic nervous system characterized by excessive sweating by the eccrine glands, responsible for temperature regulation.

Sympathetic nerve surgery has been shown to be effective in hyperhidrosis. There are different surgical techniques such as sympathectomy, sympathicolysis, sympatheticotomy, and clipping of the sympathetic chain, all of which are amenable to be performed using videothoracoscopy.

Reflex or compensatory sweating (CS) is the most frequent adverse effect after sympathetic nerve surgery, with an average incidence of 60%, regardless of the surgical technique used.

Currently, the gold standard technique is sympaticotomy, but in recent years the clipping or neurocompression of the sympathetic chain is gaining popularity because of its potential "reversibility", making it more attractive than other techniques.

Once CS is established, there are very limited treatment options for procedures that section the nerve (sympathectomy, sympathicolysis, sympaticotomy) that are considered irreversible procedures. Several authors have attempted the reconstruction of the sympathetic chain by placing intercostal or sural nerve grafts, with very different results.

J. P. Vélez (✉)
Thoracic Surgery Department, University Hospital Vall d'Hebron, Barcelona, Spain
e-mail: javperez@vhebron.net

C. Martinez-Barenys
Thoracic Surgery Department, University Hospital Germans Trias i Pujol, Barcelona, Spain
e-mail: cmartinezb.germanstrias@gencat.cat

Sympathetic chain block emerged as the only procedure that could, until now, be reversed; however, the published experience regarding the withdrawal of clips is varied and always with very few patients. Different authors have published results ranging from 52% to 100% improvement of CS.

However, it is controversial whether nerve impulse transmission can be restored after clip removal, as patients, in addition report that CS has disappeared, also report that primary hyperhidrosis has not returned, which has fueled speculation about a possible placebo effect of reversion surgery.

The evaluation of reflex sweat has been subjective in all studies, except in a Polish study by Stefaniak et al. in 2012 where it was quantified by sudometry after the removal of the clip and a decrease in the CS was demonstrated.

Clipping History

In 1994 Denny-Brown and Brenner demonstrated in experimental animals that a compressive force greater than 44 g on the nerve fiber for more than 2 weeks caused nerve conduction failures, with varying degrees of myelin loss. Based on this concept, Lin Chien, a Taiwanese surgeon, began clipping the sympathetic chain via video-assisted thoracoscopy in 1996, using an Ethicon clipping device called Ligamax® which exerts a compressive force of 150 g (Fig. 23.1).

In 1998, Lin published the first article on clipping of the sympathetic chain in the treatment of hyperhidrosis; of 326 patients who underwent sympathetic blockade by clipping, five required removal of the clips due to poorly tolerated reflex sweat, with reversibility achieved in four patients at 2 and 9 months after withdrawal.

Histopathological Alterations of the Nervous Fiber After Clipping [1]

When a nerve fiber is transected, the proximal shaft can regenerate and the distal shaft undergoes Wallerian degeneration and eventually disintegrates. As seen below, the possibility of nerve fiber regeneration depends on the degree of nerve structural damage (epineurum > perineurum > endoneurum > axon > myelin) and the distance between nerve shafts.

Depending on this structural damage there are different kinds of nerve lesions with different prognostics.

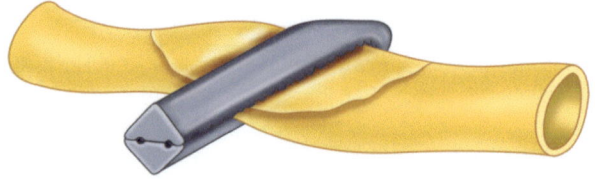

Fig. 23.1 Schematic view of nerve fiber compression with a titanium clip

The Seddon classification defines three types of nerve fiber lesions:

1. *Neuropraxia*: the reversible loss of nerve conduction, affects the myelin sheath, and keeps the axon and the surrounding connective tissue intact.

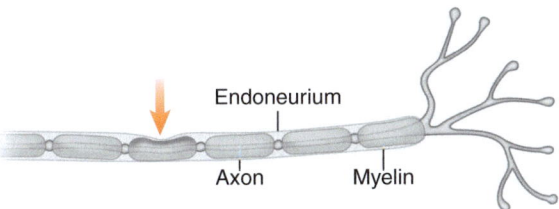

2. *Axontmesis*: nerve injury distal to injury. The regeneration of the axon is spontaneous and of good quality, affecting the myelin sheath and the axon, with preservation of the connective tissue. There is Wallerian degeneration, which can be reversible without sequelae or synkinesis.

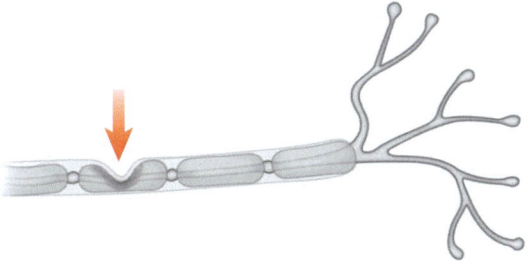

3. *Neurotmesis*: partial or complete nerve injury with complete disruption of the axon, myelin sheath, and connective tissue. There is no spontaneous regeneration and loss of nerve function is complete; therefore, it is an irreversible injury.

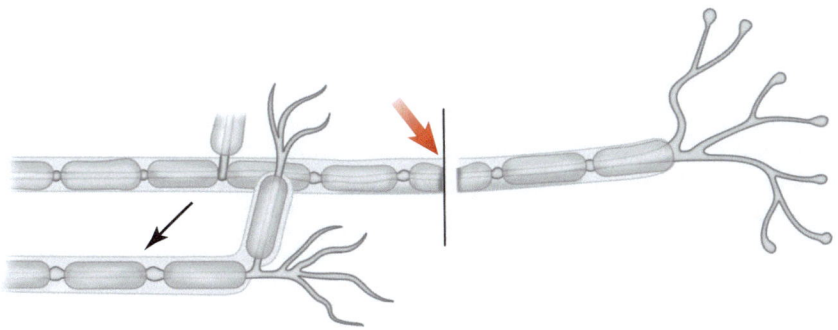

The purpose of clipping is to only block nerve conduction by affecting the myelin sheath.

According to the different results published when unclipping is performed, we believe that the Sutherland's classification of neural lesions could be more useful to explain this discordance:

- *Grade 1*: axonal conduction is blocked, biochemical disruption without anatomical lesion. Functional restoration in days or weeks without Wallerian degeneration (Seddon's neuroapraxia).
- *Grade 2*: pure axonal lesion with integrity of the endoneural sheet. There is degeneration and regeneration but with maximal options of "ad integrum" functional recovery (Seddon's axonotmesis).
- *Grade 3*: axon and endoneural sheet disrupted but with integrity of peri- and epineurum. Intrafascicular fibrosis appears but there is still some change of disorganized functional restitution (Seddon's axonotmesis/neurotmesis with axonotmesis predominance).
- *Grade 4*: disruption of all nervous layers except epineurum that ensures nerve continuity. Minimal–null restitution chance (Seddon's axonotmesis/neurotmesis with neurotmesis predominance).
- *Grade 5*: complete transection of the nerve without any chance of functional restoration (Seddon's neurotmesis).

Standard Surgical Techniques

Clipping (Sympathetic Chain Block)

Clipping is performed under general anesthesia, with sequential selective pulmonary intubation and the patient in a supine position, semi-seated with arms in abduction (semi-Fowler's position).

Two ports are used in each hemithorax; one of 5 mm in the third intercostal space anterior axillary line and another of 5–10 mm (depending on the scope diameter) in the fifth intercostal space medial axillary line. Once the sympathetic trunk is identified, the surgeon must proceed with dissection of the lateral, medial, and anterior edges of the sympathetic nerve with a harmonic scalpel in order to skeletonize the trunk at the desired level (depending on the hyperhidrosis localization) to place the titanium clip using a fireable thoracoscopic device (AcuClip™, Covidien®). Finally, transection of possible communicating branches (nerve of Kuntz) is performed by lateral extension of coagulation at the level of the corresponding rib(s) (Fig. 23.2).

If the patient develops intolerable CS during the postoperative period, a second operation is carried out in order to remove the titanium clips with a standard endodissector, simply pulling towards the contralateral side of the clip closure while taking care not to damage sympathetic trunk (Fig. 23.3).

Fig. 23.2 Titanium clip applied directly to the right sympathetic trunk, and transection of possible sympathetic communicating branches

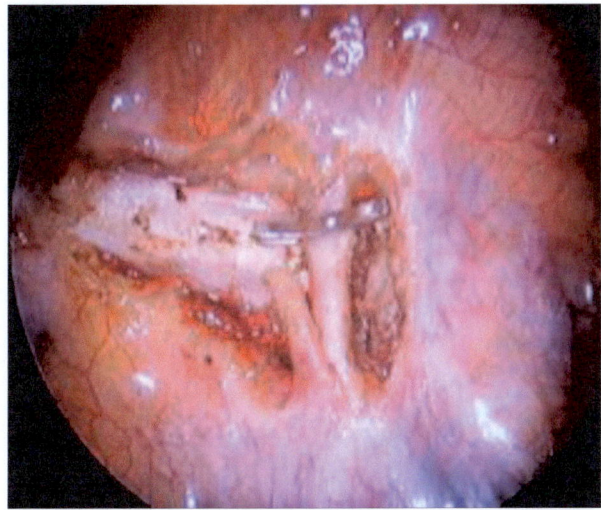

Fig. 23.3 Clip removal by pulling with a standard endo-dissector

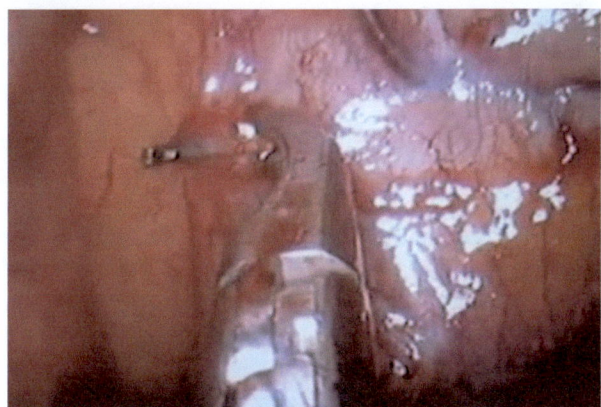

Clinical Evidence

The sympathetic chain block was first described by Lin et al. [2] in 1998, who reported a cohort of 326 patients submitted to sympathetic chain clipping for hyperhidrosis with a follow-up of 6–12 months. They demonstrated the effectiveness of the technique with good results and few complications. Only five patients required CS reversion surgery, of whom three had improved CS at 2 months, one patient at 9 months, and another showed no change after unclipping.

Since then, a solid core of publications has shown that clipping has the same effectiveness as other techniques (sympathectomy, sympathicolysis), with the appeal of being a potentially reversible technique.

Table 23.1 Summary of publications on clip removal

Authors	n	Clip removal [n (%)]	Improvement [n (%)]	Comments
Lin et al.	326	5 (1.5)	4/5 (80)	Improvement at 2 and 9 months
Reisfeld et al.	326	5 (1.4)	3/5 (60)	
Lin and Chou et al.	102	2 (2)	2/2 (100)	
Chou et al.	56	13 (23)	10/13 (77)	
Reisfeld	1274	31 (2.4)	25/31 (81)	Clip removal before 6 months
Jo et al.	87	9 (10.3)	8/9 (90)	Short-term results
Kang et al.	116	15 (12.9)	9/14 (64)	Short- and mid-term results
Reisfeld et al.	2250	36 (1.6)	13/25 (52)	Long-term results
Torn-Sen Lin et al.	16	1 (1.3)	1/1 (100)	Improvement at 2 weeks post-removal
Sciuchetti et al.	281	1 (0.4)	1/1 (100)	
Sugimura et al.	727	34 (4.7)	28/31 (90)	Long-term results
Martínez-Barenys et al.	44	1 (2.3)	1/1 (100)	Mid-term results
Findikcioqlu et al.	32	3 (9)	0/3 (0)	53 months' follow-up
Hynes et al.	82	8 (10)	5/8 (63)	Greater improvement if clips are removed during first 2 weeks

In 2009, Reisfeld [3] published the largest series of unclipping: of 2250 patients clipped, 36 (1.6%) required a reversal procedure due to CS, with good long-term results achieved in 52% of the patients.

Table 23.1 summarizes the other publications on the subject to date, showing the reversibility of the procedure ranges from 0% to 100% depending on the series; it is important to highlight that there are still very few cases and with short- and long-term follow-up periods.

Experimental Evidence

To date, there are only four experimental publications, each with different results, regarding clipping reversibility. It is important to highlight that the working methodologies used, the type of experimental animal, the type and loading force of the clip application device, and, finally, the use or not of immunochemistry techniques to evaluate nerve regeneration differ greatly between them.

The experimental work of Loscertales et al. [4], involving 30 pigs in which the clipped sympathetic chains were histologically evaluated at 10, 20, and 30 days post-clipping, showed an increasing incidence of Wallerian degeneration as the clipping period increased. They also evaluated the pigs' sympathetic chains 20 and 30 days after clip removal, finding that after unclipping the nerve appears to regain normal morphology and, although the inflammatory cells disappear, there is a notable and almost complete absence of myelinated fibers and scarcely any myelinated fibers originating above or below the clipped point, and those fibers do not cross the clipping line. They concluded that axonal regeneration was not possible and clipping cannot be considered a reversible technique.

The work of Candas et al., performed in New Zealand on 12 rabbits, showed that sympathetic nerve injury after clipping is present at 48 h and there are no signs of nerve regeneration at 45 days after clip removal.

On the other hand, two experimental studies show that clipping reversibility is possible histologically.

The hircine model used by Erol and colleagues clipped sympathetic chains for 4 weeks, with biopsy being performed immediately as well as at 4 weeks after unclipping. The immediate biopsies show the expected degeneration. At the 4-week interval, biopsies showed reaccumulation of Schwann cells, suggesting reconstitution of myelin was occurring.

The other study is that of Thomsen et al. [5] in 2014, where clipping of the sympathetic trunk was performed in adult sheep and the clip was removed after 7 days. Following another 4 weeks ($n = 6$) or 12 weeks ($n = 3$), the sympathetic trunks were harvested and analyzed using conventional and specific nerve tissue immunohistochemical stains (S100, neurofilament protein, and synaptophysin) to evaluate neural regeneration. They concluded that clipping of the sympathetic chain causes serious histological damage to the nerve, which remains visible 4 weeks after the removal of the clip; however, at 12 weeks these signs of damage clearly diminish, suggesting that the application of metal clips to the sympathetic chain is a reversible procedure if the observation period is prolonged. Unfortunately, they were unable to obtain neurophysiological measurements of nerve conduction to demonstrate conduction restoration.

Finally, one of the authors of this chapter (J. Pérez) performed an experimental work at Vall d'Hebron Hospital in Barcelona, Spain, in 2011 (unpublished data) using a porcine model that was selected because it has a sympathetic chain similar to humans in terms of distribution of nerve fibers but with a three to four times smaller diameter. This anatomical difference is related to the importance of the clip pressure over the sympathetic trunk, which is why two different clip appliers were tested: AcuClip™, Covidien® and Ligamax™ 5 Endoscopic Clip Applier, Ethicon®. Standard histological- and immunohistochemical-specific axonal regeneration techniques were used in nine pigs. Immediate changes after clipping were inflammatory. One week after unclipping, the nerve showed persistent structural injury with little regenerative activity but 2 weeks after unclipping the regenerative activity validated with specific immunohistochemical axonal regeneration techniques was very marked, suggesting a potential reversibility of the technique.

In summary, we could conclude that there is still controversy regarding the reversibility of sympathetic clipping but experimental studies show a trend towards confirming this possibility. We believe that future experimental studies require an adequate animal experimental model based on sympathetic chain anatomical similarities with the human one. There is also a lack of evidence about the maximum clipping period that should be applied, and more specifically the degree of compression that should be delivered in order to generate neuropraxia or even initial stages of axonotmesis (potentially reversible states) without reaching neurotmesis. Last but not least, neurophysiological conduction studies should corroborate that the histological reversibility translates into nerve conduction restoration.

References

1. Benedito Chuaqui. Lecciones de Anatomía Patológica. Patología celular. Capítulo 9. Pontificia Universidad Católica de Chile
2. Lin CC, Mo LR, Lee LS, Ng SM, Hwang MH. Thoracoscopic T2-sympathetic block by clipping – a better and reversible operation for treatment of hiperhidrosis palmaris: experience with 326 cases. Eur J Surg Suppl. 1998;580:13–6.
3. Reisfeld R. Sympathectomy reversal. Clamping vs nerve graft. Eighth International Symposium on Sympathetic Surgery (ISSS). New York, USA, March 25–27, 2009.
4. Loscertales J, Congregado M, Jimenez-Merchan R, Gallardo G, Trivino A, Moreno S, et al. Sympathetic chain clipping for hyperhidrosis is not a reversible procedure. Surg Endosc. 2012;26:1258–63.
5. Thomsen LL, Mikkelsen RT, Derejko M, Schrøder HD, Licht PB. Sympathetic block by metal clips may be a reversible operation. Interact Cardiovasc Thorac Surg. 2014;19(6):908–13.

Surgical Difficulties and Complications of Video-Assisted Thoracoscopic for Thoracic Sympathectomy

Laert de Oliveira Andrade Filho and Fabiano Cataldi Engel

Introduction

Endoscopic thoracic sympathectomy was initially described in 1942 by Hughes, but it was not until the 1990s that it became the best surgical choice following the development of video-assisted thoracoscopy.

Today, sympathectomy is indicated most often for the treatment of hyperhidrosis, although it is also indicated in the treatment of various organic diseases.

Hyperhidrosis has an incidence of 1% among the general population. Although it is not a life-threatening disease or one that compromises any organ-specific function, it decreases the quality of life of the affected patient by impairing social contact and creating personal suffering. Sympathectomy is the best therapeutic option, but without an accurate medical indication, it is often viewed as a cosmetic surgery.

In this context, there are a large number of patients seeking medical help for relief of symptoms, most under 30 years of age, a period during which social contact is most affected by the presence of hyperhidrosis.

The desire for surgery becomes the focus of attention of the patient with hyperhidrosis in order to solve the problem; they are motivated by information manipulated by the media, whose sources rarely report the risks inherent in the surgical procedure.

Considering these aspects, the morbidity and mortality of sympathectomy deserve special consideration. We are dealing with a young population, who are motivated and have great expectations of a positive result, but who have little information and are not really prepared for eventual failure of the surgical procedure.

L. d. O. Andrade Filho (✉) · F. C. Engel
Hospital Israelita Albert Einstein, São Paulo, SP, Brazil
e-mail: laert@einstein.br

Technical Difficulties of Thoracic Sympathectomy

Difficulties Inherent to the Operative Technique

Among the technical difficulties inherent in the surgical technique, we highlight the anesthetic difficulties and difficulties related to the video-assisted thoracoscopy system.

The first necessary condition for video-assisted thoracoscopy and good visualization of the thoracic sympathetic chain is the creation of air space within the thorax. The simplest way to create this space is through the open pneumothorax and partial collapse of the lung.

Orotracheal Intubation

Anesthetic difficulties begin at the time of intubation when opting for selective intubation system with a double-lumen probe for single-lung ventilation. This anesthetic option, when properly used, provides a complete lung collapse, which greatly facilitates the realization of the videothoracoscopic procedure and identification of the thoracic sympathetic chain, particularly when the intention is to access more segments of the chain flow such as T5. The use of a thin endoscope aids the proper positioning of the double-lumen probe, but, as it is an expensive piece of equipment, most hospitals do not have this feature and positioning the probe becomes more difficult.

Intubation with a simple probe facilitates the work of the anesthetist and lessens the impact on the patient because it is a thinner probe. The anesthesiologist should be more attentive to the surgical procedure when opting for the creation of open pneumothorax because the surgeon will need apneal moments to create the necessary space for video-assisted thoracoscopy and adequate visualization of the thoracic sympathetic chain.

Video-Assisted Thoracoscopy Equipment

The video-assisted thoracoscopy equipment must be of good quality and in good condition. The optics, camera, and video system are the eyes of the surgeon. A blurry image due to dirt, poor-quality optics, or deregulation in the camera and video system can negatively affect the result of surgery.

Endoscopic Surgical Instruments

Besides the optic system, the other instruments used for the sympathectomy should be adequate and of good quality.

Some perform the sympathectomy with an electric scalpel while others use a harmonic scalpel. The harmonic scalpel allows a limited lesion of the sympathetic chain, which does not occur with the electric scalpel as it dissipates current beyond the intended limits, although it is a considerable addition to the costs of the procedure. Particularly when handling the cranial portion of the chain, T2, limited damage provides more safety regarding prevention of stellate ganglion injury which can lead to Horner syndrome.

Difficulties Inherent to Anatomical Variations

The anatomical variations in the thorax, whether congenital or acquired, can interfere with the accomplishment of the sympathectomy by videothoracoscopy and its final result.

Pleural Adhesions

The most common finding creating difficulty in performing sympathectomy is the presence of pleural adhesions. The presence of adhesions prevents the collapse of the lung and the visualization of the thoracic sympathetic chain. The technique of videoàssisted thorascopy sympathectomy is designed to be the least invasive possible, using a few unique thin and optical input ports to perform the sympathectomy. When adhesions are firm, or with secondary vascularization, this more simplified approach of video-assisted thoracoscopy may be insufficient to adequately release the adhesions, making it impossible to perform the desired procedure without extending it to other access points and using other instruments. Sometimes the endoscopic procedure is impossible, requiring open surgery on one or both sides.

The frequency of the presence of pleural adhesions in the reports of sympathectomy in the literature reaches 6.5% of the cases. A prior history of pneumonia, tuberculosis, bronchitis, or recurrent pulmonary infections may be a warning for the possibility of pleural adhesions, but there is no imaging test to confirm or rule out such suspicion. In our series ($n = 1731$), adhesions were found in 6.7% of cases (1.6% of which were intense adhesions).

Azygos Lobe

Although it is an infrequent anatomical variation, the presence of the azygos lobe may make right thoracic sympathectomy very difficult. A chest X-ray is recommended in the preoperative evaluation of the patient. The tracing of the pleura dividing the right lung to the azygos vein, delimiting the azygous wolf, is an easily observable radiological finding and deserves the necessary care for the right thoracic sympathectomy. In these circumstances the patient should be alerted to this additional difficulty, which often entails more incisions for the greater number of entries needed to create space for the sympathectomy.

Obesity

Obese patients often have a fatty cushion over the parietal pleura that prevents correct identification of the costal arches and the sympathetic chain itself. The sympathetic chain usually has a more tense consistency and is different from the looser fat.

Scoliosis/Thoracic Aortic Aneurysm

In the left hemithorax, the T2 ganglion is identified in the intercostal space just above the aortic arch. The presence of elongated aorta can be avoided by the use of angled optics (30 ° or 45 °).

Medial and Nerve Sympathetic Chain of Kuntz

The Kuntz nerve (branches communicating between the second intercostal nerve and the ventral branch of the first thoracic nerve in the first intercostal space) has been implicated as responsible for failure of surgery in up to 1.5% of sympathectomies. However, it is an extremely controversial subject. Rarely are they identified in videothoracoscopy, although some authors show (by anatomical dissection) that they exist in 70% of patients. Subpleural veins in the first intercostal space parallel to the Kuntz nerve function as markers of the location of this nerve.

Complications of Thoracic Sympathectomy

Immediate Complications

Intraoperative Air Fistula and Pneumothorax

Pneumothorax is the most common complication occurring in up to 25% of cases. Fortunately, less than 6% of cases require chest drainage. In our series, we had to drain in 3.5% of cases. There are two types of pneumothorax resulting from sympathectomy: residual pneumothorax due to failure of complete exsufflation of pleural cavity air and pneumothorax due to pulmonary injury (by insertion of the trocar or laceration caused by the hook or pleuropulmonary adhesions section) or rupture of subpleural blebs or emphysematous blisters during positive pressure ventilation.

The residual cavity can be avoided by placing a thin tubular drain through the trocar into the pleural cavity. The drain is aspirated at the same time as the anesthesiologist manually inflates the lungs. Another alternative would be to dip the distal end of this drain into a water seal. At the end of the pulmonary insufflations or when the bubbling of air in the water seal stops this drain is removed. Sometimes on the chest X-ray we notice a small residual pneumothorax, which is not functionally translated and after a few days is reabsorbed without sequelae.

Pneumothorax resulting from lung injury is most often identified when there is continuous bubbling when inflating the lung at the end of surgery and is treated with maintenance of thoracic drainage. Occasionally, if there is persistent air fistula, there may be a need for pleurodesis.

Subcutaneous Emphysema

Subcutaneous emphysema occurs by air entering the pleural cavity through the intercostal opening created by the trocar. Usually, it is only noticed in the chest radiography, with or without pneumothorax but without any clinical repercussion. The use of 5 mm rather than 10 mm trocars minimizes the problem. We commonly perceive the radiographic presence of small subcutaneous emphysema in our patients without physiological repercussions.

Atelectasis

Atelectasis is very rare, and usually improves with analgesia and respiratory physiotherapy. It is due to problems with intubation and exaggerated secretion in the postoperative period as a result of inadequate preparation and/or respiratory infection.

Pleural Effusion
Pleural effusion is usually small, with no clinical significance and no need for treatment. Its incidence is as high as 1% of cases. Some authors believe that the incidence may be higher if the patient is discharged early. We have not observed this complication in our patients.

Hemothorax
Arterial bleeds are rare and usually occur due to subclavian or intercostal artery laceration by the hook. Arterial bleeds may require open surgical correction if massive bleeding occurs. Venous bleeds occur more frequently and can occur as a result of trocar insertion or dissection of the sympathetic chain leading to intercostal vein injury. Normally, bleeding is controlled by the endoscopy route by cauterization, tamponade, or clipping of the vein. Bleeds of 300–600 mL of blood occur in up to 5.3% of cases. In our practice, the incidence of bleeding is only 0.7% of cases (intercostal vein lesion), all controlled with clipping or cauterization.

Chylothorax
Chylothorax is extremely unusual, and can occur on the right or left side. Treatment requires thoracic drainage and a low fat diet. Occasionally there is a need for clipping of the thoracic duct or pleurodesis. We have had no complications of this nature.

Hematomas and Incisional Infections
As in any surgical procedure, hematomas and incisional infections may occur, but there are no data in the literature. This is probably because it is a minimally invasive surgery, with small incisions and very short surgical time.

Severe Pain
Thoracic sympathectomy usually causes moderate pain (in the retrosternal and upper dorsal region) that lasts for approximately 2–4 weeks, requiring only simple analgesics and anti-inflammatory drugs. However, between 0.6% and 2% of patients report severe pain, especially intercostal or ulnar neuralgia lasting up to 6 months. The use of minor trocars, anesthetic infiltration prior to trocar introduction, and the use of the single trocar technique may minimize the problem. In our series, 2.6% of patients experienced severe pain lasting more than 15 days.

Intraoperative Cardiac Arrest
Cardiac arrest and/or ventricular fibrillation may occur as a result of exaggerated sympathetic stimulation of the left star ganglion. Transient bradycardias or those requiring atropine are also reported.

Brachial Plexus Injury
Brachial plexus injury is rare and can occur due to distension as a result of poor patient positioning or direct injury. Using the thoracoscopic approach, direct injury is extremely rare, but was more common when a supraclavicular approach was used. In this case, there may be a failure to identify the sympathetic chain in relation to the costal arcs.

Excessive abduction of the upper limb during patient placement may lead to paresthesia, paresis, or temporary paralysis of the upper limb. It may occur in up to 4.6% of patients. Upper extremity paresthesia occurred in 2% of our patients.

Brain Complications

Cerebral edema can occur due to insufflation of CO_2; pulmonary thromboembolism have been rarely described.

Late Complications

Compensatory Hyperhidrosis

Compensatory hyperhidrosis is by far the most common and labor-intensive complication. It was first recognized in 1933 by Ross: "Some of our patients said that sweat has been considerably higher in areas not affected by the operation. At first, we were inclined to consider this only as an observation error, with the usual amount of sweat considered excessive when contrasted with the completely denervated area. However, the observation has been so commonly made, and it has been possible to observe the increase in sweat so often that the possibility of compensatory sweating can not be excluded".

Compensatory sweating may be defined as sweat production in areas that showed no abnormal sweating preoperatively and to a higher degree than required for heat-setting.

Compensatory sweating occurred in 92% ($n = 1115$) of our patients (quantified in the thirtieth postoperative period); in the literature, its prevalence ranges from 86% to 100%.

The most affected sites are the dorsum, abdomen, thighs, and popliteal fossa. The incidence of compensatory sweating is the main reason for regret in patients who have undergone sympathectomy (in our sample 2.5% regretted surgery). Of these, 2.2% had the same quality of life as before surgery, 0.6% a little worse, and 0.9% a lot worse.

There is a consensus in the literature that compensatory hyperhidrosis depends on the level or the extent of sympathectomy. The mechanism for compensatory hyperhidrosis to occur depends on thermoregulatory mechanisms after sympathetic denervation and/or neuro-mediated reflexes that rely on positive and negative feedback mechanisms from the hypothalamus.

In thermoregulation after high thoracic sympathectomy, there is loss of upper-limb sweat gland function, leading to greater activation of residual sweat glands in the trunk, leading to compensatory hyperhidrosis.

The regulating center of the sweat is in the hypothalamus. Sympathetic efferent discharges must be controlled by negative or positive feedback mechanisms from sympathetic afferent pathways. The T2 sympathectomy would block the negative feedback of the afferent stimuli to the hypothalamus, since it would cut off practically all the afferent pathways, and favor the appearance of compensatory hyperhidrosis in the periphery, due to the continuous release of efferent stimuli by the hypothalamus. Sympathectomy below this level would cut off a number of afferent pathways, avoiding a feedback block and decreasing compensatory hyperhidrosis.

Selective sympathectomy (ramicotomy) was used in an attempt to avoid compensatory hyperhidrosis. In this type of procedure, the communicating branches are sectioned, preserving the sympathetic chain. However, due to the high relapse rate, the procedure was abandoned.

Clamping (clipping) of the sympathetic chain has also been used. In this situation, if the patient develops compensatory hyperhidrosis, there is the possibility of reversing the surgery by removing the clips. However, while some authors report reversion of symptoms within 2 months, others have not been successful.

The treatment of compensatory hyperhidrosis is multidisciplinary. It often involves psychologists, psychiatrists, neurologists, dermatologists, endocrinologists, dietitians, physical education teachers, and thoracic surgeons. Non-medication measures may be fundamental: weight loss, non-thermogenic diet, physical exercise, climate change, use of dry-fit clothing; drug measures (application of topical, intradermal, or oral medications); and surgical treatments (lumbar sympathectomy and re-innervation of the sympathetic chain).

Gustatory Sweating

Gustatory sweating is the occurrence of craniofacial sweating when eating spicy or acidic foods. The pathophysiology of this complication is uncertain, but it is thought that the sympathectomy causes parasympathetic stimulus on the salivary glands (innervation of the salivary glands would not be totally parasympathetic).

The incidence varies greatly in studies (0–38%), and treatment involves oral anticholinergics, injectable botulinum toxin applications, or topical applications of anticholinergics. In our patients, there was a 19.3% incidence.

Horner Syndrome

Horner syndrome (palpebral ptosis, pupillary myosis, enophthalmia, and anhidrosis) was considered previously as the marker of sympathectomy success, but today it is considered a serious complication. Temporary palpebral ptosis can occur in up to 1% of cases, usually resolving in weeks or a few months. Not using the electrocautery near the star ganglion is a way to avoid this complication.

Rhinitis

The effect of sympathectomy on the subject with rhinitis is controversial. Some authors describe the onset of rhinitis with an incidence of up to 10%, while others recommend sympathectomy for the treatment of chronic rhinitis. The effect of sympathectomy on bronchial reactivity (asthma) is also unclear. In our patients, the incidence of rhinitis was 5.6%.

Ghost Sweat

Ghost sweat is a phenomenon that is little mentioned in the literature. The patient has the sensation that he will sweat, but the sweating does not occur; this situation occurs soon after the sympathectomy, is triggered by the same stimuli that would cause localized hyperhidrosis, and lasts for a few seconds. Over time this symptoms tends to improve.

Bradycardia

The sympathetic ganglia T2 and T3 are involved in cardiac sympathetic innervation. Sympathectomy at these levels has a β-blocking activity. This leads to a decrease in the heart rate and diastolic pressure is decreased on the dynamometer. Patients who are athletes should be warned about this effect of sympathectomy. In our series, 0.2% of patients had these complications.

Rare Complications

Cold intolerance, chronic pain, loss of libido, photophobia, lethargy, weight gain … these and other odd symptoms are rarely described, and many are not reported in the medical literature but instead found in depositions placed on the internet by dissatisfied patients with effects they attribue to the sympathectomy.

Mortality

There are no published reports in the literature of sympathectomy-related deaths. However, deaths due to massive hemorrhage as a result of injury to the intercostal vessels or laceration of the subclavian artery are known informally. In addition, problems in selective intubation or insufflation with CO_2 leading to hypoxia and cardiac arrest and death or severe cerebral ischemia are real.

Fortunately these fatal cases are few, but, simple as thoracic sympathectomy may seem, there is a need for adequate training so that the skilled surgeon can pay attention to the anesthetic, technical, and perioperative details, thus minimizing morbidity and mortality.

Conclusion

Thoracic sympathectomy by videothoracoscopy is widely used as a treatment for localized hyperhidrosis. It is a relatively safe, easy, and quick surgery. However, it is necessary to ensure adequate instrumentation, skilled training (surgical and anesthetic staff), and careful selection of patients (attention to adequate weight and history of respiratory infections) to reduce the inconvenience of this surgery. In addition, patients should be fully informed about the potential adverse effects and complications before they are operated.

Suggested Reading

Adar R, Kurchin A, Zweig A, Mozes M. Palmar hyperhidrosis and its surgical treatment: a report of 100 cases. Ann Surg. 1977;186:34–41.

Andrade Filho LO, Kuzniec S, Wolosker N, Yazbec G, Kauffman P, de Campos JRM. Technical difficulties and complications of symphatectomy in the treatment of hyperhidrosis: an analysis of 1731 cases. Ann Vasc Surg. 2013;27(4):447–53.

Andrews BT, Rennie JA. Predicting changes in the distribution of sweating following thoracoscopic sympathectomy. Br J Surg. 1997;84:1702–4.

Asking B, Svartholm E. Degeneration activity; a transient effect following sympathectomy for hyperhidrosis. Eur J Surg Suppl. 1994;572:41–2.

Atherton WG, Morgan WE. False aneurysm of an intercostal artery after thoracoscopic sympathectomy. Ann R Coll Surg Engl. 1997;79:229–30.

Atkins HJB. Sympathectomy by the axillary approach. Lancet. 1954;1:538–9.

Cameron AEP. Complications of endoscopic sympathectomy. Eur J Surg Suppl. 1998;580:33–5.

de Campos JRM, Kauffman P, Werebe EC, Andrade Filho LO, et al. Quality of life, before and after thoracic sympathectomy: report on 378 operated patients. Ann Thorac Surg. 2003;76:886–91.

de Campos JRM, et al. The body mass index and level of resection. Predictive factors for compensatory sweating after sympathectomy. Clin Auton Res. 2005;15:116–20.

Chiou TS-M, Chen S-C. Intermediate-term results of endoscopic transaxillary T2 sympathectomy for primary palmar hyperhidrosis. Br J Surg. 1999;86:45–7.

Drott C, Claes G, Gothberg G, Paszowski P. Cardiac effects of endoscopic electrocautery of the upper thoracic sympathetic chain. Eur J Surg Suppl. 1994;572:65–70.

Duarte JBV, Kux P. Efficacy of endoscopic thoracic sympathectomy along with severing the Kuntz nerve in the treatment of chronic non-infectious rhinitis. Ann Chir Gynaecol. 2001;90:189–92.

Dumont P. Side effects and complications of surgery for hyperhidrosis. Thorac Surg Clin. 2008;18:193–207.

Dumont D, Denoyer A, Robin P. Long-term results of thoracoscopic sympathectomy for hyperhidrosis. Ann Thorac Surg. 2004;78:1801–7.

Franz Marhold F, Izay B, Zacherl J, Tschabitscher M, Neumayer C. Thoracoscopic and anatomic landmarks of Kuntz's nerve: implications for sympathetic surgery. Ann Thorac Surg. 2008;86:1653–8.

Gossot D, Grunenwald D, et al. Early complications of thoracic endoscopic sympathectomy: a prospective study of 940 procedures. Ann Thorac Surg. 2001;71:1116–9.

Gossot D, Galetta D, et al. Long-term results of endoscopic thoracic sympathectomy for upper limb hyperhidrosis. Ann Thorac Surg. 2003;75(4):1075–9.

Gossot D, Grunenwald D, et al. Long-term results of endoscopic thoracic sympathectomy for upper limb hyperhidrosis. Eur J Cardiothorac Surg. 2005;27:741–4.

Herbst F, Fugger R, Fritsch A, et al. Endoscopic thoracic sympatectomy for primary hyperhidrosis of the upper limbs. A critical analysis and long-term results of 480 operations. Ann Surg. 2002;89:158–62.

Hughes J. Endothoracic sympathectomy. Proc R Soc Med. 1942;35:585–6.

Kauffman P, Wolosker N, de Campos JRM, Yazbec G, Jatene FB. Azygos lobe: a difficulty in video-assisted thoracic sympathectomy. Ann Thorac Surg. 2010;89(6):57–9.

Kopleman D, Bahous H, Assalia A, Hashmonai M. Upper dorsal sympathectomy for palmar hyperhidrosis. Use of the harmonic scalpel *versus* diathermy. Ann Chir Gynaecol. 2001;90:203–5.

Lai YT, Yang LH, et al. Complications in patients with palmar hyperhidrosis treated with transthoracic endoscopic sympathectomy. Neurosurgery. 1997;41:110–3.

Lai CL, Chen WC, Liu YB, Lee YT. Bradycardia and permanent pacing after bilateral thoracoscopic T2sympathectomy for primary hyperhidrosis. Pacing Clin Electrophysiol. 2001;24:524–5.

Lange JF. Inferior brachial plexus injury during thoracoscopic sympathectomy. Surg Endosc. 1995;9:830.

Lin CC. http:// www.sweathand.com.

Lin TS, Fang HY. Transthoracic endoscopic sympathectomy in the treatment of palmar hyperhidrosis—with emphasis on perioperative management (1,360 case analyses). Surg Neurol. 1999 Nov;52(5):453–7.

Lin CC, Telaranta T. Lin-Telaranta classification: the importance of different produce of for different indications in sympathectomy surgery. Ann Chir Gynaecol. 2001;90(3):161–6.

Lin C-C, Mo L-R, Hwang M-H. Intraoperative cardiac arrest: a rare complication of T2,3-sympathicotomy for treatment of hyperhidrosis palmaris. Two case reports. Eur J Surg Suppl. 1994;572:43–5.

Lin CC, Lee LS, et al. The haemodynamic effect of thoracoscopic cardiac sympathectomy. Eur J Surg Suppl. 1998a;580:37–8.

Lin CC, et al. Thoracoscopic T2-sympathetic block by clipping – a better and reversible operation for treatment of hyperhidrosis palmaris: experience with 326 cases. Eur J Surg Suppl. 1998b;580:13–6.

Ojimba TA, Cameron AE. Drawbacks of endoscopic thoracic sympathectomy. Br J Surg. 2004;91(3):264–9.

Ramsaroop L, Partab P, Singh B, Satyapal KS. Thoracic origin of a sympathetic supply to the upper limb: the 'nerve of Kuntz' revisited. J Anat. 2001;199(Pt 6):675–82.

Ramsaroop L, Partab P, Singh B, et al. Anatomical basis for a successful upper limb sympathectomy in the thoracoscopic era. Clin Anat. 2004;17:294–9.

Reisfeld R. http://www.sweaty-palms.com/reversal_ets.html.

Riet M, et al. Prevention of compensatory hyperhidrosis after thoracoscopic sympathectomy for hyperhidrosis. Surg Endosc. 2001;15:1159–62.

Ross JP. Sympathectomy as an experiment in human physiology. Br J Surg. 1933;21:5–19.

Shachor D, Jedeikin R, Olsfanger D, Bendahan J, Sivak G, Freund U. Endoscopic transthoracic sympathectomy in thetreatment of primary hyperhidrosis. A review of 290 sympathectomies. Arch Surg. 1994;129:241–4.

Telaranta T. Secondary sympathetic chain reconstruction after endoscopic thoracic sympathectomy. Eur J Surg. 1998;164(Suppl 580):17–8.

Telaranta T. Reversal surgery for reducing the side-effects of ETS. A case report. Ann Chir Gynaecol. 2001;90:175–6.

Telaranta T. http://www.privatix.fi.

Zacherl J, Herbst F, et al. Video assistance reduces complication rate of thoracoscopic sympathectomy for hyperhidrosis. Ann Thorac Surg. 1999;68:1177–81.

Outpatient Clinic Treatment for Patients with Hyperhidrosis

Camilo Osorio Barker

Videothoracoscopic sympathectomy for the treatment of primary hyperhidrosis in the hands, face, or underarms, and/or pathological facial flushing is a procedure performed in the majority of cases in young and healthy people with no significant co-morbidities or risk factors. These circumstances make it manageable on an outpatient basis.

Risks such as the presence of postoperative pneumothorax or bradycardia following sympathectomy have made some surgical groups opt for postoperative management with hospital admission.

In order to clarify this disjunction between postoperative out- or inpatient management, we submitted our series of 1251 patients who underwent bilateral videothoracoscopic sympathectomy to a retrospective analysis, from the date we began performing this procedure on 23 March 2001 until a cut-off date of 30 June 2016 (15 years).

Hospitalized management of sympathectomy was in many cases a product of the current protocol, especially in the early years of the procedure, where the short level of experience and learning curve dictated prudence that recommended leaving thoracic drains and patients being hospitalized for at least the first 24 h post-surgery. In addition, there were no representative series available within the operated patients that allowed use of their experience to define specific behaviors with respect to the surgery technique itself and its general management.

Between 23 March 2001 and February 2003, the first 46 patients, who underwent a bilateral resection of the sympathetic T2 and T3 ganglia, were operated without considering the particular symptomatology of each patient. Ports of 11 mm and optics of 10 mm at 30 ° were used at that time. All patients underwent general anesthesia through selective bronchial intubation.

C. O. Barker
Universidad Pontificia Bolivariana, Medellín, Antioquia, Colombia
e-mail: camilo.osorio@unisabana.edu.co; caol@une.net.co

During the period between March 2001 and December 2003, all patients undergoing surgery were hospitalized in the postoperative period as per protocol. At this time, 42 patients (82.3% of the total hospitalized in the series) were involved.

Regarding management of the thoracic drainage tube (thoracostomy) during that period, 27 patients were left to drain for the first 24 postoperative hours and 15 were left with drainage only during the immediate postoperative period (2 h).

From 2003 onwards, the ambulatory management for all patients was standardized in our series, using 5 mm ports (two on each side), with 5 mm and 30 ° optics. The total expansion of the lung parenchyma was verified under direct vision, and no pleural drainage tube was left in. We continued with selective bronchial intubation for general anesthesia.

After 2008, we began to use the harmonic scalpel (Jonson & Johnson) for pleural dissection and resection of sympathetic nodes, with a decrease in surgical time and the need for hemostasis in pleural dissection.

In 2013 we chose to replace conventional bronchial intubation with conventional tracheal intubation, improving the pharyngolaryngeal pain produced by the double-lumen tube. We also began to use CO_2 within the pleural cavity, at a pressure of 6–8 mm, which allows sufficient work vision within the pleural cavity. In addition, we stopped excising the nerve, only sectioning the chain at a defined level and performing fulguration of the required sympathetic ganglia, which further diminished the risk of bleeding.

All patients remained under observation 2–3 h after the procedure, with monitoring of oximetry, blood pressure, heart rate, and electrocardiogram. During this period, chest X-rays were obtained to confirm pulmonary expansion. Patients were only allowed to go home when they were fully recovered, and had oral and pain tolerance.

Home pain management was performed with opioids plus acetaminophen every 6 h orally.

Patients were followed up by telephone 12 and 24 h after surgery. Postoperative visits occurred following the first week, the first month, and the third month.

The patient and his family were informed of warning signs and given the surgeon's telephone number with 24-h availability for urgent consultations.

Results

During the 15 years of our series, 1252 patients underwent bilateral videothoracoscopic sympathectomy due to primary palmar, axillary, or facial hyperhidrosis or pathological facial flushing. Of these, only 52 were hospitalized after surgery (4.15%).

Excluding those hospitalized by protocol, a total of ten patients were hospitalized, corresponding to only 0.8% of the total number of surgeries. The reasons for not being allowed to leave the hospital after the procedure were as follows:

- Eight patients required an admission of 1–4 days for air leak in the postoperative period.
- Two patients were hospitalized for other causes: one for pulmonary edema after intubation and the other because of the patient's own decision.

- Four patients needed to be re-hospitalized after discharge (0.3% of the total number of patients) due to the following causes:
  - Residual right pneumothorax: 2 days of hospitalization.
  - Coagulated hemothorax: the patient required surgical management with thoracotomy and 8 days of hospitalization.
  - Coagulated hemothorax: the patient required video-assisted thoracoscopy and 3 days of hospitalization.
  - Right hemothorax of 1000 cc: handled with a drainage tube and 3 days of hospitalization.

No patient in the series had bradycardia or other cardiac rhythm disorders in the early postoperative period.

One patient experienced delayed a cardiac rhythm disorder and required implantation of a pacemaker, although it is not clear whether it was caused by the sympathectomy.

Four patients had a residual pneumothorax in the immediate postoperative period, which was evacuated with pleural needle puncture, without requiring hospitalization.

The postoperative satisfaction of hospitalized patients was 96.5/100, similar to the overall series.

Hospitalized Versus Ambulatory Management

Although most published articles on sympathectomy do not mention whether the management was ambulatory or hospitalized, some comment that their management was ambulatory, such as endoscopic thoracic sympathectomy (ETS) for primary hyperhidrosis in a 16-year follow-up study [1] that included 51 patients with ambulatory management.

In a study in children, the authors clearly describe hospitalized management, with an average length of 2 days (range 1–5) [2].

In a study that showed the safety and effectiveness of the procedure without tracheal intubation, even after surgical management with only deep sedation and flexible thoracoscopy (ETS with flexible thoracoscopy under deep sedation without intubation is a safe and effective method) the patients were discharged from the hospital at the second postoperative day [3].

Why Ambulatory Management in Videothoracoscopic Sympathectomy?

The reasons for ambulatory management in videothoracoscopic sympathectomy are as follows:

- It is definitely more comfortable for the patient and his family not to have to remain hospitalized after the surgery, being able to have guaranteed safety in their home with this ambulatory management.

- The reduction of the cost of hospitalization is evident if the patient is treated on an outpatient basis after the procedure.

Problems Attributed to Ambulatory Sympathectomy

In contrast to the postoperative management of the videothoracoscopic sympathectomy, some problems are associated with ambulatory sympathectomy, such as:

- Postoperative pain can be intense, especially in the first 24 h.
- The fear of some surgeons regarding the threat of the patient presenting symptomatic changes in cardiac or respiratory physiology in the early postoperative period such as bradycardia or hypotension.
- The possibility of pneumothorax, either residual or any lung parenchyma lesion not evidenced during surgery.
- Unpleasant postoperative symptoms such as vomiting caused by anesthesia or pain medication.

Several studies have shown the cardiovascular effect of sympathectomy.

Fiorelli et al., in a study in 2012 [4], concluded that "Sympathectomy may result in a disturbance of bronchomotor tone and cardiac function. Such changes remained at a sub-clinical level and seemed directly correlated with the extent of denervation".

Zhang et al. [5] analyzed the effects of thoracic sympathectomy on heart rate variability in patients with palmar hyperhidrosis and concluded the following: "There was a significant improvement in HRV (Heart rate variability, especially used by athletes) in patients with palmar hyperhidrosis after thoracic sympathotomy. This may be attributable to an improvement in autonomic nervous system balance and parasympathetic predominance in the early postoperative stage".

In a study on autonomic function following endoscopic thoracic sympathotomy for hyperhidrosis, the authors conclude that "ETS changes cardiac autonomic modulation of HR [heart rate] to levels similar to controls. Despite the minimally destructive nature of ETS, HRV effects are consistent with previously reported post-sympathectomy blunting of exaggerated sympathetic control associated with hyperhidrosis. No significant changes in the baroreflex indices suggest that ETS did not significantly affect blood pressure regulation".

Another study on hemodynamics following endoscopic thoracic sympathotomy for palmar hyperhidrosis concludes that sustained exercise capacity suggests modest clinical consequences [6].

Ambulatory Strategy

Patient Selection

Adequate patient selection of those undergoing sympathectomy due to palmar, axillary, or facial hyperhidrosis or pathological facial flushing is essential, and even more so regarding those who may receive outpatient management.

The patient selection criteria for ambulatory management should be as follows:

- Patients must be healthy people, not necessarily young, with no co-morbidities and no history of important pulmonary pathologies.
- They must have an adequate social level to be able to understand what the ambulatory management of the procedure means and the alarm signs.
- The patient must have adequate anxiety management. Patients with complex personalities or suspected behavioral disorders should be excluded, as their results will not be adequate with surgery.
- Healthcare centers must be easily accessible from the patient's home.

Physician–Patient Relationship

From the initial consultation, it is necessary to develop trust and easy communication pathways between the patient and the surgeon.

Surgery Factors

The ideal anesthesia for this type of procedure is intravenous, since it makes fast recovery at the end of the procedure possible, allowing the patient to be discharged early.

I suggest that orotracheal intubation with a single light tube always be used as it presents less discomfort and local pain in the postoperative period than the double-lumen tube with selective intubation, which also increases the cost of the procedure.

The 5 mm ports with their minimal trauma help decrease subsequent pain.

Insufflation of CO_2 in the thoracic cavity simplifies the procedure and reduces surgical time. Adequate monitoring of capnography should be performed and the gas must be completely removed at the end of the procedure on each side, allowing total lung expansion and reducing postoperative pain.

The use of the harmonic scalpel facilitates the procedure, shortens the surgical time, and reduces the risk of bleeding.

Evolution of the learning curve will allow less surgical time, tissue trauma, and complications.

Post-Surgical Observation

Close monitoring of the patient, especially oximetry and heart rate, is essential during the immediate postoperative period.

Oxygen saturation lower than 95% in a patient receiving supplemental oxygen by mask or nasal cannula should cause suspicion that the patient has a pneumothorax, which should be studied with chest X-ray.

Although it is very rare, heart rate monitoring is essential for early diagnosis of bradycardia and subsequent treatment.

In our series, time in the postoperative service before the patient leaves is 2 h, although this may be longer depending on the patient's total recovery, including oral tolerance, pain control, or other symptoms such as vomiting.

The need for control chest X-rays at the end of the procedure can be controversial. In the first 14 years of our series we routinely performed chest X-rays in all patients; however, we found that the vast majority of studies were completely normal. We currently reserve chest X-ray for patients in whom there are special circumstances, either in the transoperative or in the postoperative period, such as an oximetry less than 95% despite receiving complementary oxygen through nasal cannula or Venturi mask.

Pain Control

Pain is a real discomfort in the postoperative period for the majority of patients undergoing videothoracoscopic sympathectomy. Thus, we must give great importance to its prevention and control.

With respect to prevention, it is essential to begin with the complete evacuation of the CO_2 (which we use) or the pneumothorax in both cavities. The presence of even minimal amounts of residual pneumothorax is associated with greater pain in the immediate postoperative period.

Supplemental oxygen should be administered by nasal cannula or Venturi mask in the period during which the patient remains in recovery, for at least 2 h.

In our series we used several analgesic regimens, the most effective being the combination of codeine 30 mg plus acetaminophen 500 mg orally every 6 h, interposed with dipyrone 0.5 g also every 6 h.

> "The postoperative intercostal pain was present in all patients (100%) with mean duration of 21.88 days but in 72.6% of cases it did not require any medication as early as 48 h after surgery" [7].

Early Troubleshooting

Problems such as finding residual pneumothorax in the immediate postoperative period must be solved immediately, as this allows the ambulatory management plan to be continued. Evacuation with a No. 16 venous catheter placed in the pleural cavity and connected to a simple water trap is usually a suitable solution.

Other symptoms such as vomiting or severe pain should be checked before the patient leaves.

Easy Communication and Availability for the Patient

The patient and his/her family should have an easy means of communication (mobile phone) 24 h a day with the surgical team after leaving the hospital, so they can clarify any doubts or alarm signs.

Written Instructions

Instructions must be written using clear language, avoiding technical terminology. The written instructions given to the patient's relative or companion are fundamental in the ambulatory management of this procedure. They should include not only the signs and symptoms that occur during the immediate postoperative period but also the ones that may occur in the following days up until the post-surgical review. Ideally, they should also be sent via a service such as Chat or WhatsApp to the patient's mobile phone before surgery.

References

1. Askary A, Kordzadeth A, Lee GH, Harvey M. Endoscopic thoracic sympatectomy for primary hyperhidrosis: a 16 years follow up. Surgeon. 2013;11:130–3.
2. Sinha CK, Kiely E. Thoracoscopic sympathectomy for palmar hyperhidrosis in children: 21 years of experience at a tertiary care center. Eur J Pediatr Surg. 2013;23(6):486–9.
3. Tang H, Wu B, Xu Z, Xue L, Li B, Zhao X. A new surgical procedure for palmar hyperhidrosis: is it possible to perform endoscopic sympathectomy under deep sedation without intubation? Eur J Cardio Thor Surg. 2014;46(2):286–90; Discussion 290.
4. Fiorelli A, D'Aponte A, Canonico R, Palladino A, Vicidomini G, Limongelli F, Santini M. T2-T3 sympathectomy versus sympathicotomy for essential palmar hyperhidrosis: comparison of effects on cardio-respiratory function. Eur J Cardiothorac Surg. 2012;42(3):454–61.
5. Zhang TY, Wang L, Xu JJ. The effects of thoracic sympathotomy on heart rate variability in patients with palmar hyperhidrosis. Yonsei Med J. 2012;53(6):1081–4.
6. Wehrwein EA, Schmidt JE, Elvebak RL, Pike TL, Atkinson JL Fealey RD, Eisenach JH. Hemodynamics following endoscopic thoracic sympathotomy for palmar hyperhidrosis. Clin Auton Res. 2011;21(1):3–10.
7. Stefaniak TJ, Cwigon M. Long-term results of thoracic sympathectomy for primary hyperhidrosis. Pol Przegl Chir. 2013;85(5):247–52.

Management of Compensatory Hyperhidrosis

Dafne Braga Diamante Leiderman, Guilherme Yazbec, and Nelson Wolosker

Introduction

The first description of compensatory hyperhidrosis (CH) occurred in 1935. It is defined as a change in the quantitative distribution of sweat in response to external heat, with a compensatory increase of sweating in regions of the body not denervated by sympathectomy in order to maintain body thermoregulation. It is considered the most common and most feared adverse effect of thoracic sympathectomy, usually beginning in the first to fifth postoperative period.

For many decades, cervicothoracic sympathectomy was the gold standard in the treatment of hyperhidrosis, and with the modernization of the technique after the development of assisted video surgeries it became a safe and widely performed procedure after the 1990s. Consequently, CH was observed more frequently and with an incidence greater than 98% according to the world literature.

The pathophysiology of CH is uncertain, but it is currently believed that postsympathectomy sweating is a reflex phenomenon moderated by a self-regulating mechanism between the center of hypothalamus sweating, body heat reflectors, and sweat glands. The preoptic region in the anterior portion of the hypothalamus

D. B. D. Leiderman
Department of Vascular and Endovascular Surgery, Hospital Israelita Albert Einstein, São Paulo, SP, Brazil

G. Yazbec
Department of Vascular and Endovascular Surgery, A.C. Camargo Cancer Center, Liberdade, São Paulo, SP, Brazil

N. Wolosker (✉)
Department of Vascular and Endovascular Surgery, Hospital Israelita Albert Einstein, São Paulo, SP, Brazil

receives afferent temperature information from central and peripheral thermoreceptors and releases an efferent thermoregulatory boost to the glands.

Before sympathectomy, the temperature influences the thermoreceptors of the skin, which would trigger a response from the thermoregulatory center located in the hypothalamus. The sympathetic tone of the hypothalamus would induce sweat through synapses in the sympathetic ganglia, which triggers afferent sympathetic stimulation afferent to the hypothalamus after the synapse (Fig. 26.1). In the cases of sympathectomy at the second (G2) or third (G3) thoracic ganglion level, the sympathetic efferent stimulation is amplified by the interruption of the afferent fibers into the hypothalamus, and there is no sympathetic negative stimulus. Because the amplified sympathetic stimulus does not reach sympathectomized areas, sweating occurs in other parts of the body (Fig. 26.2).

In cases of sympathectomy at the fourth thoracic ganglion (G4) level, the majority of the afferent fibers responsible for the sympathetic negative stimulus are preserved and, therefore, severe compensatory sweating does not occur. Sympathectomy at the G2 level causes a complete interruption of negative feedback to the hypothalamus, contributing to the more frequent onset of severe CH.

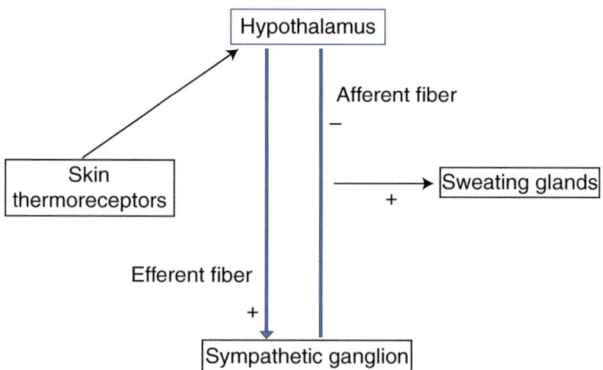

Fig. 26.1 Hypothalamic control—before sympathectomy

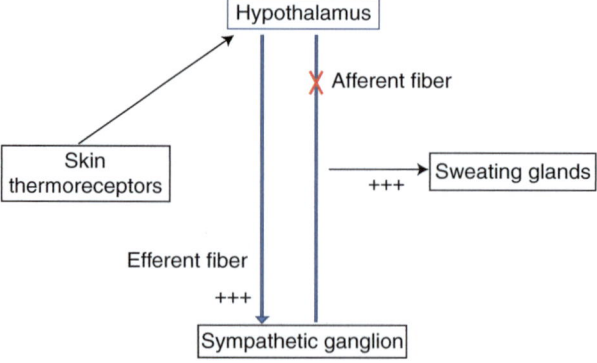

Fig. 26.2 Hypothalamic control—after sympathectomy

CH occurs mainly in the abdomen, back, thorax, and thigh, and less frequently in the feet, being commonly observed in the combination of two or more sites. It is usually symmetrical and is worse on hot days and during physical activity or emotional stress and anxiety. The symptoms may decrease over time or the patient may become accustomed to them, being usually tolerable and without major impact on quality of life; in children the CH is better tolerated and less severe. There are studies that show that more than 11.6% of patients develop severe CH with a social impact as bad or worse than their preoperative status, requiring frequent changes of clothes and avoidance of the use of colored clothing. The patient's dissatisfaction with HC is not infrequent, even going so far as to reveal regret in having undergone the surgical procedure.

In more extreme cases, complete isolation from a social point of view may occur.

Classification

Several authors have proposed classifications for CH, most of which described three or four different levels of CH intensity: mild, moderate, severe, and/or incapacitating according to the impact of excessive sweating on the patient's quality of life. There is discordance in the literature about whether small changes in the location and severity of sweating, such as sweating during hot weather and during exercise, that do not express significant concern in patients should be considered CH or only non-pathological compensatory sweating, a fact that must be taken into account in Brazil, a tropical country of high temperatures. Moderate or disturbing CH is usually considered present when patients reported visible and embarrassing sweating. Severe or incapacitating CH refers to patients who report major interference or feel incapacitated with regards to their social and professional activities (such as the need for successive changes of clothing caused by sweating) at the same intensity as their main preoperative hyperhidrosis, but in other sites (Fig. 26.3).

Yazbek et al. defines severe CH as one in which excessive sweating is visible causing embarrassment or requiring more than one change of clothing during the day.

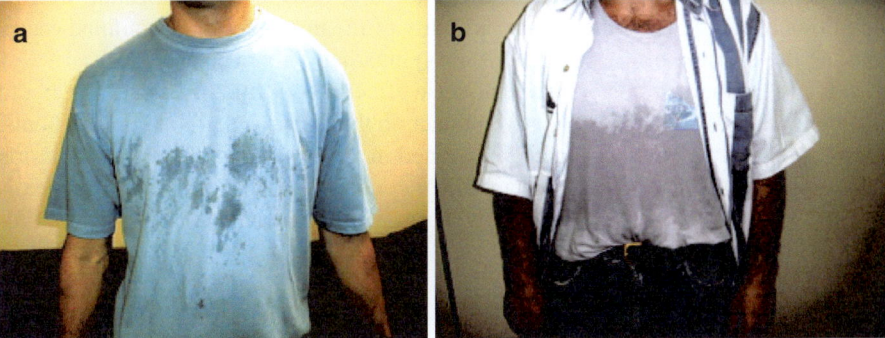

Fig. 26.3 (**a**) Moderate hyperhidrosis. (**b**) Severe hyperhidrosis

Prophylaxis

The most known risk factors for CH are the extent and level of sympathectomy and the patient's body mass index (BMI). In the more extensive denervations (G2–G4), about 40% of the body surface stops sweating, contributing to all patients having compensatory sweating in non-denervated areas. Studies show that the higher the level and the greater the extent of the sympathectomy, the more severe is the CH, justified by the greater absence of negative feedback to the hypothalamus causing it to further stimulate sweating.

CH is more pronounced when patients are operated at the G2 level, where there is an increasing convergence of afferent pathways to the hypothalamus. Some authors suggest that the preservation of the afferent pathway, which is responsible for negative feedback to the hypothalamus, would be the key factor in reducing postoperative CH rates. Therefore, denervation of a single ganglion should be performed for each site of hyperhidrosis and be performed at lower ganglion levels.

The single level G4 for axillary hyperhidrosis and G3 for palmar has been shown to be effective in the treatment of the main complaint, developing moderate or severe CH in a smaller percentage of the patients, around 3%, leading to an impressive improvement in quality of life compared with the preoperative period.

The relationship between sweating and BMI has been investigated before. It was observed that overweight or obese individuals (BMI >25.0 kg/m^2) had more severe sweating than the general population. The obese or overweight individual has a thicker layer of adipose tissue in the subcutaneous than normal, presenting greater difficulty in heat loss through irradiation, with evaporation being the main mechanism for regulating body temperature. After sympathectomy, areas of the body are denervated and cease to perspire, as previously explained, causing in the obese patient excessive sweating as a supra-regulated compensatory mechanism. For these reasons, there is a recommendation to operate only in patients classified as having a normal BMI in order to prevent severe cases of CH, in addition to technically facilitating the procedure.

The influence of the surgical technique used for sympathetic denervation, whether cut or pinched, remains controversial, despite the fact that both methods have good results if the level of approach is correctly achieved. Robotic surgical systems have the advantage of enhancing three-dimensional visualization in high definition and increasing the maneuverability of the instrument in a confined space, making the division of the postganglionic sympathetic fibers possible.

CH is a permanent postoperative adverse effect that occurs in all patients, but to different degrees and with a negative impact on the quality of life of some patients, requiring that it be emphasized and explained in detail before the patient's decision about sympathectomy. This important factor coupled with the efficacy of drug treatment caused the protocol of "primarily pharmacological treatment" for hyperhidrosis to be instituted.

Treatment

Early diagnosis and multidisciplinary treatment are important in the prevention or reduction of psychological trauma and better quality of life of patients with CH.

Non-pharmacological Treatment

1. Maintain normal BMI (<25.8 kg/m² for women and <26.4 kg/m² for men).
2. Decrease consumption of thermogenic foods that stimulate the sympathetic system: chocolate, coffee, tea, pepper, cinnamon, ginger, milk.
3. Cooler environments with low humidity and good ventilation decrease excessive sweating.

Pharmacological Treatment

- *Topical agents*: 15–25% aluminum chloride hexahydrate can treat large surface areas when applied once a night and washed in the morning (increasing frequency if necessary), but the main limitation is skin irritation and unsatisfactory results. Topical glycopyrrolate is a topical anticholinergic with slower penetration, producing fewer adverse effects typical of this class of drug.
- *Intradermal botulinum toxin*: acts by inhibiting the release of acetylcholine at the neuromuscular junction of the sympathetic nerves of the sweat glands with improvement of sweating. The main limitation is the need for frequent applications, since its effect varies from 4 to 17 months, increasing the costs of the treatment, in addition to making it uncomfortable for patients with large areas of sweating involved for the injectable treatment.
- *Systemic anticholinergics*: the most studied drug is oxybutynin, which has been shown to be effective in the treatment of CH, as it develops on large body surfaces and usually occurs in more than one site simultaneously. There are reports in the literature of a 70% improvement in the quality of life of these patients after 6 weeks of medication use. The adverse effects and contraindications are the same when the drug is used in the treatment of primary hyperhidrosis (dry mouth, constipation, urinary retention, and visual changes resulting from paralysis of accommodation—blurred or blurred vision). The alternative medication is oral glycopyrrolate. There are studies showing the positive impact of the association of oxybutynin with botulinum toxin for the treatment of severe CH.

Surgical Treatment

- *Clip removal*: the use of surgical clips instead of sympathetic fiber sections has been shown to be effective in the treatment of hyperhidrosis, and the surgical technique is possibly reversible when patients develop disabling CH with worse postoperative quality of life experienced than in the preoperative period. Removal of the clips will lead to the return of initial complaints, with improvement of CH, although the beneficial effect of this procedure is not yet fully assured. In the world literature a higher success rate is described in the reversal of CH following staple removal the earlier it is performed, varying from 48% (reversion with 11 months) to 78% (1 month after the first surgery), and the smaller the number of clips used in the initial surgery.

- *Reconstruction of the sympathetic chain*: techniques such as sural nerve grafting, intercostal nerve transposition, and use of an autogenous vein graft used as a nerve conduit were reported in the literature as showing improvement of symptoms in a portion of the patients after 1 year following the procedure. The difficulty and technical complexity of these procedures limits their wide implementation.

Conclusion

CH is the most feared and permanent adverse effect that occurs in all patients undergoing sympathectomy for the treatment of primary hyperhidrosis, with a variable impact on the quality of life of these patients. With the development of effective pharmacological treatment and improvement of surgical techniques, we can better select the cases indicated for the surgical treatment, as well as perform the procedures with more effectiveness and less collateral effect, contributing to the progressive reduction of cases of severe CH. The pharmacological treatment of CH is similar to the treatment of the primary form of the disease and the surgical reversion is of complex technique and does not have well-established efficacy.

Suggested Reading

de Campos JR, Wolosker N, Takeda FR, et al. The body mass index and level of resection: predictive factors for compensatory sweating after sympathectomy. Clin Auton Res. 2005;15(2):116–20.

Gong TK, Kim DW. Effectiveness of oral glycopyrrolate use in compensatory hyperhidrosis patients. Korean J Pain. 2013;26(1):89–93.

Lowe N, Campanati A, Bodokh I, et al. The place of botulinum toxin type A in the treatment of focal hyperhidrosis. Br J Dermatol. 2004;151(6):1115–22.

Milanez de Campos JR, Kauffman P, Gomes O Jr, Wolosker N. Video-assisted thoracic sympathectomy for hyperhidrosis. Thorac Surg Clin. 2016;26(3):347–58.

Prouty ME, Fischer R, Liu D. Glycopyrrolate-induced craniofacial compensatory hyperhidrosis successfully treated with oxybutynin: report of a novel adverse effect and subsequent successful treatment. Dermatol Online J. 2016;22(10):15.

Teivelis MP, Varella AY, Wolosker N. Expanded level of sympathectomy and incidence or severity of compensatory hyperhidrosis. J Thorac Cardiovasc Surg. 2014;148(5):2443–4.

Teivelis MP, Wolosker N, Krutman M, et al. Compensatory hyperhidrosis: results of pharmacologic treatment with oxybutynin. Ann Thorac Surg. 2014;98(5):1797–802.

Wolosker N, Yazbek G, Ishy A, et al. Is sympathectomy at T4 level better than at T3 level for treating palmar hyperhidrosis? J Laparoendosc Adv Surg Tech A. 2008;18(1):102–6.

Wolosker N, Teivelis MP, Krutman M, et al. Long-term results of the use of oxybutynin for the treatment of axillary hyperhidrosis. Ann Vasc Surg. 2014;28(5):1106–12.

Yazbek G, Wolosker N, Kauffman P, et al. Twenty months of evolution following sympathectomy on patients with palmar hyperhidrosis: sympathectomy at the T3 level is better than at the T2 level. Clinics (Sao Paulo). 2009;64(8):743–9.

Endoscopic Lumbar Sympathectomy in the Treatment of Hyperhidrosis: Technical Aspects

27

Marcelo de Paula Loureiro, Paulo Kauffman, Rafael Reisfeld, and Roman Rieger

Introduction

The Plantar Hyperhidrosis Problem

Severe palmar and plantar hyperhidrosis (PHH) affects about 1.5–2% of the general population. Obviously, palmar hyperhidrosis is much more noticeable in affected individuals than PHH; however, as PHH affects an area covered by shoes and other garments, it can be as socially and functionally disturbing as palmar hyperhidrosis. Moderate to severe cases of both types of hyperhidrosis (palmar and plantar) can pose functional and social problems. For PHH, these can include foot odor, cold feet, skin lesions and infections, unstable foothold, either in shoes or in walking barefoot, and a frequent need to change socks and shoes. In addition, sweaty feet can also be problematic for individuals at a higher intimacy level.

Medical treatment of both palmar hyperhidrosis and PHH with oxybutynin has appeared in many publications. It has been effective for some patients, but with high dropoff rates due to collateral effects or the need for life-long treatment. Since the mid-1990s, the development of both the internet/social media and advancement of endoscopic techniques has given patients and surgeons alike the ability to replace open operations with less invasive endoscopic operations. Patients are able to

M. P. Loureiro (✉)
General Surgery and Biotechnology, Positivo University and INC Hospital, Curitiba, PR, Brazil

P. Kauffman
Department of Vascular and Endovascular Surgery, University of São Paulo School of Medicine, São Paulo, SP, Brasil

R. Reisfeld
The Center for Hyperidrosis, Beverly Hills, CA, USA

R. Rieger
Surgical Department, Salzkammergut-Klinikum Gmunden, Gmunden, Austria

educate themselves about this technique, not by seeing a physician but by researching information available on the internet.

The open surgical technique for the treatment of palmar hyperhidrosis was common up until the mid-1990s, but was eventually replaced by endoscopic thoracic sympathectomy (ETS) for the treatment of severe palmar hyperhidrosis.[1] ETS produced excellent results for the treatment of palmar hyperhidrosis, and despite certain adverse effects such as compensatory sweating, it remains a popular procedure.

The level of success in treating PHH with ETS, however, has been somewhat disappointing. In the early days of performing ETS for PHH, surgeons were telling their patients they might get a 50% improvement of their sweaty feet. According to some authors, 80% of patients had at least some improvement in their plantar symptoms after undergoing ETS, but a much smaller percentage were actually cured. However, as time went on, it became apparent that the improvement with plantar sweating after ETS was approximately 30% because, for many, the improvement was only transient. Some other patients develop PHH later in life, even after undergoing ETS, because maturation of the plantar sweat glands tends to occur somewhat later in life and not during adolescence.

Lumbar sympathectomy was in the past used primarily for patients with Buerger's disease, Raynaud's disease, and reflex sympathetic dystrophy, with poor long-term results.

From the inception of videolaparoscopic surgery, in the late 1980s, many open surgery techniques were performed by this new access route. Retroperitoneal surgeries followed this trend. Lumbar sympathectomy was one of the open surgical techniques performed via the laparoscopic approach. The first series of endoscopic lumbar sympathectomy(ELS) was published by Hourlay et al. in 1995. From 2002 and on, endoscopic (laparoscopic) approaches for the treatment of PHH were developed in some countries across Europe as well as in South America.

These new approaches opened a window for an effective minimally invasive endoscopic treatment that can be accomplished on an outpatient basis with a great deal of success. Those studies and others show that endoscopic lumbar sympathectomy (ELS) can be safe and effective for the treatment of severe PHH.

Lumbar sympathectomy performed via minimally invasive access has been of increasing interest among patients who are affected by PHH as well as in physicians involved in the treatment of HH.

Lack of information on the adverse effects of lumbar sympathectomy in this group of PHH patients provoked certain skepticism among doctors, who saw a potential source of undesirable consequences in this surgery. Patients seeking out their previous surgeons (who performed their previous ETS) and reporting the permanence of plantar sweat are generally informed of the absence of treatment for the condition, or even discouraged to undergo lumbar sympathectomy, despite the access pathway.

---

[1] Note: the term endoscopic, in this context, refers to the laparoscopic and thoracoscopic techniques.

In this chapter, we discuss the technical details associated with the surgical treatment of PHH by means of ELS. The anatomical rationale of ELS for HH is well-described in the chapter 17 on the anatomy and physiology of the sympathetic system.

Surgical Techniques

There are many different methods to perform ELS. Different surgeons have developed different approaches and techniques based on their preferences and experience. The one piece of advice that should be given to any surgeon who attempts to perform ELS is to get proctored by an experienced surgeon because the learning curve might be somewhat difficult.

Three surgical techniques are presented in this chapter, and they have been performed by the authors of this chapter for over 10 years. The differences between techniques as used by the different authors are identified by their names—Loureiro (LO), Rieger (RI), and Reisfeld (RE)—and they are highlighted when necessary.

Anesthesia

All procedures were carried out under general anesthesia with endotracheal intubation in supine position with hyperextended flank.

Patient Positioning

The arms are tucked alongside the body.

The patient is rotated with one side up, at about 25 °, giving access to where the operation is going to be performed.

Additional Preparation

Markings can be applied to the skin at the hip bone and the rib cage; exactly in between these markings, the middle incision is made on the very lateral aspect of the abdominal wall. (RE) (Figs. 27.1 and 27.2).

In order to facilitate the localization of the various levels of the lumbar sympathetic trunk and its ganglia, the projection of the lumbar vertebral bodies onto the anterior abdominal wall can also be marked with fluoroscopy (RI) (Fig. 27.3).

Surgical Team Positioning

The surgeon and assistant surgeon as well as the scrub nurse place themselves on the same side that will be operated. The screen will face them on the opposite side (Fig. 27.4).

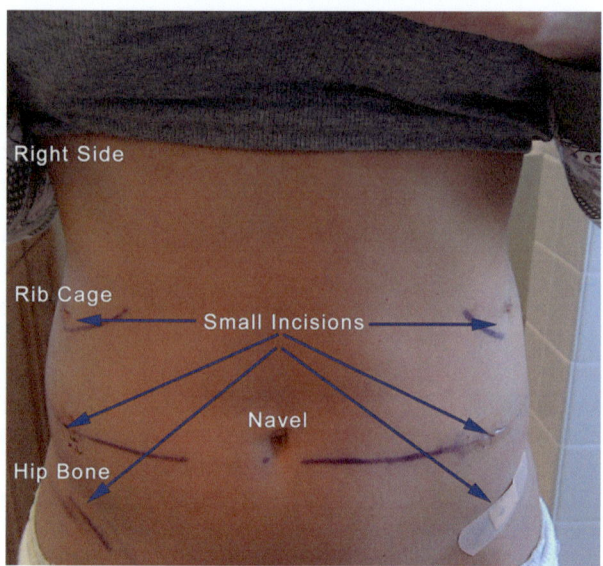

Fig. 27.1 Markings on the skin to guide the incisions

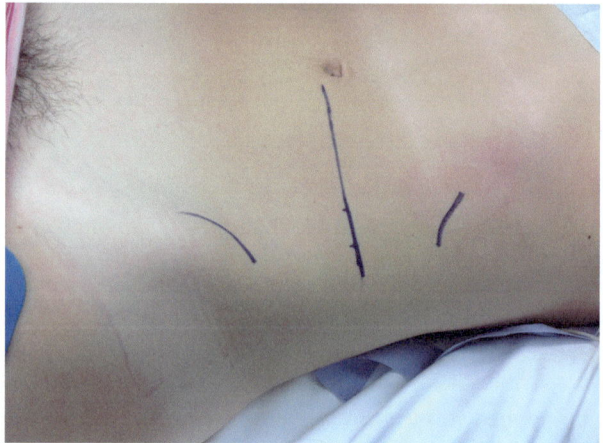

Fig. 27.2 Markings on the skin to guide the incisions (lateral view)

Tactics to Approach the Retroperitoneal Space

Space Maker

The first incision is transverse at the flank. It is about 15 mm longer and possibly, on a heavier patient, this incision might be slightly larger. The skin and the subcutaneous tissues are cut sharply, then the Scarpa's fascia is cut, and the external

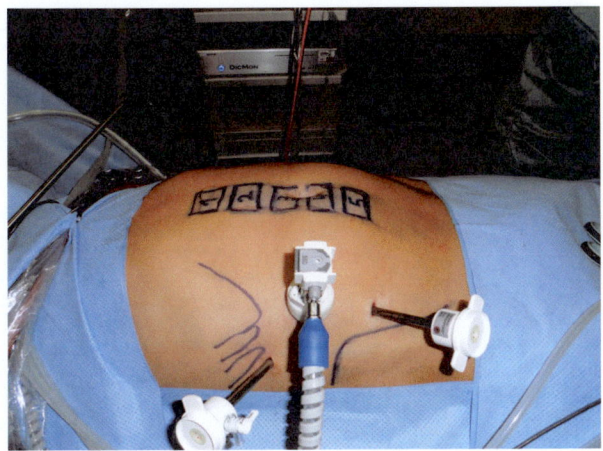

Fig. 27.3 Markings on the skin to project the lumbar vertebra; right-sided lumbar sympathectomy; the lumbar vertebral bodies are marked on the abdominal wall. One 10 mm trocar and two 5 mm trocars are placed in the flank

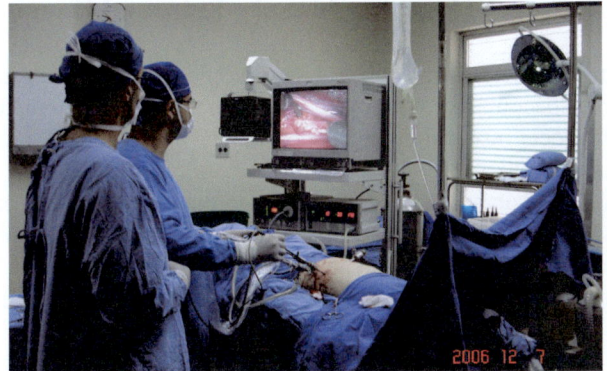

Fig. 27.4 Patient and surgical team positioning for left endoscopic lumbar sympathectomy

oblique fascia is cut along the fibers. With the help of a pean clamp, the external oblique muscle, the internal oblique muscle, and the transversalis muscle are split (not cut) between their fibers, so access into the retroperitoneal space is established. Then, space is created by a sweeping of the finger to push the peritoneum medially, with due care so to keep it as laterally as possible. Once an appropriate space is made, a balloon space maker trocar is inserted (Fig. 27.5), thus helping to create a bigger space for further dissection. The balloon space maker is inflated with the scope in it, enabling direct visualization of the slow development of the space. While doing so, one can see the abdominal muscles separating themselves from the peritoneum. When appropriate space is created, the balloon space maker is taken out, and further development of the space is created with CO_2 insufflation.

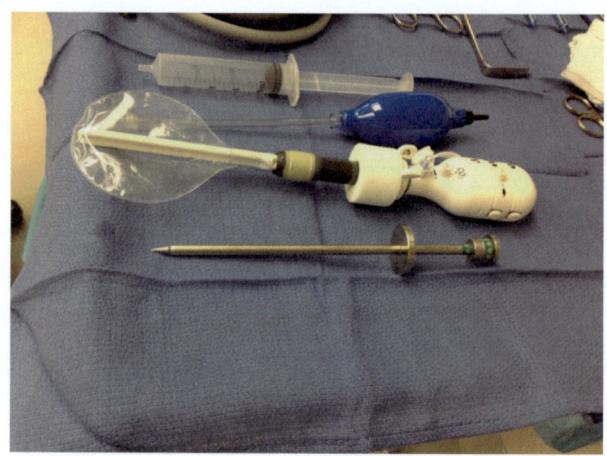

Fig. 27.5 Space maker

Combined Approach (Transperitoneal + Retroperitoneal)

There are some alternatives to achieve laparoscopic access to the retroperitoneum without using a space maker balloon, one of which is the combined approach. It uses a standard trocar inserted in the retroperitoneal space guided through an intraperitoneal laparoscopy.

The first step is to do a laparoscopic access to the intraperitoneal cavity through the umbilicus. The laparoscope is directed to the flank where the retroperitoneal trocar will be placed. At that point the initial skin incision is made. Then a blunt dissection is performed until the pre-peritoneal tissue is identified under the laparoscope vision.

Following that, a 10 mm trocar is placed and advanced up to that specific pre-peritoneal level, still under laparoscopic vision.

Once the retroperitoneal trocar is placed, the inflation tube is repositioned from the umbilical port to the retroperitoneal port.

The surgeon can still follow the initial retroperitoneal space expansion by means of CO_2 inflation. Then the intraperitoneal space is emptied while the retroperitoneum is inflated.

Initial dissection is carried out by smooth movements of the laparoscope surfing in a soft and dilatable retroperitoneal space. After achieving a sufficient lateral space, two 3 or 5 mm trocars are inserted to perform a needlescopic lumbar sympathectomy (Fig. 27.6).

Two accessory 3 or 5 mm trocars are inserted under direct vision (Fig. 27.7). Via those side ports, other instruments are inserted such as a hook cautery and Endo Peanut™ devices.

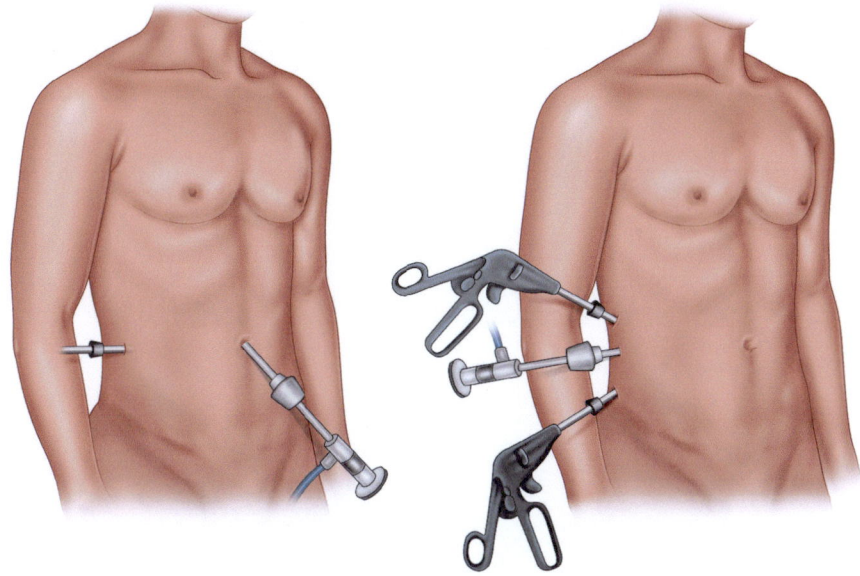

Fig. 27.6 Combined approach to reach the retroperitoneal space with the laparoscope

Fig. 27.7 Additional working trocars

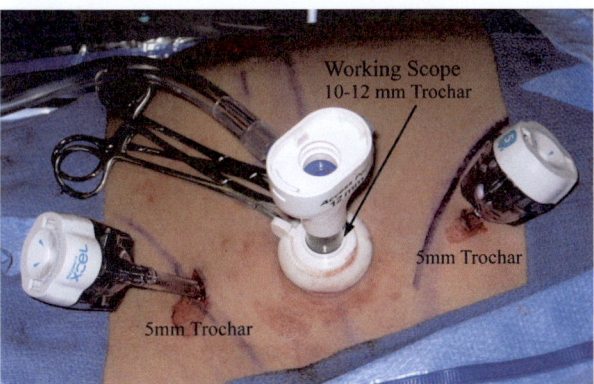

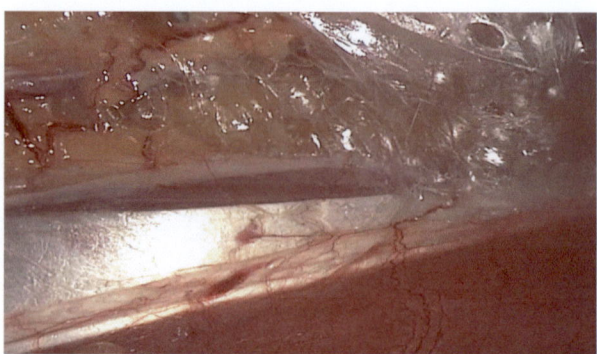

Fig. 27.8 Psoas muscle and the correct plane to the column

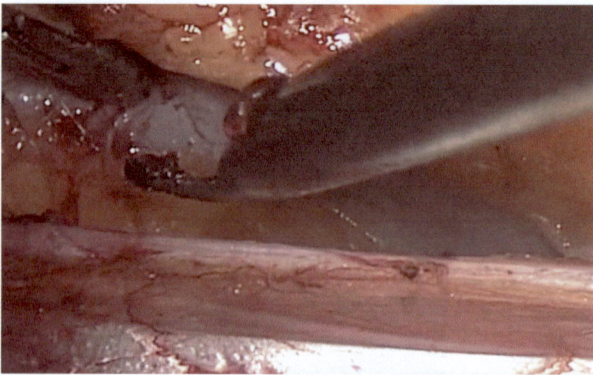

Fig. 27.9 Genitofemoral nerve under the hook

The retroperitoneoscopy is carried out with three trocars in the flank and continuous CO_2 insufflation.

Further Dissection of Retroperitoneal Space Until Sympathetic Chain Visualization is Reached

With trocars in place, the next step is to expose the psoas muscle (Fig. 27.8). Care must be taken to keep in contact with the psoas and avoid getting into the wrong plane of the quadratus lumborum. From the psoas, the dissection continues toward the lumbar vertebra. Along the way, the genital femoral nerve and the ilioinguinal nerve must be identified (Fig. 27.9). The ureter is also kept in sight and protected. In the space in between the ureter and the medial aspect of the psoas muscle, there is an areolar tissue plane that has to be opened, and the sympathetic chain is usually lying in that space (Fig. 27.10).

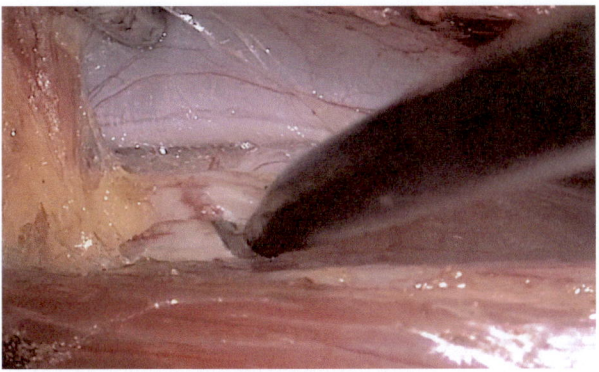

Fig. 27.10 Sympathetic trunk under vena cava being pulled and cut by the hook

Fig. 27.11 Titanium clips applied at the sympathetic lumbar chain

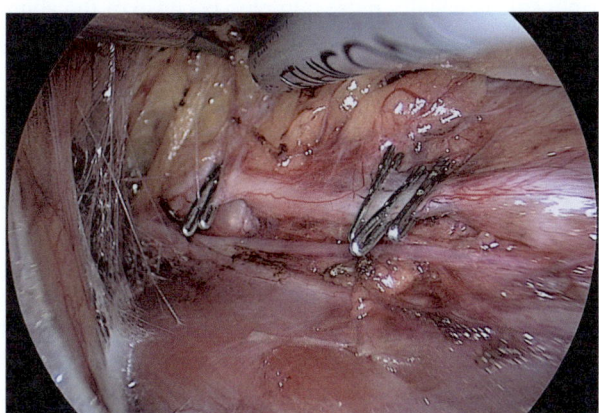

The second lumbar sympathetic ganglion (LG2), when present, is located in the space in between the second and the third lumbar vertebrae (LV2 and LV3) and below the lower renal pole. It is usually the most constant ganglion, and there are no more communicating branches below it. The third (LG3) ganglion, on the other hand, is the most easily visualized in ELS. At the right side there is the vena cava, always completely covering the sympathetic chain. There is clearly a special concern to dissect the nerve from the vein. The surgeon must always be very cautious to dissect as much of the nerve as necessary in order to resect at least one major ganglion, and no more than this if the anatomy is particularly dangerous (Fig. 27.10).

Sympathectomy or Clipping of the Sympathetic Trunk

Once the sympathetic chain is seen, it is cleared from the surrounding tissues; at a certain location (once the nerve is freed) titanium clips can be applied if the clipping technique is chosen (RE and RI) (Fig. 27.11). The location of the titanium clips is around lumbar vertebrae 2 and 3 (LV2, LV3) (RE). RI prefers to place the clips at the level of LV3 and LV4 and resect the nerve between them, with the intention of resecting the third and/or fourth lumbar ganglion. Care must be taken not to have any bleeding from lumbar veins, which can make the procedure somewhat more difficult. Once the first clip is applied, the position is checked with fluoroscopy to verify the exact location of the clip (RE). Once the location is satisfactory, two more clips are applied to block a segment of approximately 2 cm.

LO does not use the vertebra as an anatomical landmark but rather the inferior pole of the kidney and the navel. The rationale behind it is that a perpendicular approach, coming from the flank to the vertebra column, will reach the targeted segment of the sympathetic nerve. If we stay away from the first ganglion (above the renal vein) and resect one major ganglion below it, this would be sufficient to achieve the anhidrotic effect.

Basically, the same technique is applied to both the right and the left side. The right side is usually more complex because of the abundance of large lumbar veins and the proximity of vena cava, which can cause significant bleeding if injured.

Common Drawbacks and Special Tips and Tricks

A somewhat common technical issue can arise if a defect in the peritoneum is made inadvertently, which will cause air to escape from the retroperitoneal space into the abdominal cavity. Depending on the pressure build-up in the abdomen, one can remedy this problem by inserting a 3 mm trocar or a Veress needle into the abdomen, allowing intra-abdominal air to escape and to continue with the procedure.

The genitofemoral nerve on both sides can be very close to the sympathetic chain, and it can be clipped or cut inadvertently if one does not recognize it properly. The surgeon must keep in mind that the genitofemoral nerve and the ilioinguinal nerve go from the lateral aspect of the psoas medially, whereas the sympathetic chain always runs parallel to the psoas muscle and in close contact with the vertebra.

Another anatomical fact that can help identify the sympathetic chain is the appearance of ganglia, which makes it unique to the sympathetic chain. Its location between the psoas and the lumbar column is typical due to its hardness to dissect, because it is a fixed structure. It is always very important to identify those ganglia, and if the surgeon decides to use the resection technique, the specimen can always be checked by histological analysis.

Another important drawback is the need to avoid lesions to big lymphatic vessels. Sometimes they are present and very close to the sympathetic chain. They must be clipped, not coagulated, if their dissection is necessary.

There are also some particularities of using the clipping technique. Intraoperative and postoperative verification of the location is always available. Sometimes, a difference in the placement of the clips is not avoidable and it is usually the result of anatomical structures that surround the sympathetic chains (i.e., lumbar arteries and lumbar veins). Freeing the sympathetic chain from the underlying areolar tissues allows for an easier application of the clips. Once the sympathetic chain is freed from

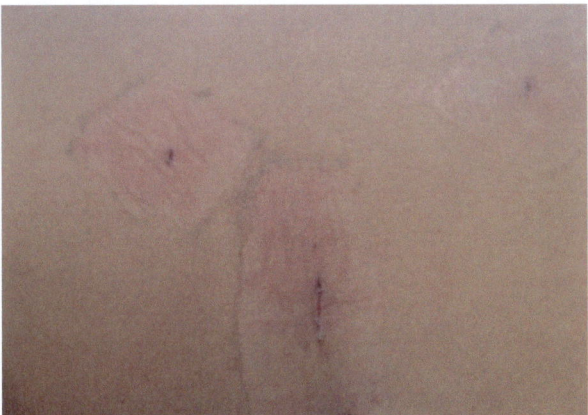

Fig. 27.12 Scars after 1 month

the surrounding tissues, one can use a hook to pull on the chain so the clips can be applied in a very precise fashion. As the application of the clips is completed, and fluoroscopic verification of the clip location is satisfactory, the surgery is completed.

As explained before, the right side can be challenging, not only because of the lumbar veins but also because of the proximity to the vena cava. Remember that a lumbar vein bleed can be dangerous, especially because those veins can easily retract inside the muscle, making hemostasis very difficult. Patients with very well-developed psoas muscles can pose another difficulty because the nerve can be buried underneath muscle fibers. Creating a decent sized retroperitoneal space allows for better spatial orientation and dissection in order to ascertain the location of the sympathetic chain. At the end of the surgery the external oblique fascia is closed with one absorbable suture and skin is also closed with absorbable sutures. If needlescopic graspers and trocars are used, very subtle scars are expected (Fig. 27.12).

Suggested Reading

Reisfeld R, Berliner KI. Evidence-based review of the non surgical management of hyperhidrosis. Thorac Surg Clin. 2008;18:157–66.
Hourlay P, Vangertruyden G, Verduyckt F, Trimpeneers F, Hendrickx J. Endoscopic extraperitoneal lumbar sympathectomy. Surg Endosc 1995;9(5):530–3.
Loureiro MP, Cury AM, Bley AG. Simpatectomia lombar retroperitoneal endoscópica. Rev Col Bras Cir. 2004;31(4):274–5.
Rieger R, Pedevilla S. Retroperitoneoscopic lumbar sympathectomy for the treatment of plantar hyperhidrosis: technique and preliminary findings. Surg Endosc. 2007;21:129–35.
Loureiro MP, de Campos JR, Kauffman P, Al e. Endoscopic lumbar sympathectomy for women: effect on compensatory sweat. Clinics (Sao Paulo). 2008;63:189–96.
Reisfeld R. Endoscopic lumbar sympathectomy for focal plantar hyperhidrosis using the clamping method. Surg Laparosc Endosc Percutan Tech. 2010;20:231–6.
Reisfeld R, Pasternack G, Daniels P, Basseri E, Nishi G, Berliner K. Severe plantar hyperhidrosis: an effective surgical solution. Am Surg. 2013;79(8):845–53.

Endoscopic Lumbar Sympathectomy in the Treatment of Hyperhidrosis: Results and Complications

28

Marcelo de Paula Loureiro, Rafael Reisfeld, Eraj Basseri, Gregg Kai Nishi, Roman Rieger, and Karina Wurm-Wolfsgruber

Introduction

Endoscopic lumbar sympathectomy (ELS) is one of the possible treatment modalities for plantar hyperhidrosis (PHH). Despite the excellent results of this technique for controlling PHH, there is still some skepticism regarding possible complications. Consequently, only a small number of surgeons currently perform ELS. In addition, the general experience is somewhat limited, and there are very few data available to support it as the treatment of choice for PHH. Nevertheless, results have been collected by few authors for the past decade.

The objective of this chapter is to present and discuss some of the largest experiences published on this subject. In order to do so, we have collected data from Dr. Reisfeld from the USA, Dr. Rieger from Austria, and Dr. Loureiro from Brazil. We have decided to join all of our available data together to bring as much light as possible to this subject and clarify all doubts and questions regarding results and complications of ELS.

This mission was not so difficult because, indeed, we are also good friends. We, Dr. Rafael Reisfeld, Dr. Roman Rieger, and myself (Marcelo Loureiro) first met during the World Congress of the International Society of Sympathetic Surgery (ISSS), which was held in the city of Recife, Brazil, back in 2007. Since that time we have been collaborating with each other, visiting each other's

M. P. Loureiro (✉)
General Surgery and Biotechnology, Positivo University and INC Hospital, Curitiba, PR, Brazil

R. Reisfeld · E. Basseri · G. K. Nishi
The Center for Hyperhidrosis, Beverly Hills, CA, USA

R. Rieger · K. Wurm-Wolfsgruber
Surgical Department, Salzkammergut-Klinikum Gmunden, Gmunden, Austria

facilities and exchanging doubts and information about our patients. We have also published some data together, so the process of writing this chapter in fact began at that time.

We work in three different countries, with different cultures and weather conditions. This obviously has a potential impact on the evaluation of our results, considering that PHH is a disease closely related to temperature and psychological conditions. We have been performing ELS with slight technical differences, which may also have impacted results, but, in general, our techniques have been equivalent so far.

Differences are highlighted in the text with reference to the author: Loureiro (LO), Rieger (RI) and Reisfeld (RE).

Patients and Baseline Characteristics

Between June 2002 and November 2016, 601 patients (165 from LO, 184 from RI, and 252 from RE) underwent bilateral ELS, which represents about 1202 procedures (Table 28.1). Almost all patients had tried conservative measures such as aluminum chloride lotion, iontophoresis devices, anticholinergic medications, or Botox® injections, with limited or short-lived success. The age range was 11–69 years (mean of 31.6 years among RE's patients, 34 among RI's patients, and 28 among LO's patients). The majority of RE and LO's patients were female (80.5% and 90.9%, respectively) but male for RI (56%). The vast majority (80%) of the patients had had previous endoscopic thoracic sympathectomy (ETS) (except for RI's—30%), which had not relieved their PHH. There was an unusual subset of patients that had isolated PHH with no evidence of palmar hyperhidrosis. There were also some patients with palmoplantar HH but whose plantar symptoms were much more bothersome. For those cases, ELS was offered instead of ETS. The time interval between ETS and ELS ranged from 6 months to 10 years. Follow-up of the patients represented in this group ranged from 3 months to 10 years.

All patients underwent preoperative evaluation with a more extensive evaluation for patients over the age of 50 years. A detailed discussion was carried out between the surgeons and the patients regarding risks and benefits. Preoperative PHH was graded as light, moderate, or severe; and severe cases were deemed as those in which patients needed to change their socks a few times a day, had to change shoes often, and had social and functional problems related to their PHH.

All but a few patients described their symptoms as severe.

Table 28.1 Differences between authors' patients

Author	Year	Patients (N)	F/M	Age	Previous ETS (%)
Loureiro	2002–2016	165	150/15	28 (11–56)	89
Rieger	2005–2015	184	81/103	34 (13–69)	30
Reisfeld	2007–2016	252	123/31	31 (15–68)	94

ETS endoscopic thoracic sympathectomy, *F* female, *M* male

Differences in Technique

There are slight differences in the technique used by these three surgeons; they are explained in detail in Chap. 27. Localization and technique of interruption of sympathetic flow is worth highlighting. RE uses the clamping method, with no resection of the sympathetic ganglia. RI uses the resection between clips applied in the level of the third and fourth lumbar vertebra body. LO does not use the vertebra as an anatomical landmark, rather the inferior pole of the kidney and the navel. The rationale behind this is that a perpendicular approach, coming from the flank to the vertebra column, will reach the targeted segment of the sympathetic nerve. The lumbar sympathetic carries out one of the most important variations of the standard anatomy of the body (it is possible to find from one to seven paravertebral ganglia in the lumbar sympathetic trunk). So, if we stay away from the first ganglion (above the renal vein) and resect one major ganglion below it, this would be sufficient to achieve the anhidrotic effect.

Outcomes

Outcomes for the Clamping Method (RE)

The ELS clamping procedure was performed at level of lumbar vertebra 3 (LV3) in about 68% of the cases, and the remaining cases were performed at the level just above that, LV2. Clip position was confirmed by a postoperative X-ray; RE does not use the X-ray for preoperative localization, only for postoperative confirmation of clip positioning. The rate of success for curing PHH after ELS is 98% in his experience. For cases in which the patients complain about post-ETS inner thigh and buttock sweating, he clips the sympathetic chain as high as possible, and in some cases one can recognize the medially running side branches of the sympathetic chain, which supply with sympathetic innervation to those mentioned locations. Thus, the patients will experience improved compensatory sweating (CS) in those locations.

Outcomes for Clamping and Resection (RI)

As previously stated, RI uses X-ray to determine the intended resection level of lumbar sympathectomy. Clips are applied to indicate the section points; so all clips were applied at the same level. The success rate for curing PHH immediately after ELS was 100% in his experience (368/368 ft). He does not use a special approach for controlling thigh HH.

Outcomes of Endoscopic Lumbar Sympathectomy Resection Without Clips (LO)

The immediate control of PHH among 165 patients (330 ft) was obtained in 328 ft (99%). One of the unsuccessful cases was clearly the misinterpretation of lumbar by the genital femoral nerve, which was resected instead.

Table 28.2 Operative complications

Complication	Frequency	Guidance/treatment
Conversion to open	LO (0); RI (0); RE (6)	Mentoring
Genitofemoral nerve resection/clipping	LO (1); RE (1)	Genitofemoral nerve has no ganglia
Lumbar vessels lesion	L (1); RO (0); RI (0)	Clip/coagulate/surgical
Inferior vena cava lesion	0	Don't play with vena cava!
Ureter	0	Always identify it
lymphatic vessels	LO (1); RO (1)	Clip big linfatics

LO Loureiro, *RI* Rieger, *RO* Raphael Reisfeld

Perioperative Complications

Overall occurrence of complications has been minimal for all of us. There was no mortality in our series of patients. Perioperative complications are in general minor and are related to one of the following situations: opening of the peritoneal tendon that supports the extra-peritoneal space; misidentification of the sympathetic trunk; inadvertent lesion of lymphatic ducts; and bleeding from lumbar vessels. Some major complications can occur and are described in the literature as ureter or vena cava injures, but this is considered extremely rare. These are the major reasons for a conversion to open surgery. Perioperative complications and their treatment are shown in Table 28.2. Conversion was only necessary for six of RE's patients, and mostly occurred at the beginning of his experience.

Misidentification of the Genitofemoral Nerve

In situations in which the anatomy is unclear, the genitofemoral nerve may inadvertently be confused with the lumbar sympathetic trunk and then be mistakenly clipped or resected. If this occurs, the result can be easily recognized in the recovery room as the patient will still have a sweaty foot and also have numbness of the inner thigh on the same leg. The great benefit of placing clips as opposed to cutting the nerve is that the patient can be returned to the operating room immediately, the clip removed, and new clips can be placed appropriately after the sympathetic chain is correctly identified.

Lymphatic Duct Injury

Occasionally, the lymphatic ducts may be injured during the retroperitoneal dissection. It should be noted that small injuries to the lymphatic channels are usually of no consequence and are not a reason for aborting the procedure. Once the procedure is completed and the retroperitoneal space is deflated, the lymphatic leak resolves on its own.

Peritoneal Tear

Another pitfall is that the peritoneum can occasionally be torn inadvertently. This results in an air leak from the retroperitoneal space to the intra-abdominal space, which in turn collapses the retroperitoneal working space. This can be controlled by inserting a Veress needle or a 3 or 5 mm trocar into the intra-abdominal space to relieve the pressure and allow work to continue in the retroperitoneal space. A peritoneal tear can make this retroperitoneal approach very difficult. Depending on the size of the tear, one should go for a trans-peritoneal approach or even abort the procedure and reschedule it for 1 month later.

Postoperative Complications

We have had some general postoperative complications such as wound hematomas in six patients (1%), a pneumonia, one left leg thrombosis, and one pulmonary embolism (0.15% each). Some patients have complained about obstipation, which is self-limited and respond to laxatives. Specific ELS complications are related to post-surgical pain, retrograde ejaculation, edemas, and compensatory sweat (CS).

Pain

As described by the majority of the patients, pain after ELS is much lower than after ETS. The retroperitoneal space is particularly painless, especially when compared with the chest. Neuralgia or local back pain is reported by more or less one-quarter of the patients. This is usually of short duration, and we have noticed that excessive use of electrocautery around the sympathetic chain in the lumbar region, which is densely populated with fine sensory nerve fibers in the cartilage/bone surroundings, can produce long-term pain. For this reason, we employ the least amount possible of electrocautery in the process of dissecting out the nerve. Ultrasonic energy is an alternative, and so can be even the use of mini-laparoscopy with a low-power blended electrocautery. In some patients, uncomfortable pain may recur even after some weeks. We use only oral analgesics for postoperative pain management and reassure patients of its self-limited character.

Pain in the lower legs can rarely occur in young athletic individuals who resume heavy physical activity in a very short time after the procedure. The hypothesis for the cause of this pain is an increase in blood flow to the lower legs, which in turn causes a mild form of compartment syndrome in the lower extremities. Other possible causes are genitofemoral neuralgia due to some kind of neuropraxia during retroperitoneal dissection or even a retrograde degeneration of pre-ganglionic fibers. No matter the cause, no treatment is needed, and simply reassuring the patient and advising them to reduce their physical activity is adequate.

Retrograde Ejaculation

Lumbar sympathectomy was feared by some surgeons as having the possibility of causing retrograde ejaculation. This fear was based on the knowledge that previous open lumbar sympathectomies performed many years before for ischemic legs (and not for PHH) caused retrograde ejaculation. We know now that performing the ELS below L2 level will not cause retrograde ejaculation. So far, this particular anatomical fact has allowed us to perform the operation on younger male patients without the fear of causing sterility. No incidents of retrograde ejaculation were reported among male patients in both the series from RE and LO. RI operated many more male patients and, among them, there were three out of 105 (2.9%) transient ejaculatory disturbances.

Swelling

Some patients can experience swelling in the operative area, evidenced by an asymmetry between the right and left flank. This is very usual, and in general it is absolutely self-limited as well as painless. It is a consequence of the dissection of the retroperitoneal space and occasionally a lesion to lymphatic tissue.

Another common swelling is in the ankle and feet associated with an increase in local temperature. This happens in the immediate postoperative period and can persist for some weeks. This is a result of the increased blood flow to the lower extremities; another self-limited consequence of an increase in the arterial flow. If it represents some discomfort to the patient, symptoms can be released by cold-pack application.

Compensatory Sweating

As in the case of ETS, one can expect transient early recurrence of feet sweating 3–4 days after ELS. This occurs only in a small number of patients but, nevertheless, patients should be warned and educated about it so to prevent unnecessary angst.

As we know from the experience with ETS operations, CS is a byproduct of ETS and it affects 100% of patients. The vast majority will have CS on a mild to moderate level that is considered by the patient to be preferable to the alternative of having extremely sweaty hands. Nevertheless, 3–5% of the patients who had ETS will describe their CS as much more than they expected to experience. However, even in this group of patients, it is rare that they seek their ETS to be reversed. Patients who had ETS and are considering ELS should anticipate CS to continue at least at the same degree as before the ELS. Physiologically speaking, this should not be a real problem because the main culprit for CS is blocking of the sympathetic chain within the chest cavity. By performing ETS, one blocks the afferent pathways that come from the lower body toward the brain. Theoretically, adding two to three more levels of the sympathetic chain or sympathetic blocks in the lumbar region should not contribute to more CS than that created by the previous ETS. General experience with patients who had only undergone ELS has shown that the amount of CS is very well-tolerated and patients do not complain too much about it.

As previously mentioned/explained, occasionally, when the anatomical presentation is such that there are medial branches from the sympathetic chain that innervate the groin and area of the buttocks, such patients may benefit from the lumbar sympathectomy at those sites. In essence, CS is the result of obstruction of the afferent information from the lower parts of the body to the upper parts of the body. We do not yet have the exact explanation for this adverse effect, and hopefully the future will bring some breakthrough findings and an ability to predict and prevent those severe cases of CS. In RI's series of patients, 67% noted development or increase in CS (60% mild, 40% strong); 32% neither developed it nor had an increase of it; and for 1% of the patients, it was not clear. RI considers that the CS level after ELS did show fluctuations, especially in the early few months after the operation, but this eventually settled down to the previous level before ELS was performed.

Among LO's patients, the CS developed or increased in 52% of the patients. Just 2% of them considered that it became strongly increased. In RE's series, there was no difference regarding CS after ELS, whether the ELS was performed at VL2 or VL3.

Therefore, to summarize CS, one should expect some fluctuation in the level of CS after ELS but, generally speaking, with the passing of time it goes back to the level it had reached before ELS was performed.

Other Uncommon Adverse Effects

Post-ELS orthostatic hypotension can happen very rarely, and again the reason is believed to be due to the increased bloodflow to the feet. Therefore, patients are instructed in the first 2–3 days after the operation to exercise caution when sitting up or standing from a laying position. Long-lasting orthostatic hypotension is extremely rare and it may be explained by an over-resection of both ETS and ELS, causing a kind of dysautonomia due to insufficient sympathetic innervation.

Very few patients complained about transient constipation. There is no anatomical support to this adverse effect because paravertebral lumbar nerve fibers are different from the pre-vertebral lumbar plexus. None of those patients altered their bowel habits definitively after surgery.

Another possible adverse effect would be a decrease of vaginal lubrication, following the same principle of possible sexual disorder that could happen in male patients. Few female patients complain about it, but in all of them this is transient. Table 28.3 summarizes postoperative complications.

Table 28.3 Differences in results among the three authors

Complication	Frequency	Guidance/treatment
Foot and ankle edema	LO (5)	Ice-bag on ankle
Compensatory sweat	LO (52%); RI (67%); RE (?%)	–
Palmar sweat	LO (4); RE (3)	Self-limited
Back and leg neuralgia	LO (22%); RI (39%); RE (18%)	NSAIDs/hot packs
Ejaculation disorders	RI (3)	Wait … (2 months)
Vagina dryness	LO (1) temporary	Wait …
Hypotension	LO (1); RE (3)	–
Pneumonia	RI (1)	Antibiotics
Thrombosis/embolism	RI (2)	Anticoagulants
Immediate recurrence	LO (2)	Review recorded surgery (genital femoral nerve)

LO Loureiro, *RI* Rieger, *RE* Reisfeld

Follow-Up Results

Follow-Up, Quality of Life, and Recurrence

LO's long-term follow-up data had too many losses. The majority of patients came from the private sector, which makes their long-term follow-up almost impossible. On the other hand, data from the first year were available for most of those patients (138 of 165 [83%]).

During the first-year follow-up, PHH was improved or eliminated in 135 patients (97.8%). There were two early (immediate), and one late (6 months) total recurrence of one of the feet. Partial recurrence was not identifiable during the first year of follow-up, but there were few patients complaining about it later on.

Quality of life during first-year follow-up improved among all patients that experienced a positive result of PHH control, except for one patient with CS. Due to the self-limited time of adverse effects, when they happened, only two of those patients considered not repeating the surgery if they needed it. In one patient that was because of persistent PHH in one of the feet; and the other because of troublesome compensatory sweat.

Better follow-up data collection came from RI's patients. His follow-up data were available for 89% (164) of the patients. Medium follow-up was 52 months (range 1–120 months). Among those patients, PHH was eliminated in 102 patients (62%), improved in 55 (33.5%), and recurred in seven (4.3%); 118 (72%) of the patients considered themselves *very satisfied*, while 34 (20.7%) were *limited satisfied*, and 12 (7.3%) were *unclear* or *not satisfied*.

Regarding quality-of-life analysis, this improved in 84.2% (138) of the patients; 5% responded that it worsened and for 8.5% it was unclear. Four patients did not answer this question.

When asked if they would repeat the operation, 78.7% answered *yes*, 10% *not sure*, 8% *no*, and 3% *did not answer*.

Recurrence after ELS rarely happens. We should divide it into early recurrence and late recurrence.

Early recurrences, meaning within days or weeks, can be due to technical reasons such as inability to identify the sympathetic chain or mistaking other structures for the sympathetic chain. This will occur less frequently as the surgeon gains experience. The genitofemoral nerve is the structure most commonly misidentified as the sympathetic trunk. The most important difference between them is that the sympathetic trunk has ganglia, and ganglia are a fixed element that bridges it to the spinal cord. So, if you find something you believe is the sympathetic trunk, try to dissect it before putting a clip or removing it. If it is too loose, it is not the correct structure.

As with ETS, a 1.5–3% rate of late recurrence is expected, no matter what method is used. The exact reason for recurrence has yet to be found. It must be emphasized that all methods used in ETS, such as resection, coagulation, and the clamping method, have the same rate of recurrence. There are a few theories about the nature of the recurrence, including recanalization and creation of new pathways within the spinal cord that bypass the areas where the sympathetic ganglia were excluded. Recurrence after ELS is even more perplexing because all of the fibers that go below GL2 are fibers that are going down to the feet without any more feeding ganglia. Plantar recurrence can be total or partial in certain parts of the feet.

Recurrences can be an indication for redoing the operation. However, it should be noted that a repeated operation in the lumbar region is extremely difficult due to early scar and adhesion formation in the retroperitoneal space. Total recurrence is extremely rare. RE also defends the clamping method in order to allow for fluoroscopic confirmation of the level at which the clips are placed during ELS. This would facilitate the redo approach.

Final Aspects

There are several other modalities that can be tried before choosing lumbar sympathectomy for treating PHH. Botox®, anticholinergics, iontophoresis, and topical agents, or even procedures such as computed tomography (CT)-guided chemical sympathectomy are within that list. Unfortunately, the results are not comparable with ELS. Even if they seem to be less invasive, they remain poorly effective in the long-term, and are also related to specific complications.

The medical community interested in the treatment of HH is always struggling to find better treatments for this troublesome disease. Unfortunately, PHH has been neglected for a long time. The majority of patients are convinced by their physicians that there is not a real possibility for treating their excessive foot sweat, other than palliative treatments.

ELS is a difficult procedure to master, but the results are clearly very convincing. A larger follow-up with more patients involved and more controlled studies are necessary to definitively state that ELS is the gold standard to treat PHH but, so far, this is the best technique available.

Take-Home Messages

ELS is the most effective treatment for PHH and, if performed correctly by a well-trained surgeon, provides excellent short-, medium-, and long-term results. Like any treatment, there are some risks and complications involved, but in general they are minor and temporary.

Suggested Reading

Hourlay PG, Vangertruyden F, Verduyckt F, Trimpeneers JH. Endoscopic extraperitoneal lumbar sympathectomy. Surg Endosc. 1995;9(5):530–3.
Loureiro MP, Cury AM, Bley AG. Simpatectomia lombar retroperitoneal endoscópica. Rev Col Bras Cir. 2004;31(4):274–5.
Loureiro MP, de Campos JR, Kauffman P, Al e. Endoscopic lumbar sympathectomy for women: effect on compensatory sweat. Clinics (Sao Paulo). 2008;63:189–96.
Neumayer C, Panhofer P, Zacherl J, Bischof G. Effect of endoscopic thoracic sympathetic block on plantar hyperhidrosis. Arch Surg. 2005;140:676–80.
Nicolas C, Grosdidier G, Granel F, et al. Endoscopic sympathectomy for palmar and plantar hyperhidrosis: results in 107 patients. Ann Dermatol Venereol. 2000;127:1057–63.
Pedevilla S. Retroperitoneoscopic lumbar sympathectomy for the treatment of plantar hyperhidrosis: technique and preliminary findings. Surg Endosc. 2007;21:129–35.
Reisfeld R. Endoscopic lumbar sympathectomy for focal plantar hyperhidrosis using the clamping method. Surg Laparosc Endosc Percutan Tech. 2010;20:231–6.
Reisfeld R, Berliner KI. Evidence-based review of the non-surgical management of hyperhidrosis. Thorac Surg Clin. 2008;18:157–66.
Reisfeld R, Pasternack G, Daniels P, Basseri E, Nishi G, Berliner K. Severe plantar hyperhidrosis: an effective surgical solution. Am Surg. 2013;79(8):845–53.
Rieger R, Pedevilla S. Retroperitoneoscopic lumbar sympathectomy for the treatment of plantar hyperhidrosis and preliminary findings. Surg Endosc. 2007;21:129–35.
Rieger R, Cheshire NJ, Darzi AW. Retroperitonesocopic lumbar sympathectomy. Br J Surg. 1997;84:1094–5.
Rieger R, Pedevila S, Pochlauer S. Endoscopic lumbar sympathectomy for plantar hyperhidrosis. Br J Surg. 2009;96:1422–8.
Rieger R, Loureiro MP, Pedevilla S, Oliveira RA. Endoscopic lumbar sympathectomy following thoracic sympathectomy in patients with palmoplantar hyperidrosis. World J Surg. 2011;35(1):49–53.
Wolosker N, Yazbek G, Milanez de Campos JR, et al. Evaluation of plantar hyperhidrosis in patients undergoing video-assisted thoracoscopic sympathectomy. Clin Auton Res. 2007;17:172–6.

Part IV

Blushing

Facial Blushing: Psychiatric Management

29

Enrique Jadresic

Introduction

Blushing refers to the transient redness of the face that is easily triggered by emotional and social situations. It is a universal experience, found in all cultures. Contrary to reddening of the face caused by conditions such as heat, alcohol, or specific dermatological diseases such as rosacea, which should be called *flushing* as it is devoid of a psychological component, blushing is accompanied by feelings of embarrassment and disruption of mental function. It is often considered to be an undesirable, involuntary response, which individuals try to conceal. Lay people and even physicians rarely view it as a disabling condition. However, this is changing as more blushers seek help from health professionals.

Most people blush infrequently, mainly in certain social contexts (mishaps, public recognition), and are not limited by their occasional episodes of facial reddening. This might be termed *normal blushing*. Frequent or severe social blushing, on the contrary, seen often in individuals who request medical assistance, may cause distress and impede a person's social interactions. Sometimes this type of social reddening is named *pathological blushing*.

Excessive or frequent blushing often leads to fear of blushing (erythrophobia) and avoidance of social situations. Precisely because of this fear, for blushers it is very difficult to admit that they suffer from the condition. When they demand treatment it is usually after an internet search, and commonly they have not shared information about their ailment with close relatives despite the fact that fear of blushing has impaired their social lives for many years.

E. Jadresic
Department of Psychiatry, Faculty of Medicine, University of Chile, Santiago, Chile

From the point of view of its speed of appearance and location, two types of facial blushing have been described: first, the typical rapid onset blush, which appears within seconds on the face, neck, and ears, and spreads uniformly over the affected areas; and second, the slowly emerging "creeping blush", which is blotchy rather than uniform in color, that appears first as red splotches, usually on the upper chest or lower neck, and then spreads upward onto the upper neck, jaws, and cheeks.

Blushing and Self-Conscious Emotions

The blush can be considered a bodily change that can accompany a range of self-conscious emotions, most commonly embarrassment but also shame, guilt, and pride. These emotions are grouped together because of the central role that self-appraisal plays in each of them. They also have been termed higher, or secondary, emotions because they are presumed to require more extensive processing by the cerebral cortex than do basic, lower, or cognition-independent emotions, such as fear and sadness.

Several of these self-conscious emotions depend in part on what the person experiencing them thinks about others, but they also hinge on what that person believes others are thinking about him or her. For example, embarrassment is an unpleasant emotional state that we experience when we know that we have been caught in an individual act or condition that is socially or professionally unacceptable. Embarrassment is similar to shame, except that we can feel ashamed of something that we alone know about ourselves, while embarrassment requires the presence of another person. That is to say, blushing is necessarily a social phenomenon. In addition, embarrassment is generally understood to be brought on by an action that is merely socially unacceptable rather than one that is morally reprehensible.

Evolutionarily, it has been assumed that blushing acts as an involuntary social apology and that, like the other self-conscious emotions, its function is to motivate us to adhere to social norms. Empirical evidence supports the hypothesis that the facial reddening that accompanies embarrassment may soften a negative evaluation from those around us. In keeping with this, it has been said that the blushing response emerges not so much as a reaction to danger but as an attempt to prevent danger from rising.

It could be understandably asked why, if blushing serves to defuse a threat, people so want to avoid it. The answer is that, regrettably, usually the distinction between normal and pathological blushing is not made, and it is wrongly assumed that blushers who ask for help do so because of normal blushing. That is not the case because, as we have seen earlier, blushing is common and a universal phenomenon, but it can also be a symptom of psychopathology. Indeed, most patients who seek help from health professionals do so not because of normal, occasional facial reddening, which we know is a natural part of life, but because they blush excessively and at socially inappropriate times, and because the experience turns disabling and undermines their quality of life.

Blushing and Social Anxiety Disorder

Blushing excessively and/or very easily often leads to fear of blushing (erythrophobia), a condition described within the group of social phobias by Pierre Janet in 1903. Current psychiatric classifications state that "blushing is a hallmark physical response of social anxiety disorder (SAD)", formerly known as social phobia. SAD is a disorder characterized by the presence of persistent and marked fear or anxiety about one or more social situations in which the individual is exposed to possible scrutiny by others. The individual fears that he or she will act in a way, or show anxiety symptoms (i.e., blushing, trembling, sweating), that will be negatively evaluated (i.e., will be humiliating or embarrassing; will lead to rejection or offend others). This disorder affects 13% of the population at some time in their lives. It has been found that up to 50% of SAD patients say they blush frequently. In other words, not all patients with SAD blush. But those who do complain of facial reddening blush more often and/or have greater overall arousal in social situations than those who do not complain of blushing. Among blushers who seek medical help because of their blushing, 90% suffer from SAD. Recently, several authors have hypothesized that autonomic hyperarousal, and blushing in particular, plays an etiological role in the development of some cases of SAD.

Psychopharmacological Treatment

Selective Serotonin Reuptake Inhibitors

Besides sympathetic activation, there is some evidence that the serotonin system is also involved in the mediation of blushing. Cutaneous flushing in patients with serotonin-related carcinoid syndrome supports this view. In line with this, it should be borne in mind that so far the only double-blind, placebo-controlled evidence for the efficacy of any treatment for blushing comes from a study from Connor et al. with sertraline, a selective serotonin reuptake inhibitor (SSRI) which was US Food and Drug Administration (FDA) approved for the treatment of SAD in 2003. These researchers found that SAD patients report specific effects of sertraline on blushing, but not on trembling and sweating. Our own study compared the efficacy of endoscopic thoracic sympathectomy (ETS) and sertraline in blushers requesting treatment. We found improvement in both groups. While in the sertraline-treated group the pre- and post-treatment scores in the blush item of the Brief Social Phobia Scale (BSPS) were 3.4 (0.7) and 1.5 (1.2), respectively, in the ETS-treated group pre- and post-treatment scores were 3.6 (0.5) and 1.5 (1.2), respectively. Though the reduction in score in the blush item was greater with ETS—2.2 (1.3) versus 1.9 (1.3)—the difference did not reach statistical significance.

In addition, another study showed that fluvoxamine, also an SSRI, was superior to a placebo for treating facial blushing associated with anxiety disorders in children. As regards fear of blushing, French authors found significant reductions after

4 weeks of treatment with escitalopram, again an SSRI. In this case the results were more pronounced at the end of a 12-week treatment, with patients experiencing a 60% decrease in their symptoms.

β-Blockers

β-Blockers (i.e., propranolol) have been used for blushing as the acute stage of blushing is regulated primarily by β-adrenergic sympathetic nerves, which are responsible for the dilation of blood vessels in the face. Several β-blockers, including propranolol and atenolol, have been somewhat more effective than placebo in individual controlled studies, and are widely believed to be useful in allaying anxiety during speaking or performing in public. These medications can be employed on an ongoing basis (atenolol, metoprolol, propranolol) or for occasional use only (propranolol). In our experience, 20–40 mg of propranolol, taken along with 0.25 mg of alprazolam 40–60 min prior to a situation that typically triggers blushing, is usually quite effective in individuals who may be incapacitated by blushing and severe performance anxiety. It is a good treatment option, but it has the drawback that if patients are able to deal successfully with social situations, they tend to attribute the success to the medication rather than taking the credit themselves. In other words, it is a strategy that reinforces the use of drugs, in comparison to cognitive–behavioral techniques, which, advantageously, involve learning processes.

Other Drugs

Clonidine, a selective α_2-adrenergic agonist, has been used to treat facial blushing, menopausal flushing, and facial flushing redness associated with rosacea. Its major adverse effects include dry mouth, sedation or fatigue, and hypotension. These effects are often poorly tolerated by anxious patients. Likewise, anticholinergics have been occasionally used for facial blushing as an alternative to surgical intervention. Data in this respect are very scarce. Interestingly, a recent study suggests that ibuprofen, a widely used anti-inflammatory, reduces blushing (arising in situations of discomfiture or embarrassment) when applied to the cheeks in gel form. It also seems to help control flushing caused by exertion. Ibuprofen works by decreasing the formation of prostaglandins, which contribute to the inflammatory processes in the face that result in blushing.

Psychological Treatment

Two cognitive–behavioral treatments (Clark and Wells 1995; Rapee and Heimberg 1997) have shown good to excellent efficacy in SAD, although sometimes response and remission rates are unsatisfactory. In blushing patients with fear of blushing (who, as mentioned earlier, generally meet criteria for SAD) these psychotherapeutic approaches are a good option but require well-trained specialists, which are not always available. There are very few therapies specially designed to treat fear of blushing. They, rather than trying to decrease the intensity and/or frequency of the episodes of facial blushing, focus on controlling the fear of blushing, or erythrophobia. This process indirectly helps people to blush less, as the expectation of blushing has been proven to act as a self-fulfilling prophecy and can actually lead to facial reddening.

Task Concentration Training

The task concentration training (TCT) technique, developed by Bögels and colleagues, is the most widely known psychological therapy for fear of blushing. It is based on the idea that people who blush are too self-conscious during social interactions (excessively focused on their emotions, behavior, physical appearance, and level of activation) and pay little attention to the tasks at hand, the other(s) involved, and their surroundings. In these individuals, any sign of activity in their sympathetic nervous system, such as a faster heartbeat, perspiring hands, and—especially—warm cheeks, increases their focus on themselves. As their blushing becomes clearly visible to others, they become even more self-conscious.

TCT therapy consists of teaching patients to direct their attention away from themselves when they blush and to focus on the tasks involved in the specific social interaction (e.g., waiting on customers) rather than on themselves. The therapy consists of three stages: (1) becoming familiar with the processes of paying attention and becoming aware of the negative effects of increasing one's attention on oneself; (2) focusing one's attention away from oneself in non-threatening situations (such as watching television, making a phone call, walking in the park, or listening to the lyrics of a song); and (3) focusing one's attention away from oneself in threatening situations.

In the first stage, the patient learns how blushing and attention on oneself reinforce each other and how this interaction begins to produce anxiety, negative thoughts about oneself, problems concentrating, and awkwardness. Next, patients are shown how, by focusing their attention outward (toward the tasks involved in the social action and their surroundings) rather than inward, they can begin to break the vicious circle that perpetuates their blushing. Patients are asked to keep a daily record of their blushing episodes, noting how anxious they were and estimating what percentage of concentration was on themselves, on the interaction, and on their surroundings at that time. Patients do concentration exercises under the guidance of the therapist that involve both listening and telling stories. Later, these daily records are used in "homework" assigned by the therapist.

During the non-threatening focusing exercises, patients are told, for example, to walk through a (quiet) park paying attention to all of the stimuli around (visual, auditory, olfactory, kinesthetic) and in their own body. Patients are instructed to focus first on one aspect at a time, and then on all stimuli simultaneously (integrated attention). One homework assignment frequently given is to have a telephone conversation and then to summarize it.

To practice threatening situations, patients make a list of around ten social situations that are important in their life and that trigger blushing. The list is organized in an increasing hierarchy, in which the first item is the least threatening for the patient. The goal is for patients to concentrate on the task involved in each situation and to return their focus to the task every time they become distracted by (thinking of) blushing or by focusing on themselves. Whenever possible, these more complex exercises are practiced first in the therapist's office, but they later become homework assignments of which patients keep written records. Any difficulties that arise are discussed with the therapist in the following session.

Learning to concentrate on the task at hand is considered a coping strategy, and it must be taught by a properly trained therapist. The training is generally done in six to eight weekly sessions lasting 45–60 min each.

Cognitive–Behavioral Therapy for Fear of Blushing

Once TCT has been completed, generally another six to eight weekly sessions are given on cognitive behavioral therapy (CBT). The procedure is similar to that used with patients suffering from SAD/social phobia, but special attention is paid to the safety-seeking behaviors that people adopt when they fear blushing but that are generally counterproductive. The therapy seeks to change these behaviors, which are generally things the person does, or does not do, in order to remain calm or to keep the blushing down, or at least less visible. One of the most common, of course, is avoiding or minimizing social contact, perhaps, for example, by sitting in the last row in a conference thinking that one might need to get up to go to the restroom. Other strategies are to use makeup, cover the face with the hair, stand against the light, wear sunglasses, or grow a beard (for men). Others are more complex, such as trying to control every aspect of a presentation one is going to make: learning it by memory, making sure that the room is as dark as possible, taking a tranquilizer beforehand, and so on.

While these safety-seeking behaviors may provide some short-term relief for people who blush, in the end they are counterproductive because, if the catastrophes that the patients anticipate do not occur, they attribute it to these behaviors instead of concluding that the situation was less threatening than they had thought. In other words, these behaviors keep them from learning that the consequences they fear are actually distorted ideas, and it prevents them from adopting coping strategies that are more productive. Several techniques are used to reduce these behaviors, such as practicing with simulations or re-creations of each problematic situation before trying the skills learned in real-life circumstances.

Other therapies used with people who fear blushing are social skills training, mindfulness-based cognitive therapy, and paradoxical intention. Likewise, in an interesting open study, an intensive weekend group intervention, specifically designed for individuals with fear of blushing, was assessed. Treatment was well accepted and consisted of a combination of attention training and behavioral therapy. At 6-month follow-up, nearly two-thirds of the participants achieved significant changes in fear of blushing. In another study, a psychoeducational group intervention for fear of blushing, that followed a cognitive–behavioral approach, but in a course setting (with "participants" and "teachers" instead of "patients" and "therapists"), the results showed that the intervention was effective in reducing fear of blushing as well as symptoms of social anxiety.

Length of Treatment

There is no scientifically based answer to the question about how long drug treatment (i.e., SSRIs) should be maintained. Clinical practice, however, tends to show that blushers who stop taking the medication are more likely to have the symptoms recur than those who continue with the drug for longer periods of time.

Concerning TBT and CBT, as described earlier, they are short-term treatments usually lasting only a few months. Since they involve learning processes, they have the advantage of providing longer-lasting results.

One option to consider, since patients tend to respond more quickly to medication than to CBT, is to begin treatment using both methods simultaneously and, after a time, to gradually decrease the use of drugs. Another alternative is to begin with a course of drug therapy, cut back gradually after a time, and then immediately begin CBT to prevent symptoms from recurring.

Conclusion

Since the advent of the internet, blushers, previously too embarrassed to ask for help, increasingly seek assistance from health professionals. In exchange, researchers now attend more to blushing in its own right or as part of SAD. There is the need to differentiate between the blushing that is expected in certain contexts and does not limit the individual and blushing that causes emotional pain and greatly interferes with a person's academic/occupational functioning or interpersonal relationships. The latter type of blushing motivates patients to seek help from health professionals. When systematically psychiatrically screened, 90% of these consulting blushers are found to suffer from SAD, a condition for which evidence of treatment efficacy, both pharmacological and psychological, is widely available. When assisting blushing patients who ask for treatment, these same therapeutic strategies for SAD should always be tried before attempting surgical options. Pharmacological and psychological treatments specifically aimed at helping blushers have been much less studied but are also available and efficacious.

Sources of Financial Support None.

Suggested Reading

Bögels SM. Task concentration training versus applied relaxation, in combination with cognitive therapy, for social phobia patients with fear of blushing, trembling and sweating. Behav Res Ther. 2006;44:1190–210.

Chaker S, Hofmann SG, Hoyer J. Can a one-weekend group therapy reduce fear of blushing? Results of an open trial. Anxiety Stress Coping. 2010;23(3):303–18.

Clark DM, Wells A. A cognitive model of social phobia. In: Heimberg R, Liebowitz M, Hope DA, Schneier FR, editors. Social phobia: diagnosis, assessment, and treatment. New York, NY: Guilford Press; 1995. p. 69–93.

Connor KM, Davidson JR, Chung H, Yang R, Clary CM. Multidimensional effects of sertraline in social anxiety disorder. Depress Anxiety. 2006;23(1):6–10.

Crozier W. Blushing and the social emotions. Basingstoke: Palgrave Macmillan; 2006.

Crozier WR, de Jong PJ. The psychological significance of the blush. Cambridge: Cambridge University Press; 2013.

Dijk C, Buwalda FM, de Jong PJ. Dealing with fear of blushing: a psychoeducational group intervention for fear of blushing. Clin Psychol Psychother. 2012;19:481–7.

Jadresic E, Suárez C, Palacios E, Palacios F, Matus P. Evaluating the efficacy of endoscopic thoracic simpathectomy for generalized social anxiety disorder with blushing complaints: a comparison with sertraline and no treatment. Innov Clin Neurosci. 2011;8:24–35.

Leary MR, Cutlip WD II, Brito TW, Templeton JL. Social blushing. Psychol Bull. 1992;3:446–60.

Rapee RM, Heimberg RG. A cognitive-behavioral model of anxiety in social phobia. Behav Res Ther. 1997;35(8):741–56.

Patient Selection for Endoscopic Thoracic Sympathectomy for Facial Blushing

Claudio Suárez Cruzat and Francisco Suárez Vásquez

Introduction

If endoscopic thoracic sympathectomy (ETS) has more than 95% success in the treatment for palmar hyperhidrosis, why are the results different for facial blushing?

Blushing surgery results in a long follow-up and shows a 73% satisfaction rate and 13% regret rate [1].

This question moved us to read, research, and think more about blushing, from the beginning.

Charles Darwin described blushing in 1872 as "the most peculiar and the most human of all expressions" [2]. There are differences between the normal blushing described by Darwin, which is associated with emotional distress, appears occasionally and everybody presents it, and the blushing that occurs in situations of mild emotional distress such as encountering another person, being observed, or alluded to by another. This kind of blushing appears frequently and is invalidating, is accompanied by a sense of shame and even mental block, and limits the normal social, emotional, and occupational development, producing psychological pain. This is called "pathological blushing", as described by Jadresic et al. [3, 4].

Facial flushing can be produced by heat, temperature changes, solar exposure, and multiple dermatological (rosacea), tumors (carcinoid), hormonal (menopause), allergic, drug or drug reactions, and autoimmune (dermatomyositis and systemic lupus erythematosus) etiologies, but none are associated with an emotional triggering factor, which is the hallmark of pathological blushing.

Patients suffering from blushing have sudden redness, with an ascending, rapidly progressive sensation of heat that sometimes also presents with redness of the neck and

C. S. Cruzat (✉) · F. S. Vásquez
Thoracic Surgery Department, Clínica Santa María, Santiago, Chile

Thoracic Surgery Program, Universidad de Los Andes, Santiago, Chile
e-mail: fsuarez@clinicasantamaria.cl

© Springer International Publishing AG, part of Springer Nature 2018
M. P. Loureiro et al. (eds.), *Hyperhidrosis*,
https://doi.org/10.1007/978-3-319-89527-7_30

upper part of the thorax, related to an emotional stimulus, which can sometimes be minimal. The production mechanism is not clear, but its frequent association with upper-limb hyperhidrosis suggests that the origin might be due to an excessive response to the stimulus, with facial vasodilatation and closing of the postcapillary sphincter, secondary to the activation of the cervical branches of the nervous sympathetic system [5].

There are different kinds of patients who consult for blushing; some people could have adequate response to selective serotonin reuptake inhibitors (SSRIs), psychotherapy, and be managed in a conservative way, and other patients will require surgery. On the other hand, there are mental and social disorders that can cause blushing, and those diseases are not improved with ETS; on the contrary, ETS may add compensatory sweating to their problems, so caution in the indication is advised. In this chapter we try to show why and how we select patients for ETS due to blushing.

Patient Selection

First, it is very important to understand that patients unhappy with ETS results occur due to two problems: compensatory sweating and lack of blushing control. We seek to select patients who will have good results with surgery and differentiate them from those who will not in the short- and long-term. Discontent increases and satisfaction decreases with greater follow-up. Thus, many authors report initial satisfaction of 95% and regret of 1–2%, but groups with prolonged follow-up show that these numbers tend to worsen over the years [1, 6]; this has led some groups to look for reversible operations or sympathetic reconstructions for patients who regret having surgery [7, 8].

Compensatory sweating is the main undesirable side effect of this surgery; there is no difference between different techniques: ETS T2, R2–3, or R2. More than 80% of operated patients will have severe or moderate body sweating during exercise, warm weather, or sudden temperature changes. This is the cause of regret in up to 13% of patients in different series (Licht et al. [9]); therefore, it is very important to explain to candidates for surgery that in most cases they will present compensatory sweating, about 30% will have gustatory sweating, and that there is the remote possibility of postoperative Horner syndrome. It is also important to tell the patient that blushing will not always disappear with the operation, and always inform them that there are other treatments before surgery, which is reserved only for some candidates.

We believe that ETS should only be performed on patients with severe, rapid-onset facial blushing, with ascending heat sensation, which is associated with social phobia or severe anxiety disorder, and without other mental illnesses.

Blushing and Endoscopic Thoracic Sympathectomy (ETS)

The first publication about surgery in facial blushing was by Wittmoser in 1985 [10], but only after the publication of Drott from Boras Hospital, Sweden, in 1998 [6] did the number of patients treated around the world by ETS increased rapidly. Telaranta proposed selection of patients with social phobia in 1998 [11].

Initially, reported patient satisfaction was about 85–88%, but this decreased to 75% in the long-term follow-up, and the regret rate increased to 13.5% [1, 6]. The causes for this were compensatory sweating, which affected 90% of operated patients, being severe in about 10–15% of the cases, and the occurrence of mild blushing over the years.

There were no controlled studies until 2011, when our group (Jadresic et al. [12]) published a prospective, observational, open-label clinical study. They compared medical treatment (sertraline, an SSRI) and ETS, showing 89% satisfaction with ETS and 59% with sertraline. With these results, they recommended selection of patients for surgery with previous medical treatment with sertraline for at least 3 months and operation only the patients with no response to an SSRI. Doing so allows a diminished regret rate to 4% in long-term follow-up [12]. The last follow-up, presented at a local meeting in Chile, showed that our regret rate is now 7%, including early patients who underwent ETS without SSRI treatment or social phobia evaluation. We still need some time to accurately evaluate these data and compare these two groups.

Licht et al. published a randomized trial that compared R2 versus R2–3 sympathectomy, with a response rate of 93%, 85% satisfaction, and a regret rate of 13% at 1-year follow-up [9]. Basically, with a minimum follow-up of 1 year, there were no significant differences regarding the control of blushing and the degree of compensatory sweating. However, in the group of exclusive R2, mild blushing recurrence at the year of surgery was slightly higher.

The recommendation to start the treatment for blushing with an SSRI was confirmed in a psychiatric publication by Pelissolo and Moukheiber in 2013 [13].

Patient Evaluation

Based in the aforementioned publications, our group indicates surgery after psychiatric evaluation and social phobia questionnaires.

We use two questionnaires, the Brief Social Phobia Scale (BSPS) (0–70, diagnosis of social phobia/social anxiety disorder with 20 points or more) and Social Phobia Inventory (SPIN) (0–68, diagnosis of social phobia/social anxiety disorder with 21 points or more), considering only patients with severe or invalidating blushing (3 or 4 on a 0–4 scale) and social anxiety disorder with high scores in the questionnaires as candidates for surgery. Usually, patients with scores between 20 and 40 in BSPS and SPIN have good results with sertraline treatment.

In addition to diagnosing social anxiety disorder, psychiatric evaluation allows other mental disorders to be ruled out and assessment of the patient's ability to cope and understand the possibility of a poor outcome. This is particularly relevant, because in patients with poor quality of life and social phobia secondary to blushing, a negative result, due to failure to control the blushing, severe compensatory sweating or Horner's syndrome, could further deteriorate their quality of life, causing a severe reactive depressive disorder.

The studies of Telaranta et al. [11], Jadresic et al. [12], and Callejas et al. [3] have shown a significant decrease in social phobia with sympathectomy, demonstrating that phobia is secondary to blushing and not vice versa, nor is it an isolated or different pathology in these patients with pathological blushing.

Compensatory Sweating and Blushing Following ETS

Compensatory sweating occurs in the vast majority of patients undergoing ETS R2, R2–3, or T2, but is severe only in 10–15%. The type of surgery does not determine this; it is apparently an individual response to partial sympathetic denervation or interruption of the flow of information from the sympathetic system to the hypothalamus for thermal regulation.

Because compensatory sweating is the main cause of regret, we prefer slim patients for this surgery (body mass index [BMI] <20–22). In our experience, with a higher BMI comes more compensatory sweating. In slim patients, compensatory sweating seems to occur with higher temperatures in comparison with patients with higher BMI. This means that slim patients with severe compensatory sweating will still have severe compensatory sweating, but it will appear on fewer occasions, for example only in hot summer periods. If we manage to reduce the number of profuse sweating episodes (wet clothing, even requiring clothes to be changed), the tolerance to this unwanted side effect will be better and the patient will not regret the surgery. He will have a predictable and low-frequency problem instead of the unpredictable and frequent blushing.

The relationship between BMI and compensatory sweating was published by Ribas Milanez in 2005 [14], showing that in T2–3 and T3–4 ETS there is a difference in the severity of compensatory sweating if the patient has BMI <20, 21–25, or >25. In our experience, as we presented in the 2015 International Society of Sympathetic Surgery (ISSS) meeting in Chile, in 221 patients who underwent R2–3 ETS due to blushing, most patients with severe compensatory sweating had BMI >21, but the sample size didn't allow statistical demonstration. It seems that women have better results following ETS for blushing, with less compensatory sweating (Smidfelt and Drott, Boras Hospital [1]). Men usually have higher BMI than women, but this information hasn't been evaluated in any study with a sufficient number of patients. The Boras Hospital group also reported that compensatory sweating could significantly diminish over years. We haven't verified this yet in our experience.

It is possible that lowering the level and reducing the extent of ablation might reduce the severe compensatory sweating, but this is a matter of debate today. The ISSS queried this with Smidfelt and Drott in a letter published in the *British Journal of Surgery*, and the authors answered that they have no significant results [15], though this same opinion regarding the level of ablation and compensatory sweating severity was published by Lin and Telaranta in 2001 [16]. They reported that compensatory sweating was less prevalent in patients that underwent T3 or T4 ETS than in those that underwent T2 ETS, the latter being the one that solves the problem of blushing.

Another variable that has great influence in compensatory sweating severity is the weather of the geographical area in which the patients live. In warmer climates, the compensatory sweating will be both more frequent and severe than in colder climates.

Our Methodology

Every patient that comes for blushing should be evaluated by a psychiatrist to assess the magnitude of the problem, the intensity of the blushing, the social anxiety disorder, and rule out that the blushing is secondary to another mental disorder. Social phobia surveys are applied and the psychiatrist defines whether the patient has pathological blushing and if they require treatment.

Patients will be considered eligible for treatment if they fulfill the following criteria:

1. Rate the severity of blushing as "severe or extreme".
2. BSPS total score ≥ 20.
3. SPIN total score ≥ 21.

When the decision to treat the patient is made, we start with pharmacological treatment with an SSRI (sertraline) for 3 months. After this period, we re-evaluate the patient's condition (blushing and phobia symptoms improvement, SSRI tolerance, treatment adherence), and in our series half of the patients have significantly improved and are not candidates for surgery.

Patients with poor results following pharmacological treatment, due to lack of blushing control or severe adverse effects (erectile dysfunction, tremor, loss of libido, headache, diarrhea), are considered candidates for surgery if they meet the following criteria:

1. Understand the compensatory sweating.
2. Understand that it is advisable to remain slim to control compensatory sweating.
3. Do not suffer another mental disorder.
4. Realize that, to date, ETS is irreversible.

Conclusion

In summary, we propose considerations for selection of patients for surgery (Table 30.1), in order to obtain the best results that improve the quality of life of our patients. When the selection process is adequate, the technical and visible results (Figs. 30.1 and 30.2) will meet the patients' expectations and overcome adverse effects.

Table 30.1 Select criteria for endoscopic thoracic sympathectomy for blushing

Severe facial blushing	Score of 3–4 on a 0–4 scale
Psychiatric evaluation	Diagnosis of social phobia or social anxiety disorder
	Rule out another mental disorder
	Evaluate the capacity to understand adverse effects or bad results
Failure to sertraline treatment	At least 3 months
Body mass index < 22	To control compensatory sweating
Consider place of residence	Best in colder climate

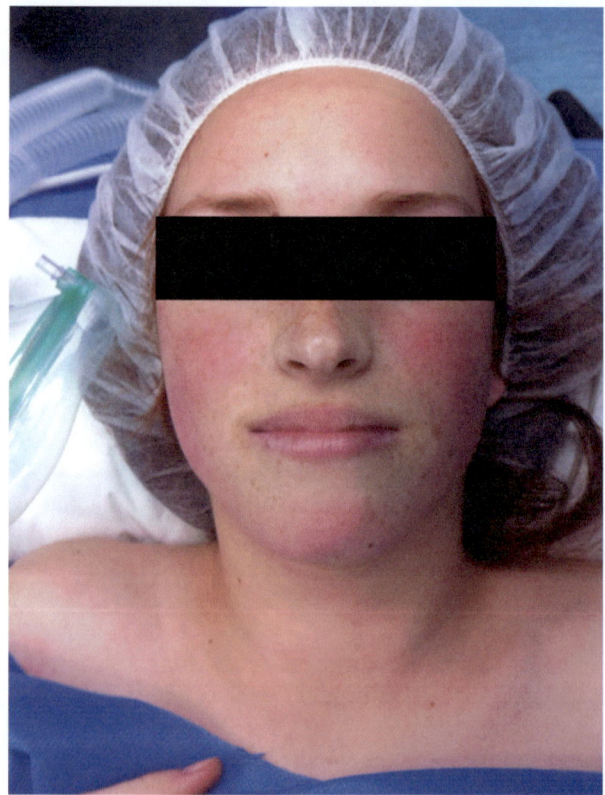

Fig. 30.1 Preoperative photograph of a young woman suffering severe blushing and social phobia

Fig. 30.2 Postoperative photograph following endoscopic thoracic sympathectomy for severe blushing

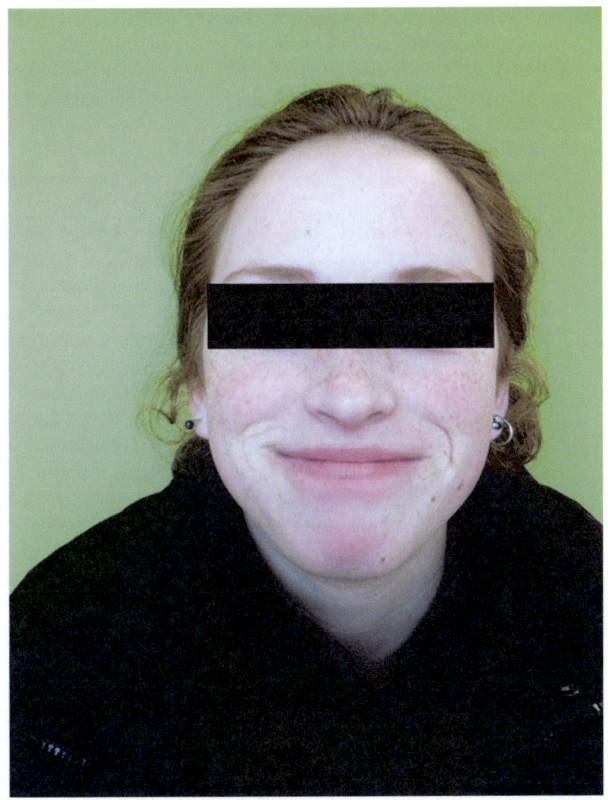

References

1. Smidfelt K, Drott C. Late results of ETS for hyperhidrosis an facial blushing. Br J Surg. 2011;98(12):1719–24.
2. Darwin C. The expression of emotions in man and animals. London: John Murray; 1872. In: Porter DM, Graham PW, editors. The portable Darwin. New York: Penguin Books; 1993. p. 364–93.
3. Callejas MA, Grimalt R, Mejia S, Peri JM. Resultados del tratamiento videotoracoscópico del blushing. Actas Dermosifiliogr. 2012;103(6):525–31.
4. Jadresic E. Is pathological blushing (PB) an illness? In: Jadresic E, editor. When blushing hurts. New York: iUniverse, Inc.; 2014. p. 19–24.
5. Callejas MA. Disfunción autonómica craneofacial. Rev Rinol. 2009;9:23–8.
6. Drott C, Claes G, Olsson-Rex L, et al. Successful treatment of facial blushing by endoscopic transthoracic sympathicotomy. Br J Dermatol. 1998;138(4):639–43.

7. Park H-S, Hensman C, Leong J. Thoracic sympathetic nerve reconstruction for compensatory hyperhidrosis: the Melbourne technique. Ann Transl Med. 2014;2(5):45.
8. Fibla JJ, Molins L, Mier JM, Vidal G. Effectiveness of sympathetic block by clipping in the treatment of hyperhidrosis and facial blushing. Interact Cardiovasc Thorac Surg. 2009;9:970–2.
9. Licht PB, Pilegaard HK, Ladegaard L. Sympathicotomy for isolated facial blushing: a randomized clinical trial. Ann Thorac Surg. 2012;94(2):401–5.
10. Wittmoser R. Treatment of sweating and blushing by endoscopic surgery. Acta Neurochir. 1985;74:153–4.
11. Telaranta T. Treatment of social phobia by ETS. Eur J Surg. 1998;580:27–32.
12. Jadresic E, Suarez C, et al. Evaluating the efficacy of endoscopic thoracic sympathectomy for generalized social anxiety disorder with blushing complaints: a comparison with sertraline and no treatment—Santiago de Chile 2003–2009. Innov Clin Neurosci. 2011;8(11):24–35.
13. Pelissolo A, Moukheiber A. Open-label treatment with escitalopram in patients with social anxiety disorder and fear of blushing. J Clin Psychopharmacol. 2013;33:695–8.
14. Ribas Milanez de Campos J, et al. The body mass index and level of resection. Predictive factors for compensatory sweating after sympathectomy. Clin Auton Res. 2005;15:116–20.
15. Hashmonai M, Licht PB, Schick C, Bishof G, Cameron A, Connery C, De Campos JRM, On Behalf of the International Society of Sympathetic Surgery. Late results of endoscopic thoracic sympathectomy for hyperhidrosis and facial blushing (Br J Surg 2011; 98: 1719–1724). Br J Surg. 2012;99:738. https://doi.org/10.1002/bjs.8769.
16. Lin CC, Telaranta T. Lin-Telaranta classification: the importance of different procedures for different indications in sympathetic surgery. Ann Chir Gynaecol. 2001;90(3):161–6.

Suggested Reading

Callejas MA, Grmalt R, Mejia S, Peri JM. Resultados del tratamiento videotoracoscópico del blushing. Actas dermosifiliogr. 2012;103(6):525–31.
Jadresic E, Suarez C, et al. Evaluating the efficacy of endoscopic thoracic sympathectomy for generalized social anxiety disorder with blushing complaints: a comparison with sertraline and no treatment–Santiago de Chile 2003–2009. Innov Clin Neurosci. 2011;8(11):24–35.
Licht P, Pilegaard H, Ladegaard L. Sympathicotomy for isolated facial blushing: a randomized clinical trial. Ann Thorac Surg. 2012;94:401–5.
Ribas Milanez JR, et al. Quality of Life, before and after thoracic sympathectomy: report on 378 operated patients. Ann Thorac Surg. 2003;76:886–91.
Smidfelt K, Drott C. Late results of ETS for hyperhidrosis and facial blushing. Br J Surg. 2011;98(12):1719–24.
Smidfelt K, Drott C. Facial blushing. Patients selection and long term results. Thorac Surg Clin. 2016;26:459–63.

Endoscopic Thoracic Sympathectomy for Facial Blushing and Craniofacial Hyperhidrosis

31

Peter B. Licht

Facial Blushing

Introduction

Sympathetic surgery for facial blushing has been performed routinely for more than three decades but the number of published papers in the literature remains low compared with research in palmar hyperhidrosis. Most of the scientific papers are single-institution case series, and there are only a few non-randomized comparative studies and one randomized clinical trial. Nevertheless, several reviews on treatment options for facial blushing have emerged, possibly due to the growing interest on facial blushing on the internet, where searches steadily increase for both non-surgical and surgical treatment options.

The Red Face

Normally, reddening of the face in flushing or blushing is part of a physiologic thermoregulatory response to hyperthermia that results from increased cutaneous blood flow caused by transient vasodilatation. Reddening of the face is also a common presenting complaint to dermatologists, allergists, internists, and family practitioners. Fever, hyperthermia, alcohol, emotional blushing, menopause, and rosacea are the most common reasons, but in some patients accurate diagnosis requires further studies to differentiate important underlying pathology such as carcinoid syndrome or pheochromocytoma.

P. B. Licht
Department of Cardiothoracic Surgery, Odense University Hospital, Odense, Denmark
e-mail: peter.licht@rsyd.dk

Although there is no consensus in the literature, reddening of the face is typically called flushing when it appears as a symptom of underlying somatic disease and blushing when it is triggered by emotion. This type of blushing is often described in the literature as erythrophobia and is characterized by frequent episodes of severe facial reddening easily elicited by emotional or social stimuli, the type of blushing that Charles Darwin described as "the most peculiar and the most human of all expressions". The exact nature of emotional blushing is unclear, but it has been described as an involuntary condition caused by autonomic dysfunction.

Social Consequences

Blushing is a common emotional response that most people have experienced occasionally, and in former times blushing was considered a sign of modesty and charm. Recent data suggest that blushing induces feelings of sympathy and trustworthiness, and therefore blushing does convey a social signal. It predominantly occurs in person-to-person contacts involving shame or embarrassment and, despite its common nature, most people consider blushing to be an undesirable response, which they often try to hide. In severe cases, blushing is associated with an intense feeling of embarrassment and shame that may lead to avoidance behavior with a negative impact on quality of life, and some individuals may experience so much distress because of blushing that they develop a phobia. From a survey of the literature, it is clear that there is a strong association between social phobia and facial blushing, but this does not necessarily imply a causal relationship. Thus, facial blushing is a cardinal symptom in the majority of patients with social phobia and often results in avoidance behavior, but not all patients with social phobia blush, and certainly not all facial blushers suffer from social phobia.

Occurrence

A national survey of 150,000 households concluded that the prevalence of primary hyperhidrosis was almost 3% in North America. There are no published estimates on the prevalence of facial blushing, but it is one of the prominent symptoms in social phobia, which has a lifetime morbid risk prevalence of up to 13%. In addition, 75% of all enquiries on a website for sympathectomy came from facial blushers compared with 25% who suffered from primary hyperhidrosis. It is likely that the incidence of facial blushing varies with geographic location. Thus, in the Nordic countries where a substantial proportion of the people are blond with fair skin, approximately half of the patients referred for sympathectomy suffered from facial blushing. The prevalence seems to be much lower in Asia, where surveys have shown that facial blushing was the indication for sympathectomy in less than 1% of patients, but this could reflect that sympathectomy for isolated facial blushing is rarely used in Asia.

Treatment

In general, patients with episodes of flushing or blushing should be first seen by a dermatologist or an internist to exclude important underlying pathology. Patients with emotional blushing triggered by emotion should be encouraged to try non-surgical options as the first line of treatment and sympathetic surgery should be the last treatment option for any patient. Pharmacologic treatment includes β-receptor blockers, anxiolytic drugs, selective serotonin reuptake inhibitors (SSRIs), and other antidepressant drugs. The effectiveness of β-blockers and topical ibuprofen gel to treat emotional blushing is largely anecdotal. SSRIs are well-documented for the treatment of social phobia but until recently the effect on facial blushing itself was not documented. A prospective study from Chile, however, demonstrated that SSRIs also have an effect on blushing, although the effect was higher in patients who underwent sympathetic surgery. There have been isolated reports of the use of intradermal botulinum toxin type A injection to treat neck and facial blushing, but this type of treatment only gives temporary relief. Some accounts in the literature mention psychotherapy such as cognitive therapy, task concentration training, psycho-educational group intervention, and cognitive–behavioral group therapy but we need more scientific research into psychological treatments for blushing per se, so that we can offer patients better information about the outcome with these treatments.

Thoracoscopic Sympathectomy

Provided non-surgical methods fail and there is still an indication for treatment, thoracoscopic sympathectomy may effectively treat facial blushing. It was first described in 1985, but it was not until 1998 that a comprehensive study was published from Sweden. Since then, several papers on thoracoscopic sympathectomy for facial blushing have emerged, but the number of papers remain much lower than that on sympathectomy for palmar or axillary hyperhidrosis. Similarly, only a few surgeons who perform thoracoscopic sympathectomy treat patients with isolated facial blushing, although more will likely begin to treat blushing as long-term follow-up studies have emerged.

Short- and mid-term results of sympathetic surgery for facial blushing are good. On average, complete satisfaction was reported in 84% of patients in a recent review of the literature. From one study it appears that the satisfaction rate declined over time and that the regret rate increased over time, which was speculated to reflect that adverse effects persist, whereas the memory of the suffering from blushing before surgery fades with time.

Patient Selection for Sympathetic Surgery for Facial Blushing

Because facial blushing is a benign condition, it is reasonable to ask if one should even attempt to treat it surgically. It is important to inform the patient about adverse effects before considering surgery, particularly compensatory sweating, which appears to be a permanent adverse effect in the majority of patients. Results from the literature indicate that sympathectomy for facial blushing is effective in more than 80% of patients despite a meticulous and critical selection process. It is likely that the rate of success will drop if patients are not selected carefully: the type of blushing likely to benefit from sympathectomy is mediated by the sympathetic nerves and is the uncontrollable, rapidly developing blush that is typically elicited by receiving attention from other people. Many patients mention a family history, either isolated facial blushing or in combination with palmar hyperhidrosis, and, although there is no data to support this, it is often the impression of sympathetic surgeons that such patients have a better outcome following surgery. In addition, and very importantly, blushing must be of major concern to the patient—enough to tolerate a substantial amount of compensatory sweating after the operation. Approximately 7% of patients in the published series regret the operation, and this figure should always be mentioned before considering surgery. Finally, it should be kept in mind that upper chest or neck blushing as well as a slowly emerging and long-lasting facial flushing respond poorly to sympathetic surgery.

Surgical Technique

The operation is performed under general anesthesia with double-lung or single-lung ventilation with or without insufflation of carbon dioxide. In an otherwise healthy patient, standard intubation with a single endotracheal tube is adequate and short periods of apnea are usually tolerated well for several minutes during identification and transection of the sympathetic chain. The patient is typically placed supine or in a semi-sitting position with abduction of both arms for bilateral access. One, two, or three ports may be used to gain access to the chest. Most sympathetic surgeons use two 5 mm ports, which are placed in the hairline in the anterior part of the axilla. Any thoracoscope may be used, but most surgeons prefer a 5 mm thoracoscope for minimal access with a 0 ° or a 30 ° optic. The latter makes it easier to visualize different parts of the pleural space. Sympaticotomy (transection of the sympathetic chain) or sympathectomy (resection) is performed by electrocautery or by an ultrasonic scalpel. The disadvantage with all of these approaches is that they are irreversible. Because of this problem, the use of clamps on the sympathetic trunk has emerged as an alternative approach. Such clamps are employed increasingly to treat primary hyperhidrosis and in facial blushing, where it appears to be at least as safe and effective as the earlier cauterization techniques and, in some patients with intolerable compensatory sweating, an increasing number of papers demonstrate that the reverse operation reduces this adverse effect.

Which Level of Sympathetic Chain for Facial Blushing?

There is no consensus on the extent of sympathectomy for isolated facial blushing, but it is generally accepted by all sympathetic surgeons who operate for facial blushing that it should be targeted where it passes over the second rib (R2). Some include the third rib (a R2–R3 procedure), but non-randomized retrospective comparative data have suggested that R2 should be the preferred method because of fewer adverse effects. Data from a randomized trial, however, did not reveal any difference in adverse effects between R2 and R2–R3 interventions.

Adverse Effects and Complications After Sympathectomy for Facial Blushing

Complications and adverse effects after sympathectomy for facial blushing are similar to those after sympathetic surgery for primary hyperhidrosis. Major surgical complications such as bleeding is extremely rare. Pneumothorax may be seen postoperatively in up to 25% of patients who are operated with simple inflation of the lung after sympathetic surgery, without leaving a chest drain in place for removal in the postoperative period. In these patients pneumothorax is an incidental a radiological finding in the vast majority because the lung did not fully expand after having been collapsed during the surgical procedure. Pneumothorax very rarely needs treatment unless the patient develops respiratory symptoms or if serial chest X-rays reveal progression of the pneumothorax. Damage to intercostal nerves depends on the operative technique and the diameter of the instruments. It is generally rarely reported but persisting pain has been seen in up to 8% of patients. Technical failure after sympathetic surgery for blushing occurs when the sympathetic chain is not completely severed—typically on one side where it results in Harlequin's phenomenon, which is treated by re-do surgery on the affected side. This should not be mistaken for recurrent facial blushing, which occurs in up to one-third of patients but is usually less severe than the original symptoms. The risk of Horner's syndrome due to damage of the stellate ganglion is higher than in sympathetic surgery for primary hyperhidrosis because the R2 level of the sympathetic chains is targeted for facial blushing. It has been speculated to occur due to thermal injury from simple cautery, and for that reason many sympathetic surgeons use ultrasonic energy to transect the sympathetic chain when operating for facial blushing. It has also been suggested that it occurs due to miscalculation of the target level, but Horner's syndrome has occurred without any good explanation as judged following analysis of videos of procedures where Horner's syndrome developed.

Adverse effects are much more common. The most frequent adverse effect after sympathetic surgery for facial blushing remains compensatory sweating, which refers to increased sweating in non-denervated parts of the body. It has been claimed to occur more frequently after surgery for facial blushing because the surgery targets the sympathetic chain at the R2 level. As with surgery for palmar hyperhidrosis, it mostly occurs on the back or the trunk, but lower limbs and the groin and other parts of the body may be affected. On average, compensatory sweating developed in 74% of the patients in a systematic review, but in one study it was as high as 99% of the patients. It may be so severe in some patients that they regret surgery and this proportion is claimed to be higher after facial blushing due to R2 interruption—on average, in a large review, less than 7% regretted surgery, but long-term follow-up indicates that regret rates increase over time. It is very important to discuss this frequent adverse effect before considering surgery for facial blushing. But it is also important to remember that previous follow-up studies only dealt with perception of increased compensatory sweating. Quantization was not performed, and whether there is an increased level of compensatory sweating or merely an increase in the subjective discomfort is not known. For example, someone with severe facial blushing cured by sympathectomy would most likely tolerate a great amount of new back sweating postoperatively, whereas someone with mild axillary sweating and the same amount of new back sweating postoperatively would not be satisfied with the result. Gustatory sweating is another common complication that, on average, affects 24% of patients who are treated for facial blushing. It is triggered by different foods or drinks, most often those that are spicy and particularly acidic (citrus), and causes increased sweating in the face. The pathophysiology of this symptom, which resembles Frey's syndrome after parotid surgery, remains unknown. Treatment options for gustatory sweating include oral anticholinergic drugs, topical application of anticholinergics or aluminum chloride, injection of botulinum toxin, or use of topical glycopyrrolate. Relative bradycardia from a decreased sympathetic cardiac tone is also seen in almost every patient if they are investigated, but it rarely leads to clinical symptoms unless the patient is a top athlete or has bradycardia preoperatively, in which case one should not perform sympathetic surgery for facial blushing. Because the upper extremity receives its sympathetic afferents through the second ganglia, most patients who undergo surgery for facial blushing develop dry hands postoperatively. This is often a desired response when the patients suffer from a combination of blushing and palmar hyperhidrosis, but dry hand can be a nuisance if they don't.

Craniofacial Hyperhidrosis

Craniofacial hyperhidrosis is a facial form of primary hyperhidrosis that results in excess sweating beyond normal physiological needs. The condition usually affects the forehead bilaterally but can also involve other regions of the face. It is claimed to be a primary condition characterized by sudomotor dysregulation stimulated by triggers such as heat and stress, and skin biopsies from patients have demonstrated that the eccrine glands are not morphologically abnormal but purely hyperactive. Craniofacial hyperhidrosis usually starts in adulthood and is less common than the axillary and palmar forms. Some claim that up to one-fifth of patients with primary hyperhidrosis are troubled by the craniofacial form, but this is likely dependent on geographical location. Thus, it is very rare in northern Europe and, although more prevalent in Asia, the craniofacial form only constitutes a fraction of patients treated surgically for palmar hyperhidrosis.

As with other forms of primary hyperhidrosis, sympathetic surgery should be the last treatment option because of adverse effects, which are similar to those of sympathetic surgery for facial blushing mentioned earlier. Dermatologists recommend topical glycopyrrolate or oral oxybutynin as first-line treatments. Intradermal botulinum toxin A may be used but, similar to other types of primary hyperhidrosis, this type of treatment only gives temporary relief and can be expensive in the long run. If non-surgical treatments fail, and provided there is still an indication for treatment, craniofacial hyperhidrosis is treated surgically in a similar manner to facial blushing by targeting the sympathetic chain at R2 or R2–R3 depending on local preferences.

The reported efficacy after surgery of craniofacial hyperhidrosis is high and varies between 70% and 100%. Adverse effects are similar to surgery for facial blushing listed earlier and in particular includes compensatory sweating in up to 95% of patients.

Suggested Reading

Girish G, D'Souza RE, D'Souza P, Lewis MG, Baker DM. Role of surgical thoracic sympathetic interruption in treatment of facial blushing: a systematic review. Postgrad Med. 2017;129:267–75.

Hartling S, Klotsche J, Heinrich A, Hoyer J. Cognitive therapy and task concentration training applied as intensified group therapies for social anxiety disorder with fear of blushing-a randomized controlled trial. Clin Psychol Psychother. 2016;23:509–22.

Kristian S, Christer D. Facial blushing: patient selection and long-term results. Thorac Surg Clin. 2016;26:459–63.

Licht PB, Pilegaard HK. Management of facial blushing. Thorac Surg Clin. 2008;18:223–8.

Nicholas R, Quddus A, Baker DM. Treatment of primary craniofacial hyperhidrosis: a systematic review. Am J Clin Dermatol. 2015;16:361–70.

Part V

Final

Quality-of-Life Evaluation During Treatment of Hyperhidrosis

32

Hugo Veiga Sampaio da Fonseca
and José Ribas M. de Campos

Introduction

"Quality of life is the general well-being of individuals and societies, outlining negative and positive features of life. It observes life satisfaction, including everything from physical health, family, education, employment, wealth, religious beliefs, finance and the environment...". So begins the definition of what quality of life (QoL) is on the free encyclopedia site https://en.wikipedia.org/wiki/Quality_of_life. In fact, it is the individual's perception of their position in life in the cultural and social context in relation to their more individual issues such as their goals, expectations, standards, and concerns. As you can see, it is a simple term to write, yet broad enough to be the focus of various areas of human knowledge (economic, social, cultural, medical, philosophical, and religious).

The World Health Organization (WHO) in 1946 defined health as "a complete state of physical, mental and social well-being and not merely the absence of disease or infirmity". This definition allows the assertion that for an individual, even without any organic change, to be considered healthy, they must live with quality. Therefore, based on this concept, the measurement of health can no longer be restricted to the absence of diseases or injuries and it becomes important to consider the different dimensions involved, as well as the repercussions of health problems in the daily lives of individuals.

H. V. S. da Fonseca (✉)
Royal Thoracic Surgery Clinic – Royal Portuguese Hospital of Beneficense in Pernambuco, Recife, Brazil

J. R. M. de Campos
Thoracic Surgery, University of São Paulo and Hospital Israelita Albert Einstein,
São Paulo, SP, Brazil
e-mail: jribas@usp.br

© Springer International Publishing AG, part of Springer Nature 2018
M. P. Loureiro et al. (eds.), *Hyperhidrosis*,
https://doi.org/10.1007/978-3-319-89527-7_32

Table 32.1 Graduation of quality of life based on the score obtained on completing the questionnaire

Before surgery	After surgery	Score
Excellent	Much better	20–35
Very good	Better	36–52
Good	Same	53–68
Bad	Worse	69–84
Very bad	Much worse	>84

But why this concern with QoL if the purpose of this chapter is to talk about the treatment of hyperhidrosis? Well, this disease can be considered a chronic disorder, accompanied by subjective suffering in a world in which abundant sweating is labeled as non-aesthetic, causes distress in social situations, and even becomes dangerous in certain professions. Transpiration is a biological function of homeothermic beings, but when it becomes exaggerated, it can cause disorders that affect the individual's QoL. In addition, the objective measurement of hyperhidrosis has failed to determine the correlation between the clinical complaint and the physiological intensity of excessive sweating.

Why Use a Quality-of-Life (QoL) Questionnaire?

The desire to measure the QoL of an individual has led the WHO to develop an instrument to evaluate QoL from a cross-cultural perspective, in an international context, which consists of 100 questions distributed in the following areas: physical, psychological, level of independence, social relationships, environmental, and spiritual aspects (religion, personal beliefs). The instrument was named the World Health Organization Quality of Life (WHOQOL-100). Other general questionnaires, such as the Short-Form 36 (SF-36), are generic instruments, and thus they are not intended to assess the dimensions normally affected by a specific health problem. However, there are other health-related QoL indicators that consider the impact of more specific conditions of different diseases such as primary hyperhidrosis (PH).

Taking these facts into account, a specific questionnaire would be necessary to accurately assess QoL in patients with PH. When elaborating a specific questionnaire for this pathology, there are four domains of skills that need to be considered: functional–social, personal, emotional, and special conditions. All of these domains have been defined taking into account the various situations in which hyperhidrosis decisively interferes in the patients' QoL. These observations were first made by Amir and were reassessed and adapted by Milanez de Campos and Wolosker to develop a specific questionnaire for hyperhidrosis and to serve as the basis for determining the best treatment from an individualized perspective (see complete questionnaire here and in Table 32.1).

HEALTH RELATED QUESTIONAIRE - HYPERHIDROSIS

NAME: ....DATE....../......./.......
Date of the Surgical Procedure: ..../........../..........

This study is RESTRICTED TO QUESTIONS CONCERNING YOUR WELL-BEING AND LIFE QUALITY, BEFORE AND AFTER SURGERY FOR CORRECTION OF HYPERHIDROSIS AND OR FACIAL BLUSHING/SWETTING. This information is important because we want to know how you feel and how well you are able to conduct your daily activities. Please answer each question marking only the answer as indicated. If you are in doubt about the answer, reread the question and try to answer to the best of your ability.

TABLE 01. Generally speaking, how would you rate your life quality BEFORE SURGERY?

Excellent	1
Very good	2
Good	3
Poor/Inferior	4
Very poor/Inferior	5

TABLE 02. Compared to the period before surgery how would you rate your life quality AT LEAST 30 DAYS AFTER SURGERY?

Much better	1
Slightly better	2
The same	3
Slightly worse	4
Much worse	5

ATTENTION: STARTING FROM THE NEXT QUETION, PLEASE ALWAYS USE THE SCALE OF VALUES USED IN THE TWO TABLES ABOVE, SELECTING ONLY ONE CHOICE FOR EACH ANSWER. THIS QUESTIONNAIRE IS CONFIDENTAL AND WILL BE UTILIZED ONLY FOR STUDY PURPOSES.

1) **FUNCTIONAL / SOCIAL DOMAIN**, with relation to the following items, how would you rate your quality of life:

	Before surgery:	After surgery:
Writing:	1 2 3 4 5	1 2 3 4 5
Doing manual work:	1 2 3 4 5	1 2 3 4 5
Doing recreation:	1 2 3 4 5	1 2 3 4 5
Doing sports:	1 2 3 4 5	1 2 3 4 5
Shaking hands:	1 2 3 4 5	1 2 3 4 5
Being with friends (public palces):	1 2 3 4 5	1 2 3 4 5
Grasping objects:	1 2 3 4 5	1 2 3 4 5
Social dancing:	1 2 3 4 5	1 2 3 4 5

2) **PERSONAL DOMAIN**, with your partner / spouse. How would you rate your quality of life:

	Before surgery:	After surgery:
Holding hands:	1 2 3 4 5	1 2 3 4 5
Intimate touching:	1 2 3 4 5	1 2 3 4 5
Intimate affairs:	1 2 3 4 5	1 2 3 4 5

3) **EMOTIONAL-SELF or OTHERS**; how would you rate the fact that after sweating/blushing excessively:

	Before surgery:	After surgery:
I always justified myself:	1 2 3 4 5	1 2 3 4 5
People rejected you slightly:	1 2 3 4 5	1 2 3 4 5

4) **UNDER SPECIAL CIRCUMSTANCES** - How would you rate your quality of life:

	Before surgery:	After surgery:
In a closed or hot environment:	1 2 3 4 5	1 2 3 4 5
When tense or worried:	1 2 3 4 5	1 2 3 4 5
Thinking about the problem:	1 2 3 4 5	1 2 3 4 5
Before an examination/meeting/speaking in public:	1 2 3 4 5	1 2 3 4 5
Wearing sandals/walking barefoot:	1 2 3 4 5	1 2 3 4 5
Wearing colored clothing:	1 2 3 4 5	1 2 3 4 5
Having problems at school/work:	1 2 3 4 5	1 2 3 4 5

Recommended by the Society of Thoracic Surgeons' consensus since 2011 and quoted in more than 100 articles related to the topic, the WHOQOL-100 is one of the most recommended specific questionnaires for treatment of PH. It has been used in the longest cohort to evaluate the correlation between bilateral videothoracoscopic sympathectomy (VTS) and QoL, and is therefore quite useful.

It consists in the scoring of 20 items predetermined by previous research and distributed among the four mentioned domains. In this way, through the sum of the points, it is possible to determine the general and specific QoL perception for each domain, as well as to understand the variation according to the time of clinical or surgical treatment.

QoL Changes with Clinical Treatment

Patients with PH have marked expression of acetylcholine receptors in the lymphatic ganglia of the sympathetic chain. Oxybutynin is an anticholinergic drug that reduces sweat excess by inhibition of sweat gland nerve stimulation through muscarinic receptors. It has been used as a medication for the initial treatment for patients with hyperhidrosis with good results in the face, hands, feet, and axillary regions. It is, therefore, a great alternative for initiating therapy for patients with PH and may be an option to improve QoL in patients who are not candidates for surgery.

In general, the use of oxybutynin as the first option in the treatment of PH is associated with an improvement in 66–75% of the patients whose QoL is most affected by hyperhidrosis: those classified as "bad" and "very bad". In fact, those who benefit most from this therapeutic option are those with the greatest negative impact on QoL before starting any treatment. Importantly, oxybutynin is a safe drug. However, closed-angle glaucoma is an important limitation to its use, as well as bowel obstruction, pregnancy, and lactation.

Interesting characteristics in patients over 40 years of age undergoing clinical treatment should be emphasized, among them the distribution of excessive sweating frequency in the body. In patients of more advanced ages, there is a higher prevalence of craniofacial hyperhidrosis, representing more than 50% of cases in patients over 50 years of age. Satisfaction compared with previous complaints shows a significant improvement, with 75–87% of patients placing themselves as better or much better than the pre-treatment condition (Table 32.2).

Table 32.2 Quality-of-life progression after treatment with oxybutynin in patients over 40 years old

Treatment result	Score	40–49 years (%)	≥50 years (%)
Much better	20–35	42	46
Better	36–51	33	41
Unaltered	52–67	24	13
Worse	68–83		
Much worse	>84		

Prospective analysis

The degree of QoL interference depends, as previously stated, on the condition's severity and the patient's ability to self-adapt, even in children. Some children with mild hyperhidrosis may report poor QoL. Others with more intense symptoms may report acceptable QoL. Oxybutynin is safe for infantile use and the contraindications remain the same, notably angle-closure glaucoma. It is an excellent alternative to surgical treatment for patients who are not yet fit for the surgical procedure.

Recent studies have shown satisfactory results in pediatric use. Improvement is observed in more than 85% of children (between 5 and 14 years), a result superior to that obtained in adults when reassessed after 6 weeks of treatment. On long-term observation, on average 2 years after starting treatment, high rates of satisfaction still remain.

QoL Changes with Surgical Treatment

Videothoracoscopic bilateral sympathectomy is the standard surgical procedure for the treatment of PH because it has the best long-term results in terms of symptomatic clinical improvement and QoL. However, it has as two major challenges: the control of compensatory hyperhidrosis (CH) and the fact that it is irreversible. In this sense, correct measurement of the impact on QoL is the main way to determine who will benefit most from this surgical procedure.

The following data refer to the largest cohort that has been evaluated regarding the long-term results of video-assisted bilateral sympathectomy in the treatment of PH. All details can be checked in the bibliographical recommendations section (item 1). The data were evaluated after 30 days, 5 years, and 10 years of follow-up and are consistent in showing the short- and long-term effect of the treatment proposed on QoL. Between 1995 and 2002, 403 patients were submitted to video-assisted sympathectomy at the Clinics Hospital of the University of São Paulo Medical School and their QOL variation was monitored according to the completion of the proposed questionnaire. The distribution of the hyperhidrosis complaint in each area of the body is shown in Table 32.3:

30 Days' Follow-Up

Patients' responses to QoL are shown in Fig. 32.1 prior to surgery and 30 days after the procedure.

Table 32.3 Hyperhidrosis complaint distribution between patients

Complaint	Distribution (%)
Palmar + plantar	57
Palmar + plantar + axillary	25
Axillary only	15.7
Craniofacial only	6.5

Of the patients who considered their QoL to be "good" before surgery, 66.7% reported it to be "much better" or "a little better". Of the patients who considered their QoL to be "bad" before surgery, 83.1% changed their answer to "much better" or "a little better". Of those who classified their QoL as "very bad", 98.3% reported it to be "much better" or "a little better". From the total sample, 92% considered their QoL to be at least "a little better" or "much better" after surgery. The worse the patient rated their QoL before surgery, the greater the patient felt the improvement to be.

5 Years' Follow-Up

Of the patients who considered their QoL to be "good" before surgery, 77% said they were "much better" or "a little better" after 5 years' follow-up. Of the patients who considered their QoL to be "bad" before surgery, 83.5% changed their rating to "much better" or "a little better". Of those who rated their QoL as "very bad", 93.2% said they were "much better" or "a little better". Of this total, 89.4% considered their QoL to be at least "a little better" or "much better" 5 years after surgery. We noticed that the worse the patient classified their QoL before operating, the greater the improvement was considered (Fig. 32.2).

Thirty days after surgery, 75.5% of patients rated their QoL as "much better"; 5 years later, this percentage decreased to 56.7%. However, 69.2% of the patients maintained their opinions in both periods, 30.8% indicated a "worse" QoL than before, and 10.4% indicated a "better" QoL. The result is highly significant ($p < 0.001$), indicating that there are differences between the two periods regarding patient responses.

It is possible to notice that the differences found are between the categories "much better" and "a little better". The number of responses of "much better" declined while "a little better" increased from one period to the next. We emphasize

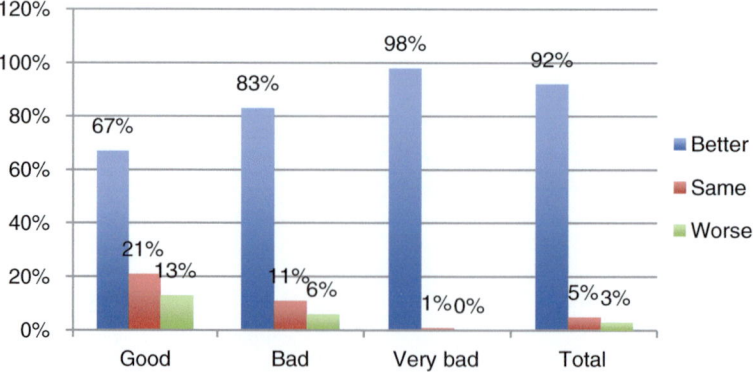

Fig. 32.1 Quality-of-life improvement 30 days after surgery compared with initial preoperative status

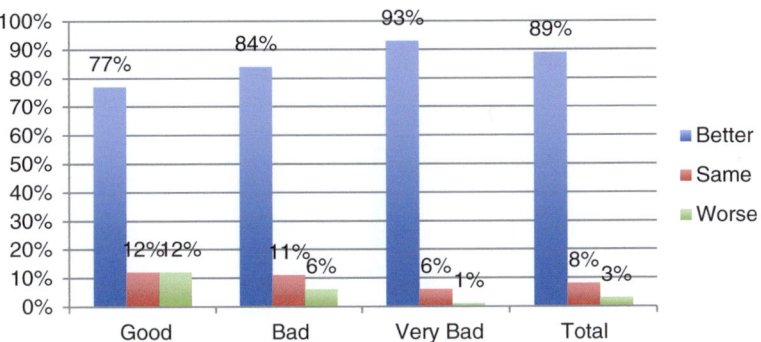

Fig. 32.2 Quality-of-life improvement 5 years after surgery compared with initial preoperative status

that if we consider only two categories of answers ("best" and "the same or worse"), we see 92% "best" answers in 30 days and 90.6% in 5 years. These numbers demonstrate that, despite the difference in the two periods, an immediate change to "better" and the continued maintenance of this QoL improvement after sympathectomy is very important.

10 Years' Follow-Up

Currently, we have more than 500 patients under follow-up who underwent surgery in the same period in which the study of 5 years was conducted. Now, after 10 years of follow-up, the results remain similar for improvement in QoL. In a total of 513 patients studied, 55.9% of patients are categorized as "much better", 34.8% as "a little better", 3.2% as "same", around 3% as "a little worse", and 3.1% as "much worse". Using these same numbers, 90.7% of the patients experience better QoL 10 years after thoracic sympathectomy. This confirms the initial improvement, which can be considered stable for patients in whom it has been achieved. On the other hand, we observe some slight changes in the results: "same" fell from 6.8% to 3.2%; "a little worse" rose from 1.1% to 3.0%; and "much worse" also rose from 1.4% to 3.1% (Fig. 32.3). These results are currently under interpretation to understand a difference found between the sexes. So far, this difference is linked to a gradual increase in body mass index (BMI) after 10 years, rather than any other studied factor.

QoL in Compensatory Hyperhidrosis

CH may occur with any level of sympathectomy and patients report different symptom intensities. When it is of low magnitude (almost all patients submitted VTS will develop it), it has no effect on the QoL questionnaire. It is necessary for CH to be intense and interfere in daily activities before it counteracts the good results related

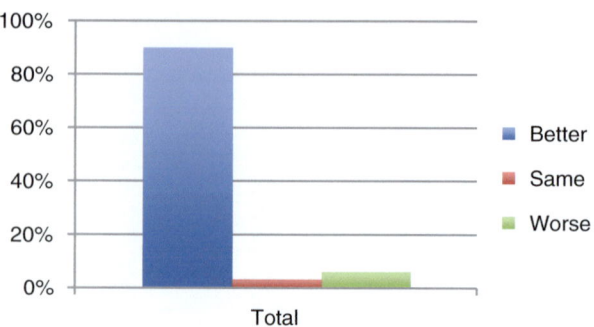

Fig. 32.3 Quality-of-life improvement 10 years after surgery compared with initial preoperative status

to the main complaint. In these cases, patients will regret the VTS, as we found in our study, in which most patients who reported no satisfaction with surgical treatment mentioned CH as the cause.

Regarding the development of CH, we found the following: 15 (3.7%) patients did not report any occurrence of CH; 57 (14.1%) reported it as mild; 174 (43.2%) as moderate; 150 (37.2%) as intense; and only seven (1.7%) patients were unhappy and reported regretting having undergone the surgical procedure. After 10 years of follow-up, these numbers are slightly higher, as suggested earlier, and to date this is believed to be the result of an increase in BMI.

Abundant compensatory sweating can be a cause of regret related to surgery, and consequently a reduction in QoL rates. In some cases, despite this manifestation, many of our patients revealed high satisfaction with VTS. There is no clinical or laboratory test that allows safe prediction of CH intensity. Hence, there is a need to warn all patients with hyperhidrosis about these unpleasant effects, which are difficult to control with currently available therapies.

Suggested Reading

Cerfolio RJ, De Campos JRM, Bryant AS, Connery CP, Miller DL, DeCamp MM, et al. The Society of Thoracic Surgeons expert consensus for the surgical treatment of hyperhidrosis. Ann Thorac Surg. 2011;91(5):1642–8.

Milanez De Campos JR, Kauffman P, De Campos Werebe E, Andrade Filho LO, Kusniek S, Wolosker N, et al. Quality of life, before and after thoracic sympathectomy: report on 378 operated patients. Ann Thorac Surg. 2003;76(3):886–91.

Milanez De Campos JR, da Fonseca HVS, Wolosker N. Quality of life changes following surgery for hyperhidrosis. Thorac Surg Clin. 2016;26:435–43.

Pompili C, Novoa N, Balduyck B. Clinical evaluation of quality of life: a survey among members of European Society of Thoracic Surgeons (ESTS). Interact Cardiovasc Thorac Surg. 2015;21(4):415–9.

Wolosker N, de Campos JRM, Kauffman P, Puech-Leão P. A randomized placebo-controlled trial of oxybutynin for the initial treatment of palmar and axillary hyperhidrosis. J Vasc Surg. 2012;55(6):1696–700.

Wolosker N, Schvartsman C, Krutman M, Campbell TPDA, Kauffman P, De Campos JRM, et al. Efficacy and quality of life outcomes of oxybutynin for treating palmar hyperhidrosis in children younger than 14 years old. Pediatr Dermatol. 2014;31(1):48–53.

Wolosker N, Teivelis MP, Krutman M, de Paula RP, Schvartsman C, Kauffman P, et al. Long-term efficacy of oxybutynin for palmar and plantar hyperhidrosis in children younger than 14 years. Pediatr Dermatol. 2015;32(5):663–7.

Ethical and Legal Aspects of the Management of Hyperhidrosis

33

Irimar de Paula Posso, Daniella Salazar Posso Costa, and Fabiana Salazar Posso

Introduction

Patients, even those from less fortunate social layers, are now fully aware of their rights and increasingly look to uphold their rights when they understand that physicians have not complied with their contractual relationship.

Changes in autonomic nervous system physiology and sweating glands bring discomfort and disorders to many people, leading them to look for medical or other professionals, the vast majority of whom are not adequately prepared to treat such a disease.

It is critical for both invasive and non-invasive therapies that well-documented clinical and laboratory diagnoses are carried out, if possible with images, as well as that patients are informed about the risks and benefits, advantages and disadvantages of any proposed therapy and, if patients agree, such information be recorded. Patients and an independent witness should then sign the consent document, because unfortunately in Brazil there is a culture that means when things happen as planned by the patients, the merit is theirs and physicians are just an agent; but when things do not go as planned, physicians are always to be blamed.

When considering ethical and legal principles guiding hyperhidrosis therapy, physicians should be technically and legally qualified to treat such a disease, and legal statutes, such as the Constitution, Civil, Criminal, Consumer Protection, and

I. de Paula Posso (✉)
Hospital Israelita Albert Einstein, São Paulo, Brazil

Study and training center, School of Medicine ABC, Santo André, São Paulo, Brazil

D. S. P. Costa
Posso Costa Associated Lawyers, São Paulo, SP, Brazil
e-mail: daniella@possocosta.adv.br

F. S. Posso
Clinic Rhinoderma, Santo André, São Paulo, SP, Brazil

Medical Ethics Codes should be followed in aspects applied to hyperhidrosis therapy.

Ethical and legal principles guiding life in society and, as it should be, the medical profession are based on the duty and liability duality, and of course ethical and legal aspects related to hyperhidrosis therapy are also based on liability and duty concepts.

Duty and Liability

Human beings are free to choose their conduct, but are also totally responsible for their actions and consequences. Liability is a notion inherent to human nature, because everyone knows that they are always responsible for any damage or loss caused by them, or by the non-compliance with a liability arising from the law or an agreement.

There are constant relationships among people when living in society, which result in duties, such as doing or not doing something. Duty means doing something, giving something, or not doing something previously established or agreed. If people do not comply with their duty, there is liability as a reaction of the law. Duty could relate to means or results.

Means duty is that where contracted parties are obliged to use with diligence, expertise, and prudence all their knowledge, insight, and experience to comply with the objective of the agreement, but without the obligation of producing a result favoring those contracting them. In result duty, contracted parties are obliged to produce a certain result, which if not obtained shall hold contracted parties responsible for damages or losses for those who have contracted them.

Physicians' Liability

Physicians' liability is always a means rather than a result liability, because biological variations, changes induced by time, and advances in technological and medical knowledge by no means assure a favorable result.

Physicians may, and should, use their technical qualification, be up-to-date, and always act with diligence, expertise, and prudence to apply their efforts to get the best result for their patients. When assisting patients, physicians should make their best efforts to obtain cure, even if not achieving it. Physicians' liability for poor results shall only be characterized when there is blame for malpractice, imprudence, or negligence.

Jurisprudence understands that when assisting patients, there is a real agreement between them and the physician, a medical liability agreement, where physicians are not committed to curing, but rather to acting according to the rules and methods of their specialty.

Although considering medical activity as an agreement, despite it likely being perceived otherwise, there is no presumed physicians' guilt despite this agreement.

Physicians' profession is ruled by the Medical Ethics Code, where duties are scope duties, allowing different interpretations, and very often are far from a concrete reality. Physicians are also subject to common right provisions, as are any other citizen; however, the Criminal and Civil Codes have some more specific provisions relating to medicine.

Guilt

Guilt is a relevant topic since malpractice, imprudence, and negligence, which may be classified as modalities of guilt, are prominently dealt with in the Civil, Criminal, and Medical Ethics Codes.

Malpractice occurs when physicians present an inability, ignorance, lack of competence, lack of theoretical or practical technical qualification, or lack of elementary and basic knowledge relating to the profession.

Imprudence assumes a hasty action, without caution, such as when physicians acts in a hasty way, adopting attitudes different from those expected or needed due to lack of foresight and attention to complying with a certain act.

Negligence may be characterized when physicians fail to take measures or to present the conduct expected for the situation, do not take due care, do not follow the act with due attention and diligence, or act with sloppiness by not taking required or needed precautions.

When the presence of one or more guilt elements is proven, and the guilt of the physician is characterized, there is the duty to undertake repair, because even without intention he has caused damage.

Physicians' ethical responsibility is based on Article 1 of the Medical Ethics Code, which provides that it is prohibited for physicians "To practice professional acts noxious to patients which could be characterized as malpractice, imprudence or negligence". Penalties to which physicians are subject vary according to the severity of the event, which may vary from a simple confidential warning in a private notice, to a confidential reprimand in a reserved notice, to a public reprimand in an official publication, to suspension of professional practice for up to 30 days, and even, in more extreme cases, cessation of professional practice.

Physicians' civil liability is based on Articles 186 and 927 of the Civil Code, which provide that "Those by volunteer action or omission, negligence or imprudence, violate rights and cause damage to third parties, even if exclusively moral, commit illicit act", and that "Those who, by illicit act (arts. 186 and 187), cause damage to third parties, are obliged to repair it".

Indemnity is calculated from an evaluation of damages, be they material or moral. It is pecuniary and should be proportional to damage, as provided in Articles 949, 950, and 951 of the Civil Code.

Physicians' criminal liability is based on Article 18 of the Criminal Code, which provides that "wrongful crime is defined when the agent has caused the result by imprudence, negligence or malpractice".

There is wrongful offense when the agent acts without due care, or does not give due attention or diligence, acting without the necessary care, and does not notice the result that could have been foreseen or, treated with proper gravity, should never be ocurred, or that it could have been avoided.

Applicable penalties to physicians in case of wrongful crime may be depriving them of their freedom or restricting their rights.

Medical Records

Medical records are a set of standardized and organized medical documents in which to record professional care given to patients; they are critical for checking medical assistance, for teaching and research, in addition to being a valuable tool in legal defense.

Medical records must be prepared by physicians, according to Articles 87 and 88 of the Medical Ethics Code, which provide that is prohibited to physicians "to fail to prepare a legible record for each patient. § 1 Records must contain clinical data necessary for the good management of the case, being filled in every evaluation, in chronological order with date, hour, signature and number of physician's registration in the Regional Council of Medicine. § 2 Records shall be kept by the physician or the institution assisting the patient", and it is also prohibited to "Deny to patients access to their records, lack to supply them copies, when asked, as well as lack of giving necessary explanations to their understanding, except when they pose risks for patients themselves or third parties".

Medical records are protected by professional or medical secrecy and should be prepared with care and legibly, and should contain the patient's identification, medical history, examinations conducted (such as laboratory and radiological, etc.), medical reasoning with diagnostic hypotheses, and the final diagnosis and therapeutic approach with a description of any surgery, prescribed drugs, and biopsy and imaging examinations reports.

Informed Consent

Informed consent is a voluntary written decision of an autonomous and capable person, made after an information process, for the acceptance of specific therapy, showing that they are aware of risks, benefits, and possible consequences.

Legal principles are delimited in Item II of Article 5 of the Federal Constitution, which provides that "No one will be obliged to do or not to do something unless if provided by law" in Article 15 of the Brazilian Civil Code, which states that "no one should be forced to be submitted of life threatening medical treatment or surgical intervention", and in Item III of Article 6 of the Consumer Protection Code, which provides that basic consumer rights are "Adequate and clear information on different products and services, with correct specification of quantity, characteristics, composition, quality, taxes and price, as well as about their risks".

Along the same lines, the Medical Ethics Code establishes in Articles 22, 24, 31, and 34, respectively, that it is prohibited for physicians "to fail to obtain patients' or their legal representatives consent after explaining the procedure to be performed, except in cases of imminent death risk"; "Fail to assure patients the exercise of the right to freely decide about their person or wellbeing, as well as to exert their authority to limit them"; "Disrespect patients or their legal representatives right to freely decide about execution of diagnostic or therapeutic practices, except in case of imminent risk of death"; and "Fail to inform patients about diagnosis, prognosis, risks and objectives of the therapy, except when direct communication may cause damage, case in which communication should be done to their legal representatives".

To be considered valid, informed consent should be prepared before the medical act, be in accordance with legal ordinance, be in accessible language, and outline procedures or therapies that will be used, as well as their objectives and background, possible discomforts and risks and expected benefits, and existing alternative treatment methods, and give signature or fingerprint identification of the patients or their legal representatives.

The informed consent shall clearly contain the patient's name, day and time of consent, the nature of the procedure, objective, risks, and alternative treatments in non-technical language, information about the non-assurance of success, identification of the physician or physicians who will assist the patient, the name of the physician who explained the treatment to the patient and/or their representative and who is obtaining the consent, a statement that the patient and/or their representative had the opportunity to ask questions about treatment and that all questions were answered, and the signature of the patient or their legal representative and of at least one witness.

Implications of not complying with ethical rules and failure to obtain the specific informed consent to perform the invasive or non-invasive procedure for hyperhidrosis may, in case of dispute be referred to the Regional Council of Medicine, characterize infringement of the Medical Ethics Code, thus generating penalties, which may vary from a confidential censorship in a reserved notice to a public censure in official publication, and even, in a more extreme case, the suspension of the professional exercise for up to 30 days.

In the civil context, failure to obtain specific informed consent for invasive or non-invasive treatment for hyperhidrosis may, in case of a lawsuit, generate pecuniary penalty for material and moral damage, in values established by the court, depending on the severity of the damage.

Although not potentially lethal, hyperhidrosis treatment may cause discomfort or deformities, so it is critical for physicians' defense to get the specific informed consent for the procedure to be performed, be it invasive or not, pointing out possible adverse events specific to each type of hyperhidrosis therapy, exemplified as follows.

Non-invasive treatment with anti-sweating agents that decrease sweating have undesirable effects such as dermatitis, skin stains, clothes stains, and the need for daily use. Anticholinergic agents have more adverse effects, such as dry mouth, blurred vision, palpitations, urinary retention, speech, taste, chewing and swallowing disorders, and do not promote the desirable reduction of excessive sweating. Sedative and psychological assistance may help decrease social phobias but have little action on hyperhidrosis.

Minimally invasive therapy with iontophoresis is not very practical, painful, may generate skin injuries, and its duration of action is short. Botulinum toxin is easy to use with topical anesthesia, local or loco-regional anesthesia or sedation; however, the therapeutic effect has a mean duration of 7 months, and it is uncomfortable due to the need for periodic repetition of injections.

Surgical treatment with subcutaneous tissue excision, skin and subcutaneous tissue excision en bloc, and skin and underlying subcutaneous tissue excision may cause unaesthetic scars and scar retraction, with possible limitation of joint mobility.

Subdermal axillary lipoaspiration ruptures the nervous supply of sweat glands and removes or destroys sweat glands, but may cause hematoma, seroma, infection, asymmetry, skin retraction, and changes in joint mobility.

Thoracic sympathectomy is a permanent treatment for hyperhidrosis, both palmar and axillary; however, it may have adverse effects such as compensatory sweating, Claude-Bernard-Horner syndrome, causalgia, incomplete results, anesthetic complications, and low satisfaction or dissatisfaction with results. Lumbar sympathectomy is a therapy for isolated or persistent compensatory plantar hyperhidrosis after thoracic sympathectomy but may have adverse effects such as injuries to adjacent sympathetic chain structures, mild abdominal distention, neuralgia, causalgia, hypoesthesia in the lower abdomen and thigh, leg movement limitation, anterolateral abdominal wall paresthesia, changes in libido, dyspareunia, pulmonary embolism, hemorrhages, arrhythmias, and cardiac decompensation.

There are numerous judgements where the lack of specific and well-developed informed consent is reason for condemnation for moral and material damage, as shown by the following compiled summary, which, although relating to plastic surgery, is a clear example of relevant jurisprudence.

TJ-DF—Civil Appeal 0003469–69.2006.8.07.0003.

> Summary: Material and moral damage. Civil liability. Hospital and physician. Esthetic surgery. ...2. The result is contract obligation for performing esthetic surgery. If result can be improved, surgery has not reached the expected satisfaction degree and if so, obligation was not complied with. 3. Imprecise and vague document, not informing patient about surgical risks, not supplying the requirement of effective informed consent...

In the same line lawsuits for moral and material damage were accepted in hyperhidrosis surgeries where informed consent was poorly developed and has not specified possible adverse effects of the technique.

TJ-PR—Civil Appeal 678.667-0—10th Appealing Civil Court of the Central Court of the Metropolitan Region of Curitiba.

> Indemnity action for material and moral damage. Performance of chest surgery to treat hyperhidrosis. Severe side effects. Compensatory sweating in other body regions. Frustrated treatment. Limitations to patient's social life. Information duty. Sentence maintained. 1.

Physicians have the duty to inform to provide patients with conditions to express their free consent to the proposed treatment, especially with regard to risks, possibilities of failure, contraindications and adverse reactions. 2. Although the forensic report concludes that medical treatment was adequate to patient, the physician shall be liable for consequences to patient due to lack of clear and precise information about surgical procedure risks, and which cannot be supplied by journal stories or scientific articles…

From the sentence, we have extracted the following text to call attention to the need for adequately informing patients:

There has been forensic proof that "more common risks were reported…" being that "… however complications such as kilothorax were not reported because they are very uncommon however subject to occur…".

It is certain that the physician knew the risks of chest surgery to treat hyperhidrosis, since he has extensive curriculum in this specialty area, as instructed in the records with technical literature in this sense. So, in face of the severity of possible and eventual adverse effects, it was up to the physician to give the patient detailed explanations and to call their attention to surgical risks and consequences. However, as recorded in the sentence by the analysis of proofs, the plaintiff was not adequately informed about tje risks and consequence of the surgery he was submitted to.

The physician–patient relationship goes beyond the use of a good technique to involve and protect the whole relationship, it being up to the physician to carry out the duty of informing the patient about the chance of healing and of pathologies which may affect the patient. In the search for the valid and effective consent, the patient should be able to self-determine using clear and accurate information provided. It is worth mentioning that the physician–patient relationship does not end in the technical dimension of applying available scientific knowledge, but also involves elementary duties of care, attention, and information. It is not enough for the physician to act defensively in the light of hypotheses made available by medicine; he should go beyond, watching over his patient, showing typical attention and care for those dealing with life, its evils, and possibilities.

As to the duty to inform, the doctrine provides that:

The duty to inform provided in art. 6, III, Consumer Protection Code, is linked to the principle of transparency and obliges the supplier to provide all information about the product or service. This principle is detailed in art. 31, which emphasizes the need for accurate, clear, precise and ostensive information about services, as well as about risks to health and safety of consumers. Also part of the information duty group there is the duty of guiding patients and their relatives about risks of treatment and drugs to be prescribed. So, there is a general duty of information of physician to patient, respecting people's autonomy, of informing in understandable language, all details about the pathology, available therapies and chances of healing, providing patients with the decision of being or not submitted to treatment and its inherent risks.

On the other hand, the presence of the term "specific consent", developed according to already detailed rules, was enough for the dismissal of a lawsuit against a physician for an unsatisfactory result after thoracic sympathectomy surgery which evolved with compensatory hyperhidrosis.

TJ-RS—Civil Appeal 70062235981.

Summary: Civil liability. Moral and material damage. Medical malpractice. Chest sympathectomy. Craniofacial hyperhidrosis. Compensatory hyperhidrosis. Conclusive forensic evidence. Fail of medical assistance not verified. Informed consent. Inadequacy of unverified procedure. Duty to compensate absent .... the author filed a claim for compensation for moral and material damages, in view of the damages experienced as a result of the surgical procedure of thoracic sympathectomy performed by the demanded physician, supposedly in a negligent way, which has led to unsatisfactory result after surgery, with compensatory hyperhidrosis.

In the circumstances of the case, this is personal liability, since plaintiff filed suit against the physician responsible for surgical thoracic sympathectomy. Physician's duty is means duty, and all available techniques should be used to treat patient; however, cure cannot be assured, because it depends on several factors. Physician's liability depends on proving guilt according to provisions of art. 14, §4, CPC....

According to forensic evidence, medical assistance was correct, with the use of available means and knowledge, not existing facts which indicate negligence, imprudence or malpractice. Testimonials collected during procedural instruction just confirm what has been described by the plaintiff about excessive sweating leading him to the medical procedure. Procedural proof is not enough to configure the duty to indemnify.

Right for information. With regard to right for information, this is a basic consumer right (art. 6, III, CPC) and aims at giving patients objective elements of reality for them to give or deny consent. Documental proof in the procedure rules out eventual failure of physician's duty to inform. Document of page 74 (Explanation, Science and Consent Term) is clear with regard to the possibility of complications associated to the procedure. Procedural elements lead to the belief that plaintiff knew about the procedure, as well as about possible side effects of the surgical intervention. Groundlessness sentence maintained. Appeal devoid of purpose.

Experimental Therapies or Those Not Approved by Science

Procedures and techniques not yet Approved by science should be avoided; however, if there is a need or indication for experimental therapy, the patient should be informed and treatment should only start if there is full agreement duly recorded in medical records and detailed in the consent term. The Medical Ethics Code provides in the sole paragraph of Article 102 that:

> The use of experimental therapy is allowed when accepted by competent bodies and with patients or their legal representatives' consent, after being adequately explained about the situation and possible consequences.

There is already jurisprudence about this, as shown below.
TJ-SP—Appeal 010345650-2006-8.26-0100.

Summary: Civil liability. Indemnity for moral and material damage. Opht[h]almic surgery. Complications not reported to patient. Lack of informed consent term. Experimental surgery. No warning to the plaintiff was seen in the procedures about the severity of her disease. She was also not warned in detail about surgery risks. As seen, not even information supposedly delivered to plaintiff would supply lack of information. Although being unable to point misuse of the practice and care of the defendant with the plaintiff, the physician cannot submit patient to the risk of still not consecrated procedure and technique, and consequently to all possible complications, without informing patient about them.

Medical Advertising and Hyperhidrosis Therapy

Hyperhidrosis is a disease which, although causing discomfort and being able to significantly impair patients' lives, is not lethal, and this is the reason why there are several therapies not discussed in the media; however, physicians should be aware that according to Articles 111 and 112 of the Medical Ethics Code, it is prohibited to physicians "to allow that their participation in the disclosure of medical subjects, in any mass communication media, lacks the exclusive character of explaining and educating society", and "to spread information about medical subject in a sensationalist, promotional or untrue content way".

Surgical Therapy for Compensatory Sweating

Reversion of hyperhidrosis therapy surgery should be indicated with care, explaining to patients that compensatory sweating is a physiological response that is not due to medical malpractice or technical failure of the surgical team performing the procedure. Techniques and possibilities of failure should be explained in detail, never compromising results, and always taking into consideration that a new surgery does not always offer satisfactory risks and results.

Sympathetic nerve reconnection surgery using an intercostal nerve graft may be performed but, if so, it should be emphasized that the risks and results are not very encouraging.

Judicialization

Another aspect that cannot be forgotten is judicialization aimed at achieving health insurance coverage for hyperhidrosis therapy, often without the required benefit being granted, as in the two following cases.

TJ-DF Decision 655166 Lawsuit 20120020240897.

> Interlocutory appeal. Obligation to do lawsuit. Tutorship anticipation. Axillary hyperhidrosis. Treatment with botulinum toxin. Denial. Unequivocal proof of verisimilitude and justified fear of irreparable or difficult to repair damage. Absence. For purposes of tutorship anticipation request it is necessary the presence of both requirements, that is, unequivocal proof of verisimilitude and justified fear of irreparable or difficult to repair damage. So, in the absence of risk of death or imminent risk to psychic health of plaintiff suffering from axillary hyperhidrosis, the decision denying anticipated tutorship should be maintained.

TJ-SC Civil Appeal 2009.052953-8

> Summary: Civil appeal. Collection action. Defense retrenchment. Anticipated judgment of the deal. Denied thesis. Medical and/or hospital assistance agreement. Hyperhidrosis. Surgical procedure. Coverage denied. Treatment with social objective. Express policy on coverage exclusion. Restrictive interpretation. Reimbursement denied. Sentence maintained. Resource devoid.

Suggested Reading

Brasil. Código Civil. Lei Nº 10.403, de 10 de janeiro de 2002. Brasília DF 2002.
Brasil. Código de Defesa do Consumidor. Lei No 8.087, de 11 de setembro de. Brasília. DF. 1990:1990.
Brasil. Código Penal. Lei n° 9.777, de 26 de dezembro de 1998. Brasília. DF. 1998.
Conselho Federal de Medicina – Código de Ética Médica. Brasília, 1988.
Kfouri NM. Responsabilidade civil do médico. 8a ed. Revista e Ampliada. Editora Revista dos Tribunais: São Paulo; 2013.

Questions and Answers on Hyperhidrosis, Its Treatment and Consequences

34

Miguel L. Tedde, Elias Albino Theophilo, and Flavio Henrique Savazzi

What is hyperhidrosis?
Hyperhidrosis is a pathologic condition of excessive sweating in amounts greater than physiologically needed for the regulation of body temperature (thermoregulation). Hyperhidrosis is a distressing condition for patients: it causes physical discomfort and social awkwardness, negatively impacts on daily activities, and results in depression and reduced levels of confidence.

How does hyperhidrosis manifest itself?
Hyperhidrosis can be generalized or focal.

The generalized form of hyperhidrosis affects the entire body and may happen without a known cause (idiopathic) or secondary to a metabolic or systemic disease, such as endocrine diseases (menopause, hyperthyroidism, diabetes), neurological disorders (Parkinson disease, peripheral neuropathies, brain lesions), congestive heart failure, neoplasias, or use of some medications (such as propranolol, tricyclic antidepressants, cholinesterase inhibitors, and opioids).

Conversely, focal hyperhidrosis, which occurs in otherwise healthy patients, involves specific sites of the body, most commonly the axilla, palms, soles, and sometimes the craniofacial area, often before the age of 25 years.

The most common cause of focal hyperhidrosis is primary idiopathic hyperhidrosis. It is important to note that primary hyperhidrosis ceases when sleeping, in contrast to night sweats, which can indicate an underlying disorder.

M. L. Tedde (✉)
Department of Thoracic Surgery, Heart Institute (InCor), Hospital das Clinicas, University of São Paulo and Hospital Samaritano, São Paulo, Brazil
e-mail: tedde@usp.br

E. A. Theophilo
Hospital Santa Catarina, São Paulo, Brazil

F. H. Savazzi
Hospital Alemão Oswaldo Cruz, São Paulo, Brazil

Is hyperhidrosis a congenital disease? Does it affect parents and children?

There is evidence for a genetic component to hyperhidrosis but it does not mean that if parents have it, children will have it too. Some genetic analysis suggests that an allele for hyperhidrosis may be present in 5% of the population, and that 25% of people with one or two copies of the allele will have hyperhidrosis, and roughly two-thirds of patients report a positive family history.

What are the treatments for hyperhidrosis?

Hyperhidrosis has a medical or non-surgical and a surgical treatment.

Patients who are overweight, have full-body hyperhidrosis, or who have secondary causes such as hyperthyroidism, hypertension, diabetes mellitus, infections, brain lesions, and other systemic medical conditions should be treated medically and should not be treated with surgery.

The non-surgical treatment includes:

(a) Antiperspirants, which are thought to work by mechanically obstructing the eccrine sweat gland ducts or by causing atrophy of the secretory cells.
(b) Systemic medical regimens may also be employed in the treatment of hyperhidrosis. Anticholinergic agents (glycopyrrolate, propantheline, oxybutynin) are sometimes used; however, the dosage required to reduce sweating also causes development of adverse effects such as dry mouth, blurred vision, or urinary retention. Another significant drawback of this kind of treatment is that the possible benefits disappears if the patient stops taking medication.
(c) β-Blockers or benzodiazepines may be useful for reducing the emotional stimulus that leads to the excessive sweating in patients with hyperhidrosis that is triggered by specific emotional events.
(d) Iontophoresis is the introduction of ionized substances through intact skin by the application of direct current and appears to alleviate symptoms in palmar or plantar hyperhidrosis. The drawback is that it is often irritating to the skin and may cause scaling and fissuring.
(e) Botulinum toxin type A (Botox®) has been shown to be effective for axillary and palmar hyperhidrosis by temporarily reducing sweat production. It usually lasts for 3–4 months; however, it can last as long as 7 months. Drawbacks include local pain (20–40 injections are needed), an abbreviated response, transient weakness of the small hand muscles, and the cost of the procedures.

There are two types of surgical treatment: local surgical treatment and sympathectomy.

The local surgical treatment for axillary hyperhidrosis is the removal of the axillary sweat glands by means of curettage or liposuction. Complications include wound infection, scar formation, skin necrosis, and skin discolorations.

Sympathectomy can be performed in several forms: the sympathetic chain can be transected, resected, ablated with a cautery, or clips can be used. No clear differences have been demonstrated among the different techniques. The important concept about nerve disruption is that there is enough separation between the ends of the chain so that regrowth is impossible.

How can we explain the disease?
Although the pathophysiology remains unknown, and it can also occur spontaneously and intermittently, the cause of hyperhidrosis appears to be an abnormal central response to emotional stress.

Which are the more frequent symptoms?
The first step in the evaluation of hyperhidrosis is to differentiate between generalized and primary (or focal) hyperhidrosis. Patients with focal hyperhidrosis have sweating involving the craniofacial region, palms, soles, or axillae, and the sweating can present in only one of these regions or in more than one.

The most common causes of generalized sweating are excessive heat and obesity. Generalized sweating also suggests a secondary etiology related to other systemic diseases.

Is it possible to measure the intensity of hyperhidrosis?
Yes, it is possible to measure the amount of sweat produced in some body areas such as, for instance, palmar or axillary regions. But it is a complicated procedure and it has no importance in clinical decisions.

The most relevant aspect when making a decision regarding whether a case should be treated is not the amount of sweat produced by the patient but how much discomfort or social awkwardness this sweat causes to the patient. For instance, palmar hyperhidrosis can be much more disturbing for someone that has a job that involves close contact with people than for a swimming teacher who spends part of the day in a swimming pool. For practical clinical purposes, any degree of sweating that interferes with the activities of daily living should be viewed as abnormal.

Will hyperhidrosis disappear if I take anxiolytic medication?
As explained before, although hyperhidrosis appears to be related to an abnormal central response to stress, it does not mean that hyperhidrosis will disappear when a patient takes anxiolytic medication. But, on the other hand, when people that present hyperhidrosis become anxious or are under emotional tension, the symptoms (sweat production) usually increase.

At which age do symptoms appear?
The palmar symptoms start in early childhood, axillary symptoms in adolescence, and craniofacial symptoms in adulthood. The symptoms often worsen during puberty.

Will these symptoms disappear over time?
There is no an answer to this question, but the low prevalence of hyperhidrosis among elderly people is thought to possibly represent regression of the disease over time.

Can hyperhidrosis be related to other diseases?
The generalized form of hyperhidrosis, which affects the entire body, can be idiopathic or secondary to a metabolic or systemic disease, such as endocrine diseases (menopause, hyperthyroidism, diabetes), neurological disorders (Parkinson disease, peripheral neuropathies, brain lesions), congestive heart failure, neoplasias, or use of some medications (e.g., propranolol, tricyclic antidepressants, cholinesterase inhibitors, and opioids).

Can hyperhidrosis be related to some kinds of food?

It's possible to sweat when you eat hot or spicy foods. If a specific food raises your body temperature, then your body will try to cool itself with sweating. But some people sweat when they eat any kind of food or sweat when they just think about food. Often called gustatory hyperhidrosis (and sometimes called Frey's syndrome), this food-related sweating can be embarrassing and uncomfortable.

Many cases of gustatory sweating appear after surgery or trauma to a parotid gland. The parotid glands are the body's largest salivary glands; if a parotid gland is damaged or if surgery to a parotid is required (damage can occur due to inflammation, infection, and mumps), then related nerves may become damaged or may regenerate in an inappropriate way. The result is that when a person is supposed to salivate, he or she may also sweat and experience facial flushing. This combination of sweating and flushing related to parotid trauma is called Frey's syndrome, and usually affects just one side of the face.

Gustatory sweating can also occur for no known reason (idiopathic) or related to another medical condition (due to conditions such as diabetes, cluster headaches, Parkinson disease, and facial herpes zoster). In these cases, the sweating is often experienced on both sides of the face.

Can the presence of axillary odor be related to hyperhidrosis?

The medical term for the presence of offensive body odor is bromhidrosis and it can cause significant social embarrassment. Bromhidrosis is due to biotransformation of odorless natural secretions into odorous molecules and is linked with excessive sweating.

The sudiferous (sweat) glands are divided into eccrine glands, found all over the body, and apocrine glands, found in the axilla, breast, and groin region. While bacterial metabolism of apocrine sweat usually causes the malodor, eccrine sweating can also become offensive after ingestion of certain foods, such as garlic and alcohol.

Which is the best age to be submitted to sympathectomy?

The first point to be keep in mind is that no patient with hyperhidrosis "needs" to be submitted to sympathectomy: people with hyperhidrosis will not live any less or will die with cancer because of it. Proceeding to surgery is not a medical decision, it is a patient decision.

When a patient feels disabled by hyperhidrosis, and since sympathectomy is the most effective way to get rid of it, the surgery can be done as soon as possible. In children it usually occurs when they begin their school life, around 7 years old. The surgical risks of sympathectomy are very low and there is nothing contraindicating surgery.

Since there is no "ideal" age to be submitted to sympathectomy, the most appropriate way forward is to discuss the timing of the surgery with your doctor.

How many days will I spend in the hospital following sympathectomy?

In most cases of video-assisted thoracic sympathectomy, the patient is discharged on the next day or even on the same day.

How many incisions are necessary in a sympathectomy?

Video-assisted thoracic sympathectomy is usually performed through only one or two incisions, and surgeons usually try to place the incision in the axillary region so the resulting scar will be hidden.

For how long do I have to avoid exercise after sympathectomy?
Your surgeon can give you a precise answer, but since the trauma resulting from video-assisted sympathectomy is minimal, exercise can be resumed shortly after the surgery.

Is there a reversible technique for sympathectomy?
For a long time it was believed that sympathectomy performed with clips could be reversible. Despite initial enthusiasm, the presumption that the patient can return for "surgical reversal" by removing the clip appears dubious. The reason for the failure of reversibility is more than likely related to perineural damage of the nerve by the clips, which is usually irreversible.

What is compensatory sweating?
Compensatory sweating is excessive sweat production from skin areas with preserved sudomotor function, such as the abdominal, lumbar, groin, thigh, and popliteal regions, and it is the most common adverse effect of sympathectomy. Its incidence is widely variable and the occurrence of severe compensatory sweating has been reported to be as high as 28%.

The etiology of compensatory sweating is currently unknown, but potentially involves a combination of physical, physiological, and psychological factors.

The most common risk factor cited in the literature for moderate to severe compensatory hyperhidrosis includes T2 ganglion interruption. The number of levels interrupted has been inconclusive as a risk factor.

Patients who are candidates for sympathectomy who are already experiencing increased sweating in the trunk, groin region, or upper thighs should be warned that they are at increased risk of developing compensatory sweating, and the patient should think twice about going forward with the procedure.

Some surgeons utilize a "clipping method" of sympathetic chain interruption as a potentially reversible technique, whereby the clip can be removed if the patient is dissatisfied due to severe compensatory hyperhidrosis. The patient should be advised that, regardless of the method of surgery, the clip procedure should be considered irreversible [38].

Which treatment is used for plantar hyperhidrosis?
When the main symptom is plantar hyperhidrosis (sweat in the feet) the treatment is lumbar sympathectomy.

In other cases in which the plantar hyperhidrosis is accompanied by palmar and/or axillary hyperhidrosis, the usual recommendation is to first treat the hands or axilla because after thoracic sympathectomy many patients present amelioration of their feet symptoms. In this situation lumbar sympathectomy is reserved for cases where there was no improvement of the foot symptoms.

What kind of anesthesia will be required during sympathectomy?
Although it is possible to carry out endoscopic sympathectomy with local anesthesia, it is much safer to do it with general anesthesia.

Should I take analgesic medication after video-assisted sympathectomy? For how long?
The range of intensity of how people experience pain varies a lot, but most people complain of pain for 2 weeks after video-assisted sympathectomy. The most

common complaint is thoracic pain in the first 3 days (perhaps related to residual air in the pleural space) and back pain for 10 days.

Your surgeon will probably prescribe some analgesic medication so you can go through this period without strong discomfort.

Suggested Reading

de Campos JR, da Fonseca HV, Wolosker N. Quality of life changes following surgery for hyperhidrosis. Thorac Surg Clin. 2016;26(4):435–43.

Cerfolio RJ, De Campos JR, Bryant AS, Connery CP, Miller DL, DeCamp MM, McKenna RJ, Krasna MJ. The Society of Thoracic Surgeons expert consensus for the surgical treatment of hyperhidrosis. Ann Thorac Surg. 2011;91(5):1642–8.

Rieger R. Management of plantar hyperhidrosis with endoscopic lumbar sympathectomy. Thorac Surg Clin. 2016;26(4):465–9.

Sternbach JM, DeCamp MM. Targeting the sympathetic chain for primary hyperhidrosis: an evidence-based review. Thorac Surg Clin. 2016;26(4):407–20.

Wolosker N, Milanez de Campos JR, Fukuda JM. Management of compensatory sweating after sympathetic surgery. Thorac Surg Clin. 2016;26(4):445–51.

Index

A
Acromegaly, 16
Adenosine triphosphate (ATP), 62
Adjustment disorder, 59, 60
Aldehydes, 76
Aluminum chloride, 75, 87
Ambulatory management
   vs. hospitalized, 191
   videothoracoscopic sympathectomy
      ambulatory sympathectomy, 192
      early troubleshooting, 194
      easy communication and availability for patient, 194
      pain control, 194
      patient selection, 192, 193
      physician–patient relationship, 193
      post-surgical observation, 193, 194
      surgery factors, 193
      written instructions, 194
Ambulatory sympathectomy, 192
Anticholinergic drugs, 76, 86, 128, 158, 185
Antiperspirants, 81, 86, 87, 272
Anxiety, 53, 56–58
   assessment, 54
   excessive sweating, 54
   prevalence, 54
   somatic symptoms, 55
   symptoms, 59
   treatment, 55
Apocrine sweat glands, 10, 11, 84
Arterial bleeds, 183
Atelectasis, 182
Autonomic nervous system (ANS), 53
   anatomy, 119, 120
   biochemical–functional level, 118
   body's vegetative functions, 117
   central control, 118
   cervical sympathetic trunk, 121, 122
   communicating branches, 125
   effects of, 119
   emotional arousal, 119
   functions, 118, 119
   Kuntz nerve, 125, 126
   lumbar and sacral paravertebral sympathetic chain, 123
   metabolic changes, 119
   neuroeffective junctions, 123, 124
   neuro-effector junctions, 120
   neurotransmitters, 123, 124
   plexuses, 121
   postganglionic fibers, 120
   preganglionic fibers, 120
   sympathetic ganglia, 121
   thoracolumbar sympathetic trunk, 122, 123
Axillary anhidrosis, 165
Axillary hyperhidrosis, 30, 42, 85, 95, 101–104, 107, 108, 149, 165
   anesthesia, 108
   antiperspirants with aluminum salts, 91
   aspiratory curettage cannula, 109, 110, 112
   blunt cannulas, 110, 111
   botulinum toxin, 91, 92
      advantages, 103
      cryotherapy, 102
      regional anesthesia, 101
      therapeutic algorithms, 103
      treatment, 104
   clinical presentation, 90
   complications, 112, 114
   compression, 112
   dermatological lasers, 92
   endoscopic thoracic sympathectomy, 103–104
   epitheliolysis and segmental necrosis, 113
   expansive hematoma, 113
   genetic analysis, 89
   glycopyrrolate, 91
   injectable treatment, 91

Axillary hyperhidrosis (cont.)
  microfocused ultrasound, 92
  microwave energy thermolysis, 92
  non-surgical treatment, 91
  oral anticholinergics, 91
  oxybutynin, 91
  physiopathology, 89
  postoperative care, 112
  during puberty, 90
  starch and iodine test, 90
  surgical positioning and preoperative demarcation, 108
  systemic treatment, 91
  topical glycopyrrolate, 91
  topical oxybutynin, 92
  vacuum curettage, 114
Axillary trichotomy, 150
Axontmesis, 173
Azygos lobe, 168, 181

B
Bacterial infection, 40
Benzodiazepines, 77, 272
Bilateral cervicothoracic sympathectomy, 65
Bilateral proptosis, 14
Bilateral thoracic sympathectomy
  axillary hyperhidrosis, 149
  craniofacial hyperhidrosis, 148
  facial flushing, 148
  long QT syndrome, 147
  outcomes, 152
  palmar hyperhidrosis, 149
  postoperative complication, 152
  post-traumatic pain syndromes, 147
  primary hyperhidrosis, 147, 150
  Raynaud's phenomenon, 149
  surgical technique, 150–152
β-Blockers, 230, 272
Botulinum toxin (BTX), 42, 78–79, 96, 97, 100, 101, 185, 266
  biological weapon, 95
  clinical use, 96
  contraindications, 97
  facial wrinkles, 96
  food poisoning, 95
  injection of, 128
  patient management, 97
  serotypes, 96
  type A (BTX-A)
    antibody formation, 97
    colorimetric response, 101
    commercial presentations, 96
    diffusion capacity, 100

immune responses, 97
injection of, 100
Botulinum toxin type A (Botox®), 91, 96, 158, 162, 216, 223, 272
Brachial plexus injury, 183
Bradycardia, 186
Brazilian Society of Angiology and Vascular Surgery, 72
Brazilian Society of Thoracic Surgery, 72
Breast cancer, 87
Brief Social Phobia Scale (BSPS), 229
Bromidrosis, 93
Bromohidrosis, 107, 114
Brown adipose tissue, 62, 63
Buerger's disease, 204
Bupivacaine, 160

C
Calcium channel blockers, 77
Carcinoid syndrome, 17
Cardiac rhythm disorder, 191
Causalgia, 147, 150, 153, 266
Central nervous system (CNS), 61
Cephalic thermogenesis, 62
Cerebral edema, 184
Cervicothoracic sympathectomy, 71, 197
Chain clipping method, 137
Children
  botulinum toxin, 42
  iontophoresis, 41
  local treatment, 41
  oxybutynin, 42, 43
  primary focal hyperhidrosis
    definition, 40
    diagnosis, 40
    emotional implications, 41
    focal hyperhidrosis, 40
    generalized hyperhidrosis, 40
    infection, 40
    medical appointments, 41
    regional hyperhidrosis, 40
  surgical treatment, 43–44
  symptoms, 39
Chylothorax, 183
Clamping (clipping), 185
Clostridium botulinum, 78
Coagulated hemothorax, 191
Coagulation disorders, 14
Cognitive behavioral therapy (CBT), 55, 56, 232
Compensatory hyperhidrosis (CH)
  classifications, 199
  complications, 184–185
  definition, 197

Index

hypothalamic control, 198
QoL, 259–260
pathophysiology of, 197
prophylaxis, 200
symptoms, 199
treatment
    non-pharmacological treatment, 201
    pharmacological, 201
    surgical, 201, 202
Compensatory sweating (CS), 161, 171, 172, 175, 184, 220–221, 238–239, 269, 275
Constraints, primary hyperhidrosis
    case study, 67
    correct diagnosis, 71–72
    emotional factor, 66
    humidity, 66
    medical recommendations, 66, 67
    social phobia, 66
Conventional tracheal intubation, 190
Corynobacteria, 84
Craniofacial hyperhidrosis (CH), 30, 31, 148, 165, 248

D

Deodorants, 86, 87
Depression, 54, 57–59
Dermatology Quality of Life Index, 156
Diazepines, 85
Diet-induced thermogenesis (DIT)
    brown adipose tissue, 62
    cephalic phase, 62
    definition, 61
    energy balance, 61
    energy content, 63
    high-carbohydrate diet, 62
    MCTs, 63
    mixed diet, 62
    monounsaturated fatty acids, 63
    polyunsaturated fatty acids, 63
    protein-rich diet, 62
    SNS, 61
    sucrose concentration, 63
    UCP-1, 62
Dysautonomia, 53

E

Eating patterns, 22, 23
Eccrine sweat glands (meroccrins), 7
    concentration, 82, 83
    description, 82
    disorders, 84

    secretory function, 82
    clear cells, 8, 10
    dark cells, 8, 10
    intraepidermal excretory portion, 10
    localized hyperhidrosis, 10
    myoepithelial cells, 8, 10
    parasympathomimetic drugs, 10
Ectoderm, 53
ELS, *see* Endoscopic lumbar sympathectomy
Emotional sweating, 28
Emotional symptoms, 59, 60
Endo Peanut™ devices, 208
Endoderm, 53
Endoscopic lumbar sympathectomy (ELS)
    anesthesia, 205
    differences in technique, 217
    drawbacks, 212–213
    follow-up, 222
    markings on skin, 205–207
    outcomes
        clamping method, 217
        resection, 217
        resection without clips, 217
    patient positioning, 205
    patients and baseline characteristics, 216
    perioperative complications
        genitofemoral nerve, 218
        lymphatic duct injury, 218
        peritoneum tear, 219
    PHH, 204
    postoperative complications, 222
        compensatory sweating, 220–221
        pain, 219
        quality of life, 222
        retrograde ejaculation, 220
        swelling, 220
        transient constipation, 221
        vaginal lubrication, 221
    recurrence, 223
    retroperitoneal space
        combined transperitoneal and retroperitoneal approach, 208, 209
        dissection, sympathetic chain, 210–211
        space maker, 206–208
    scars, 213
    surgical team positioning, 205, 207
    sympathetic trunk clipping, 211
    trocars, 208–210
Endoscopic thoracic sympathectomy (ETS), 179, 191
    axillary hyperhidrosis, 165
    axillary sweating, 158, 159
    complications and adverse effects
        compensatory sweating, 161

Endoscopic thoracic sympathectomy
(ETS) (cont.)
gustatory sweating, 162
Horner's syndrome, 162
post-ETS syndrome, 162
too dry and cracked, 162
contraindications, 166
craniofacial hyperhidrosis/facial flushing, 165, 248
difficulties
azygos lobe, 167, 168
level of costal arches, 166
pleural adhesion, 166
facial blushing
adverse effects and complications, 247–248
eligibility, 239
occurrence, 244
patient selection, 236, 245–246
patient evaluation, 237–238
red face, 243
R2 vs R2–3 sympathectomy, 237
vs. sertraline, 237
social consequences, 244
with social phobia, 236
surgical technique, 246
sympathetic chain, 246–247
thoracoscopic sympathectomy, 245
treatment, 245
general anesthesia, 164
palmar hyperhidrosis, 165, 235
patient information, 159
patient positioning, 164
preoperative assessment, 159
types of, 160
VATS, 168
Energy, types, 139, 140
Estrogen-modulated hypothalamic body temperature control dysfunction, 14
Ethical and legal aspects
compensatory sweating, 269
duty, 262
experimental therapy, 268
guilt, 263
hyperhidrosis therapy, 269
imprudence, 263
informed consent, 264–268
judicialization, 269
liability, 262
malpractice, 263
medical advertising, 269
medical records, 264
negligence, 263
physicians' liability, 262

ETS, see Endoscopic thoracic sympathectomy
Excessive sweating, 54, 55, 58, 65–68
Experimental therapy, 268
Ex-suadinha, 66
Eyelid retraction, 14

F
Facial blushing
adverse effects and complications, 247–248
eligibility, 239
occurrence, 244
patient evaluation, 237–238
patient selection, 236, 245–246
psychological treatment
cognitive behavioral therapy, 232
length of treatment, 233
task concentration training technique, 231, 232
psychopharmacological treatment
anticholinergics, 230
β-blockers, 230
clonidine, 230
ibuprofen, 230
selective serotonin reuptake inhibitor, 229
selective α_2-adrenergic agonist, 230
R2 vs. R2–3 sympathectomy, 237
red face, 243
self-conscious emotions, 228
vs. sertraline, 237
social anxiety disorder, 229
social consequences, 244
with social phobia, 236
surgical technique, 246
sympathetic chain, 246–247
thoracoscopic sympathectomy, 245
treatment, 245
Facial flushing, 31, 51, 68, 127, 147, 148, 165, 189, 190, 192, 230, 235, 246, 274
Facial hyperhidrosis, 79, 91, 152, 190, 192
Fatty acids, 62, 63
Federal University of Amazonas (UFAM), 35
Focal hyperhidrosis, 87, 157, 271
Food processing, 21, 22
Foot surgery, 71
Fungal infections, 40

G
Gastrointestinal thermogenesis, 62
General anxiety, 54
Generalized hyperhidrosis, 16, 40, 85, 271
Generalized secondary hyperhidrosis, 157

Genitofemoral nerve, 210, 212, 218
German Dermatology Society guideline, 42
Ghost sweat, 185
Glycopyrrolate, 77
Glycopyrronium bromide, 157
Graves' orbitopathy, 14
Gustatory sweating, 162, 185
Gynecological neoplasia, 14

H
Hair follicles, 5
Harmonic scalpel, 190
Healthy lifestyle, 20, 23
Hematomas, 183
Hemothorax, 183
High-carbohydrate diet, 62
High-fat diet, 62
Horner syndrome, 162, 163, 180, 185
Humidity, 66
Hyper-emotive constitution, 27
Hyperhidrosis disease severity scale (HDSS), 36, 156
Hyperhidrosis Outpatient Clinic of the Thoracic Surgery Service, 58
Hyperthyroidism, 14, 15
Hypoglycemic syndrome, 16
Hypothalamic/thermal hyperhidrosis, 86
Hypothalamus, 61

I
Immunohistochemical axonal regeneration techniques, 177
Incisional infections, 183
Indomethacin, 77
Informed Consent, 264–268
Intermittent dysautonomia, 53
International Society of Paraplegia's journal, 34
Intradermal botulinum toxin, 201
Intraoperative air fistula, 182
Intraoperative cardiac arrest, 183
Iontophoresis, 41–42, 77–78, 128, 158, 266, 272
Irritation, 87
Isocaloric diets, 63

J
Judicialization, 269–270

K
Kuntz nerve, 182

L
Life changes, 71
Life story, 69
Ligamax®, 172
Lipids, 62
Lung parenchyma, 190
Luteolin, 63
Lymphatic duct injury, 218

M
Macronutrients, 21–22, 62, 63
Mammary glands, 5
Mediastinal pleural, 151
Medical advertising, 269
Medical Ethics Code, 265
Medium-chain triglycerides (MCTs), 63
Menopausal hot flushing, 157
Menopause, 13, 14
Mesoderm, 53
Mind–body dichotomy, 45
Minimally invasive endoscopic techniques, 163
Minor starch test, 98, 99
MiraDry® microwave device, 158
Mixed diet, 62
Moderate hyperhidrosis, 199
Monounsaturated fatty acids, 63
Murray's (projective) thematic apperception test, 49

N
Nervous system, 53
Neural hyperhidrosis, 84, 85
Neuralgia/local back pain, 219
Neuroectoderm, 53
Neuroendocrine tumors, 17
Neuropraxia, 173
Neurotmesis, 173
Neutralizing antibodies (NAbs), hyperhidrosis, 97, 98
Non-neural hyperhidrosis, 85
Nutrition, 61

O
Obesity
    behavioral changes, 20
    body fat accumulation, 19
    cancer, 19
    coronary heart disease, 19
    diet planning
        energy density, 21
        food processing, 21, 22

Obesity (cont.)
　　healthy eating pattern, 22, 23
　　macronutrient composition, 20, 21
　dyslipidemia, 19
　fluid intake, 20
　health-related problems, 23
　heat loss reduction, 19
　hyperhidrosis, 19
　hypertension, 19
　nutrition therapy, 20
　patients' quality of life, 23
　physiological changes, 20
　psychosocial aspects, 20
　sebaceous glands, 20
　sebum production, 20
　skin barrier function, 20
　sleep apnea, 19
　stroke, 19
　sweat glands, 20
　thoracic sympathectomy, 181
　transepidermal water loss, 20
　type 2 diabetes mellitus, 19
　ultra-processed food, 22
　visceral adipose tissue, 19
Opioids plus acetaminophen, 190
Oral anticholinergics, 76
Orotracheal intubation, 180
Oxybutynin, 42–43, 76–77, 157

P

Palmar and plantar hyperhidrosis (PHH), 203–205, 215–217, 220, 222–224
Palmar anhidrosis, 165
Palmar hyperhidrosis, 29, 32, 41–43, 95, 104, 149, 165, 192
　botulinum toxin
　　applications, 104 (see Botulinum toxin (BTX))
　primary, 133
Palmoplantar hyperhidrosis, 40–43
Palpation, 166
Parasympathetic nervous system, 117
Paroxetine, 77
Pel-Ebstein fever of Hodgkin's lymphoma, 157
Peritoneal tear, 219
Perspiring copiously, 68–71
Pharmacological treatment
　benzodiazepines, 77
　botulinum toxin, 78
　calcium channel blockers, 77
　clonidine, 77
　glycopyrrolate, 77
　indomethacin, 77
　iontophoresis, 77
　oral anticholinergics, 76
　oxybutynin, 76, 77
　paroxetine, 77
　topical agents, 75, 76
Pheochromocytomas, 15
Physical exercise, 63, 71
Physicians' civil liability, 262, 263
Physicians' criminal liability, 263
Physicians' ethical responsibility, 263
Pigid desiderative questionnaire, 49
Plantar hyperhidrosis, 30, 41, 86, 275
Pleural adhesions, 166, 181
Pleural effusion, 183
Pleuropulmonary diseases, 166
Pneumatic calf compression devices, 160
Pneumothorax, 182
Polyunsaturated fatty acids, 63
Porcine model, 177
Prevalence, of PH, 34–36
　1977 to 2017
　　severe cases, 36
　　study evaluation, 34
　Brazil
　　Blumenau, 35
　　Manaus, 35
　　Sergipe, 35, 36
　China, 34
　Germany, 35
　Israel, 34
　Japan, 35
　Poland, 35
　USA, 34
Primary focal hyperhidrosis (PFH)
　children
　　definition, 40
　　diagnosis, 40
　　emotional implications, 41
　　focal hyperhidrosis, 40
　　generalized hyperhidrosis, 40
　　infection, 40
　　medical appointments, 41
　　regional hyperhidrosis, 40
Primary hyperhidrosis (PH), 45
　axillary, 30
　biopsychosocial problems, 33
　craniofacial segment, 28, 31
　definition, 33
　diagnosis, 32
　epidemiology, 28
　facial flushing, 31
　foot, 30
　incidence, 32

palmar, 28, 29
psychology (*see* Psychological evaluation)
Primary palmar hyperhidrosis
  bupivacaine, 160
  compensatory sweating, 161
  diagnosis, 156
  direct-vision gynecological laparoscope, 160
  ETS
    axillary sweating, 158, 159
    gustatory sweating, 162
    Horner's syndrome, 162
    patient information, 159
    post-ETS syndrome, 162
    preoperative assessment, 159
    types of, 160
  examination, 156, 157
  non-surgical options
    anticholinergic drugs, 158
    Botox®, 158
    iontophoresis, 158
    miraDry® microwave device, 158
    subdermal curettage, 158
  pneumatic calf compression devices, 160
  symptoms, 155, 156
Protein-rich diet, 62
Psoas muscle, 210
Psychiatric features, 54
  anxiety (*see* Anxiety)
  excessive sweating, 54
  social consequences, 54
Psychological evaluation
  crisis, 50
  Murray's (projective) thematic apperception test, 49
  objectives, 48
  Pigid desiderative questionnaire, 49
  psychic characteristics, 49, 50
  psychological returning, 49
  semi-directed psychological interview, 48
  WHOQOL Brief, 48, 49
Psychological returning, 49
Psychological treatment, 66
Psychosomatic disease, 27, 28
Psychosomatic patient, 47, 48, 51
Psychotherapy, 51, 60
Pulmonary diseases, 166
Pulmonary expansion and aspiration, residual air, 143

Q

Quality of life (QoL), 40, 49, 51, 54–59, 69
  clinical treatment, 254–257
  compensatory hyperhidrosis, 259–260
  definition, 253
  ELS, 222
  questionnaire, 254–256
  surgical treatment
    follow-up, 257–260
    hyperhidrosis complaint distribution, 257

R

Raynaud's disease, 149, 204
Reflex sweating, 138, 172
Reflex sympathetic dystrophy, 147, 204
Residual pneumothorax, 182, 191, 194
Retrograde ejaculation, 220
Retroperitoneoscopy, 210
Rhinitis, 185
Robotic surgical systems, 200

S

Scoliosis, 181
Sebaceous glands, 5
Second lumbar sympathetic ganglion (LG2), 211
Seddon classification, 173
Selective serotonin reuptake inhibitor (SSRI), 229
Selective sympathectomy (ramicotomy), 185
Self-esteem, 50, 53, 81
Self-rejection, 50
Semi-directed psychological interview, 48
Serotonin reuptake inhibitor medication, 55, 56
Sertraline, 55
Shoes/boots, 86
Short-Form 36 (SF-36), 254
Single trocar technique, 183
Sinus bradycardia, 166
Skin glands
  apocrine, 5
  eccrines, 5
  functions, 5–11
  types, 5–11
Social anxiety disorder (SAD), 54–56, 229
Social phobia, 50, 51, 236, 239
Social revolution, 27
Social stigma, 54
Somatic disorders, 27
Space maker, 206–208
Spices, 63
Stress, 58, 59
Stressor, 59
Suando em Bicas, 65

Subacute thyroiditis, 15
Subcutaneous emphysema, 182
Subdermal axillary lipoaspiration, 266
Subdermal curettage, 158
Subxiphoid thoracic sympathectomy, 141
Sudoripar glands, *see* Sweat glands
Superficial ectoderm, 53
Surgery, 47, 48, 50, 51
Surgical hyperhidrosis
   endoscopic thoracic sympathectomy, 118
   sympathetic chain, 117
      thoracic sympathetic chain, 118
Sutherland's classification, 174
Sweat glands, 82, 84, 85, 87
   anatomy, 3, 5
   derme, 3
   epidermis, 3–5
   heat loss by evaporation, 27
   hipoderme, 3
   sweat production, 27
Sweaty palms, 155
Sympathectomy, 65, 66, 70, 72, 127–129, 179, 189, 192, 198, 200, 211–212, 272, 275
Sympathetic chain, 163–168, 171, 172, 181, 202, 246–247
Sympathetic chain block, 172, 174, 175
Sympathetic nerve surgery
   clipping method
      clinical evidence, 175, 176
      clip removal, 175
      experimental evidence, 176, 177
      histopathological alterations of nervous fiber, 172–174
      nerve fiber compression with titanium clip, 172
      ports, 174
      titanium clip, 175
Sympathetic nervous system, 27, 53, 55, 61, 62, 117
   anatomy, 118
   skin and vessel specific aspects, 124, 125
   stimulation, 124
   sweat gland secretion control, 117
   unbalance of, 117
Sympathetic trunk, 211
Sympaticotomy, 171, 246
Systemic anticholinergics, 201
Systemic medical regimens, 272

T
Task concentration training (TCT) technique, 231, 232
Testimonials, 65, 68, 70
Thermoablation, 164–166
Thermoregulatory requirements, hyperhidrosis, 28
Thoracic aortic aneurysm, 181
Thoracic drainage tube (thoracostomy), 190
Thoracic sympathectomy, 133, 266
   anatomical variations
      azygos lobe, 181
      medial and nerve sympathetic chain of Kuntz, 182
      obesity, 181
      pleural adhesions, 181
      scoliosis/thoracic aortic aneurysm, 181
   anterior approach, 134
   chain section methods, 136, 137
   difficulties inherent in operative technique
      endoscopic surgical instruments, 180
      orotracheal intubation, 180
      video-assisted thoracoscopy equipment, 180
   endoscopic video-assisted techniques, 133
   general anesthesia, 142
   harmonic scalpel, 139, 143
   immediate complications
      atelectasis, 182
      brachial plexus injury, 183
      brain complications, 184
      chylothorax, 183
      hematomas, 183
      hemothorax, 183
      incisional infections, 183
      intraoperative air fistula and pneumothorax, 182
      intraoperative cardiac arrest, 183
      pleural effusion, 183
      severe pain, 183
      subcutaneous emphysema, 182
   incision, 142, 143
   late complications
      bradycardia, 186
      compensatory hyperhidrosis, 184–185
      ghost sweat, 185
      gustatory sweating, 185
      Horner syndrome, 185
      rhinitis, 185

lateral approach, 135, 136
mortality, 186
patient positioning, 133, 142
pleural opening, 143
posterior approach, 134, 135
rare complications, 186
surgical techniques, 133
sympathectomy, 133
sympathic chain section level, 137, 138
uniportal *vs.* multiportal, 138, 139
Thoracic sympathotomy, 192
Thoracoscopic sympathectomy, 245
Titanium clips, 211
Topical treatment, 75, 76, 86–87
Tranquilizers, 85
Transareolar uniportal thoracic sympathectomy, 140
Transumbilical thoracic sympathectomy technique, 140–141
Trauma, 46, 51
Treatment and consequences, 57–60
  age, 274
  analgesic medication, 275
  anxiolytic medication, 273
  compensatory sweating, 275
  congenital disease, 272
  craniofacial segment, 28
  definition, 271
  differential, 273
  focal form, 271
  follow-up, 274
  general anesthesia, 275
  generalized form, 271
  intensity, 273
  non-surgical treatment, 272
  offensive body odor, 274
  plantar hyperhidrosis, 275
  surgical treatment, 272
  sympathectomy, 275
  symptoms, 273
  type of food, 274
Trocars, 208, 209

U

Ultra-processed foods, 22
Unclipping, 174–177
Uncoupling protein 1 (UCP-1), 62
Unilateral sympathectomy approach, 141, 142

V

Venous bleeds, 183
Video-assisted thoracic sympathectomy, 274
Video-assisted thoracoscopic surgery (VATS), 167, 168, 180
Videoendoscopic thoracic sympathectomy, 167
Videolaparoscopic surgery, 204
Videothoracoscopic sympathectomy, 43, 129, 164, 189, 190, 257
  ambulatory sympathectomy, 192
  early troubleshooting, 194
  easy communication and availability for patient, 194
  pain control, 194
  patient selection, 192, 193
  physician–patient relationship, 193
  post-surgical observation, 193, 194
  surgery factors, 193
  written instructions, 194
Viral skin infection, 40

W

Wallerian degeneration, 176
Whole foods, 63
World Health Organization (WHO), 253, 254
World Health Organization Quality of Life (WHOQOL-100), 254, 256

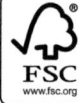

MIX
Papier aus verantwortungsvollen Quellen
Paper from responsible sources
FSC® C105338

If you have any concerns about our products,
you can contact us on
ProductSafety@springernature.com

In case Publisher is established outside the EU,
the EU authorized representative is:
**Springer Nature Customer Service Center GmbH
Europaplatz 3, 69115 Heidelberg, Germany**

Printed by Libri Plureos GmbH
in Hamburg, Germany